SANFORD GUIDE®

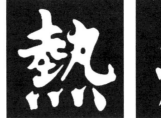

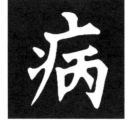

Thirty-Ninth Edition

THE SANFORD GUIDE

TO ANTIMICROBIAL

THERAPY

2009

Editors:

David N. Gilbert, M.D.
Director of Medical Education & Earl A. Chiles Research Institute
Providence Portland Medical Center
Professor of Medicine
Oregon Health Sciences University
Portland, Oregon

Robert C. Moellering, Jr., M.D.
Shields Warren-Mallinckrodt Professor of Medical Research
Harvard Medical School
Boston, Massachusetts

George M. Eliopoulos, M.D.
Chief, James L. Tullis Firm, Beth Israel Deaconess Hospital
Professor of Medicine
Harvard Medical School
Boston, Massachusetts

Henry F. (Chip) Chambers, M.D.
Professor of Medicine
University of California at San Francisco
Chief of Infectious Diseases
San Francisco General Hospital
San Francisco, California

Michael S. Saag, M.D.
Professor of Medicine & DIrector, Division of Infectious Dieases
Director, UAB Center for AIDS Research
University of Alabama
Birmingham, Alabama

THE SANFORD GUIDE TO ANTIMICROBIAL THERAPY 2009
(39ᵀᴴ EDITION)

Jay P. Sanford, M.D.
1928-1996

Editors

David N. Gilbert, M.D.   Robert C. Moellering, Jr., M.D.
George M. Eliopoulos, M.D.   Henry F. (Chip) Chambers, M.D
Michael S. Saag, M.D.

The Sanford Guides are updated annually and published by:
Antimicrobial Therapy, Inc.
P.O. Box 276, 11771 Lee Highway, Sperryville, VA 22740-0276 USA
Tel 540-987-9480 *Fax* 540-987-9486
Email: info@sanfordguide.com
www.sanfordguide.com

Acknowledgements
Thanks to Lingua Solutions, Inc., Los Angeles, CA for assistance in preparation of the manuscript; Royalty Press, Westville, NJ for printing and Fox Bindery, Quakertown, PA for finishing this edition of the Sanford Guide to Antimicrobial Therapy.

Publisher's Note to Readers
Though many readers of the SANFORD GUIDE receive their copy from a pharmaceutical company representative, please be assured that the SANFORD GUIDE has been, and continues to be, independently prepared and published since its inception in 1969. Decisions regarding the content of the SANFORD GUIDE are solely those of the editors and the publisher. We welcome your questions, comments and feedback concerning the SANFORD GUIDE. All of your feedback is reviewed and taken into account in preparing the next edition.

Every effort is made to ensure the accuracy of the content of this guide. However, current full prescribing information available in the package insert of each drug should be consulted before prescribing any product. The editors and publisher are not responsible for errors or omissions or for any consequences from application of the information in this book and make no warranty, express or implied, with respect to the currency, accuracy, or completeness of the contents of the publication. Application of this information in a particular situation remains the professional responsibility of the practitioner.

Content-related notices are published on our website at:
http://www.sanfordguide.com/notices

Printed in the United States of America
ISBN 978-1-930808-54-6
Library Edition

—TABLE OF CONTENTS—

QUICK PAGE GUIDE TO THE SANFORD GUIDE[*]

[*] Adapted from materials provided by Stephanie Troy, M.D., Stanford Univ. Med. Ctr.

3

ABBREVIATIONS

3TC = lamivudine
ABC = abacavir
ABCD = amphotericin B colloidal dispersion
ABLC = ampho B lipid complex
ACIP = Advisory Committee on Immunization Practices
AD = after dialysis
ADF = adefovir
AG = aminoglycoside
AIDS = Acquired Immune Deficiency Syndrome
AM-CL = amoxicillin-clavulanate
AM-CL-ER = amoxicillin-clavulanate extended release
AMK = amikacin
Amox = amoxicillin
AMP = ampicillin
Ampho B = amphotericin B
AM-SB = ampicillin-sulbactam
AP = atovaquone proguanil
AP Pen = antipseudomonal penicillins
APAG = antipseudomonal aminoglycoside (tobra, gent, amikacin)
ARDS = acute respiratory distress syndrome
ARF = acute rheumatic fever
ASA = aspirin
ATS = American Thoracic Society
ATV = atazanavir
AUC = area under the curve
Azithro = azithromycin
bid = twice a day
BL/BLI = beta-lactam/beta-lactamase inhibitor
BW = body weight
C&S = culture & sensitivity
CAPD = continuous ambulatory peritoneal dialysis
CARB = carbapenems (DORI, ERTA, IMP, MER)
CDC = Centers for Disease Control
Cefpodox = cefpodoxime proxetil
Ceftaz = ceftazidime
Ceph = cephalosporin
CFB = ceftobiprole
CFP = cefepime
Chloro = chloramphenicol
CIP = ciprofloxacin; **CIP-ER** = CIP extended release
Clarithro = clarithromycin; **ER** = extended release
Clav = clavulanate
Clinda = clindamycin
CLO = clofazimine
Clot = clotrimazole
CMV = cytomegalovirus
CQ = chloroquine phosphate
CrCl = creatinine clearance
CRRT = continuous renal replacement therapy
CSD = cat-scratch disease

CSF = cerebrospinal fluid
CXR = chest x-ray
d4T = stavudine
Dapto = daptomycin
DBPCT = double-blind placebo-controlled trial
dc = discontinue
ddC = zalcitabine
ddI = didanosine
DIC = disseminated intravascular coagulation
div. = divided
DLV = delavirdine
Dori = doripenem
DOT = directly observed therapy
DOT group = B. distasonis, B. ovatus, B. thetaiotaomicron
Doxy = doxycycline
DRSP = drug-resistant S. pneumoniae
DS = double strength
EBV = Epstein-Barr virus
EES = erythromycin ethyl succinate
EFZ = efavirenz
ENT = entecavir
ERTA = ertapenem
Erythro = erythromycin
ESBLs = extended spectrum β-lactamases
ESR = erythrocyte sedimentation rate
ESRD = endstage renal disease
ETB = ethambutol
Flu = fluconazole
Flucyt = flucytosine
FOS-APV = fosamprenavir
FQ = fluoroquinolone (CIP, Oflox, Lome, Peflox, Levo, Gati, Moxi, Gemi)
FTC = emtricitabine
G = generic
Gati = gatifloxacin
GC = gonorrhea
Gemi = gemifloxacin
Gent = gentamicin
gm = gram
GNB = gram-negative bacilli
Griseo = griseofulvin
HEMO = hemodialysis
HHV = human herpesvirus
HIV = human immunodeficiency virus
HLR = high-level resistance
HSCT = hematopoietic stem cell transplant
HSV = herpes simplex virus
IA = injectable agent/anti-inflammatory drugs
ICAAC = International Conference on Antimicrobial Agents & Chemotherapy

IDSA = Infectious Diseases Society of America
IDV = indinavir
IFN = interferon
IMP = imipenem-cilastatin
INH = isoniazid
Inv = investigational
IP = intraperitoneal
IT = intrathecal
Itra = itraconazole
IVDU = intravenous drug user
IVIG = intravenous immune globulin
Keto = ketoconazole
LAB = liposomal ampho B
LCM = lymphocytic choriomeningitis virus
LCR = ligase chain reaction
Levo = levofloxacin
LP/R = lopinavir/ ritonavir
M. Tbc = Mycobacterium tuberculosis
Macrolides = azithro, clarithro, dirithro, erythro, roxithro
mcg = microgram
MER = meropenem
Metro = metronidazole
mg = milligram
Mino = minocycline
Moxi = moxifloxacin
MQ = mefloquine
MSSA/MRSA = methicillin-sensitive/resistant S. aureus
NB = name brand
NF = nitrofurantoin
NFDA-I = not FDA-approved indication
NFR = nelfinavir
NNRTI = non-nucleoside reverse transcriptase inhibitor
NRTI = nucleoside reverse transcriptase inhibitor
NSAIDs = non-steroidal
NUS = not available in the U.S.
NVP = nevirapine
O Ceph 1,2,3 = oral cephalosporins—see *Table 10C*
Oflox = ofloxacin
P Ceph 1,2,3,4 = parenteral cephalosporins—see *Table 10C*
P Ceph 3 AP = parenteral cephalosporins with antipseudomonal activity—see *Table 10C*
PCR = polymerase chain reaction
PEP = post-exposure prophylaxis
PI = protease inhibitor
PIP = piperacillin
PIP-TZ = piperacillin-tazobactam
po = per os (by mouth)
PQ = primaquine
PRCT = Prospective randomized controlled trials
PTLD = post-transplant lymphoproliferative disease

ABBREVIATIONS (2)

Pts = patients
Pyri = pyrimethamine
PZA = pyrazinamide
qid = 4 times a day
QS = quinine sulfate
Quinu-dalfo = **Q-D** = quinupristin-dalfopristin
R = resistant
RFB = rifabutin
RFP = rifapentine
Rick = Rickettsia
RIF = rifampin
RSV = respiratory syncytial virus
RTI = respiratory tract infection
RTV = ritonavir
rx = treatment

S = potential synergy in combination with penicillin, AMP, vanco, teico
Sens = sensitive (susceptible)
SM = streptomycin
SQV = saquinavir
STD = sexually transmitted disease
subcut = subcutaneous
Sulb = sulbactam
Tazo = tazobactam
TBc = tuberculosis
TC-CL = ticarcillin-clavulanate
TDF = tenofovir
TEE = transesophageal echocardiography
Teico = teicoplanin
Telithro = telithromycin
Tetra = tetracycline

Ticar = ticarcillin
tid = 3 times a day
TMP-SMX = trimethoprim-sulfamethoxazole
TNF = tumor necrosis factor
Tobra = tobramycin
TPV = tipranavir
TST = tuberculin skin test
UTI = urinary tract infection
Vanco = vancomycin
VISA = vancomycin intermediately resistant S. aureus
VL = viral load
Vori = voriconazole
VZV = varicella-zoster virus
WHO = World Health Organization
ZDV = zidovudine

ABBREVIATIONS OF JOURNAL TITLES

AAC: Antimicrobial Agents & Chemotherapy
Adv PID: Advances in Pediatric Infectious Diseases
AHJ: American Heart Journal
AIDS Res Hum Retrovir: AIDS Research & Human Retroviruses
AJG: American Journal of Gastroenterology
AJM: American Journal of Medicine
AJRCCM: American Journal of Respiratory Critical Care Medicine
AJTMH: American Journal of Tropical Medicine & Hygiene
Aliment Pharmacol Ther: Alimentary Pharmacology & Therapeutics
Am J Hlth Pharm: American Journal of Health-System Pharmacy
Amer J Transpl: American Journal of Transplantation
AnEM: Annals of Emergency Medicine
AnIM: Annals of Internal Medicine
AnPharmacother: Annals of Pharmacotherapy
AnSurg: Annals of Surgery
Antivir Ther: Antiviral Therapy
ArDerm: Archives of Dermatology
ArIM: Archives of Internal Medicine
ARRD: American Review of Respiratory Disease
BMJ: British Medical Journal
BMTr: Bone Marrow Transplantation
Brit J Derm: British Journal of Dermatology
Can JID: Canadian Journal of Infectious Diseases
Canad Med J: Candadian Medical Journal
CCM: Critical Care Medicine
CCTID: Current Clinical Topics in Infectious Disease
CDBSR: Cochrane Database of Systematic Reviews
CID: Clinical Infectious Diseases
Clin Micro Inf: Clinical Microbiology and Infection
Clin Micro Rev: Clinical Microbiology Reviews
CMAJ: Canadian Medical Association Journal
COID: Current Opinion in Infectious Disease

Curr Med Res Opin: Current Medical Research and Opinion
Derm Ther: Dermatologic Therapy
Dermatol Clin: Dermatologic Clinics
Dig Dis Sci: Digestive Diseases and Sciences
DMID: Diagnostic Microbiology and Infectious Disease
EID: Emerging Infectious Diseases
EJCMID: European Journal of Clin. Micro. & Infectious Diseases
Eur J Neurol: European Journal of Neurology
Exp Mol Path: Experimental & Molecular Pathology
Exp Rev Anti Infect Ther: Expert Review of Anti-Infective Therapy
Gastro: Gastroenterology
Hpt: Hepatology
ICHE: Infection Control and Hospital Epidemiology
IDC No. Amer: Infectious Disease Clinics of North America
IDCP: Infectious Diseases in Clinical Practice
IJAA: International Journal of Antimicrobial Agents
Inf Med: Infections in Medicine
J AIDS & HR: Journal of AIDS and Human Retrovirology
J All Clin Immun: Journal of Allergy and Clinical Immunology
J Am Ger Soc: Journal of the American Geriatrics Society
J Chemother: Journal of Chemotherapy
J Clin Micro: Journal of Clinical Microbiology
J Clin Virol: Journal of Clinical Virology
J Derm Treat: Journal of Dermatological Treatment
J Hpt: Journal of Hepatology
J Inf: Journal of Infection
J Med Micro: Journal of Medical Microbiology
J Micro Immunol Inf: Journal of Microbiology, Immunology, & Infection
J Ped: Journal of Pediatrics
J Viral Hep: Journal of Viral Hepatitis
JAC: Journal of Antimicrobial Chemotherapy

JACC: Journal of American College of Cardiology
JAIDS: JAIDS Journal of Acquired Immune Deficiency Syndromes
JAMA: Journal of the American Medical Association
JAVMA: Journal of the Veterinary Medicine Association
JCI: Journal of Clinical Investigation
JCM: Journal of Clinical Microbiology
JID: Journal of Infectious Diseases
JNS: Journal of Neurosurgery
JTMH: Journal of Tropical Medicine and Hygiene
Ln: Lancet
LnID: Lancet Infectious Disease
Mayo Clin Proc: Mayo Clinic Proceedings
Med Lett: Medical Letter
Med Mycol: Medical Mycology
MMWR: Morbidity & Mortality Weekly Report
NEJM: New England Journal of Medicine
Neph Dial Transpl: Nephrology Dialysis Transplantation
Ped Ann: Pediatric Annals
Peds: Pediatrics
Pharmacother: Pharmacotherapy
PIDJ: Pediatric Infectious Disease Journal
QJM: Quarterly Journal of Medicine
Scand J Inf Dis: Scandinavian Journal of Infectious Diseases
Sem Resp Inf: Seminars in Respiratory Infections
SGO: Surgery Gynecology and Obstetrics
SMJ: Southern Medical Journal
Surg Neurol: Surgical Neurology
Transpl Inf Dis: Transplant Infectious Diseases
Transpl: Transplantation
TRSM: Transactions of the Royal Society of Medicine

TABLE 1A – CLINICAL APPROACH TO INITIAL CHOICE OF ANTIMICROBIAL THERAPY*
Treatment based on presumed site or type of infection. In selected instances, treatment and prophylaxis based on identification of pathogens *(Abbreviations on page 3)*

ANATOMIC SITE/DIAGNOSIS/ MODIFYING CIRCUMSTANCES	ETIOLOGIES (usual)	SUGGESTED REGIMENS*		ADJUNCT DIAGNOSTIC OR THERAPEUTIC MEASURES AND COMMENTS
		PRIMARY	ALTERNATIVE§	
ABDOMEN: *See Peritoneum, page 44; Gallbladder, page 15; and Pelvic Inflammatory Disease, page 23*				
BONE: Osteomyelitis. Microbiologic diagnosis is essential. If blood culture negative, need culture of bone. Culture of sinus tract drainage not predictive of bone culture. *Review: Ln 364:369, 2004.*				
Hematogenous Osteomyelitis				
Empiric therapy—Collect bone and blood cultures before empiric therapy				
Newborn (<4 mos.) See Table 16 for dose	S. aureus, Gm-neg. bacilli, Group B strep	**MRSA possible: Vanco+ (Ceftaz or CFP)**[1]	**MRSA unlikely: (Nafcillin or oxacillin) + (Ceftaz or CFP)**[1]	*Table 16 for dose.* Severe allergy or toxicity: (**Linezolid**[NFDA-I] 10 mg/kg IV/po q8h + **aztreonam**). Could substitute **clindamycin** for linezolid.
Children (>4 mos.)—Adult: Osteo of extremity	S. aureus, Group A strep, Gm-neg. bacilli rare	**MRSA possible: Vanco**	**MRSA unlikely: Nafcillin or oxacillin**	Severe allergy or toxicity: **Clinda** or **TMP-SMX** or **linezolid**[NFDA-I]. *Dosages in Table 16. See Table 10 for adverse reactions to drugs.*
		Add **Ceftaz or CFP** if Gm-neg. bacilli on Gram stain (**Adult doses below**, *see footnote*). *Peds Doses: Table 16*		
Adult (>21 yrs) **Vertebral osteo ± epidural abscess**; other sites (NEJM 355:2012, 2006)	S. aureus most common but variety other organisms. **Blood & bone cultures essential.**	**MRSA possible: Vanco** 1 gm IV q12h; if over 100 kg, 1.5 gm IV q12h	**MRSA unlikely: Nafcillin or oxacillin** 2 gm IV q4h	**Dx: MRI early to look for epidural abscess.** Allergy or toxicity: **TMP-SMX** 8-10 mg/kg per day div. IV q8h or **linezolid** 600 mg IV/po q12h *(AnIM 138:135, 2003)*[NFDA-I]. *See MRSA specific therapy comment.* Epidural abscess ref.: *AnIM 164:2409, 2004.*
Specific therapy—Culture and in vitro susceptibility results known				**Other options if susceptible in vitro and allergy/toxicity issues:** 1) **TMP/SMX** 8-10 mg/kg/d IV div q8h. Minimal data on treatment of osteomyelitis; 2) **Clinda** 600-900 mg IV q8h – have lab check for inducible resistance especially if erythro resistant *(CID 40:280,2005)*; 3) [(**Cip** 750 mg po bid or **levo** 750 mg po q24h) + **rif** 300 mg po bid]; 4) **Daptomycin** 6 mg/kg IV q24h; –clinical failure secondary to resistance reported *(J Clin Micro 44:595:2006)*; 5) **Linezolid** 600 mg po/IV bid – anecdotal reports of efficacy *(J Chemother 17:643,2005)*, optic & peripheral neuropathy with long-term use *(Neurology 64:926, 2005)*; 6) **Fusidic acid** NUS 500 mg IV q8h + **rif** 300 mg po bid. *(CID 42:394, 2006).*
	MSSA	**Nafcillin or oxacillin** 2 gm IV q4h or **cefazolin** 2 gm IV q8h	**Vanco** 1 gm q12h IV; if over 100 kg, 1.5 gm IV q12h	
	MRSA—*See Table 6, page 75*	**Vanco** 1 gm IV q12h	**Linezolid** 600 mg q12h IV/po ± **RIF** 300 mg po/IV bid	
Hemoglobinopathy: Sickle cell/thalassemia	Salmonella; other Gm-neg. bacilli	**CIP** 400 mg IV q12h	**Levo** 750 mg IV q24h	Thalassemia: transfusion and iron chelation risk factors.
Contiguous Osteomyelitis Without Vascular Insufficiency				
Empiric therapy: Get cultures!				
Foot bone osteo due to nail through tennis shoe	P. aeruginosa	**CIP** 750 mg po bid or **Levo** 750 mg po q24h	**Ceftaz** 2 gm IV q8h or **CFP** 2 gm IV q12h	*See Skin—Nail puncture, page 52.* Need debridement to remove foreign body.
Long bone, post-internal fixation of fracture	S. aureus, Gm-neg. bacilli, P. aeruginosa	**Vanco** 1 gm IV q12h + [**ceftaz** or **CFP** (*see footnote*)]. *See Comment*	**Linezolid** 600 mg IV/po bid[NFDA-I] + (**ceftaz** or **CFP**). *See Comment*	Often necessary to remove hardware to allow bone union. May need revascularization. **Regimens listed are empiric.** Adjust after culture data available. If susceptible Gm-neg. bacillus, **CIP** 750 mg po bid or **Levo** 750 mg po q24h. For other S. aureus options: *See Hem. Osteo. Specific Therapy, above (Table 1(1)).*

* **DOSAGES SUGGESTED** are for adults (unless otherwise indicated) with clinically severe (often life-threatening infections. Dosages also assume normal renal function, and not severe hepatic dysfunction.

§ **ALTERNATIVE THERAPY INCLUDES** these considerations: allergy, pharmacology/pharmacokinetics, compliance, costs, local resistance profiles.

[1] Drug dosage: **ceftazidime** 2 gm IV q8h, **CFP** 2 gm IV q12h

TABLE 1A (2)

ANATOMIC SITE/DIAGNOSIS/ MODIFYING CIRCUMSTANCES	ETIOLOGIES (usual)	SUGGESTED REGIMENS*		ADJUNCT DIAGNOSTIC OR THERAPEUTIC MEASURES AND COMMENTS
		PRIMARY	ALTERNATIVE§	
BONE/Contiguous Osteomyelitis Without Vascular Insufficiency/Empiric therapy (continued)				
Osteonecrosis of the jaw	Probably rare adverse reaction to bisphosphonates	Infection is secondary to bone necrosis and loss of overlying mucosa. Treatment: minimal surgical debridement, chlorohexidine rinses, antibiotics (e.g. PIP-TZ). NEJM 355:2278, 2006.		
Prosthetic joint	See **prosthetic joint**, page 30			For details: CID 44:913, 2007.
Spinal implant infection	S. aureus, coag-neg staphylococci, gram-neg bacilli	Onset within 30 days culture, treat & then suppress until fusion occurs	Onset after 30 days remove implant, culture & treat	
Sternum, post-op	S. aureus, S. epidermidis	**Vanco** 1 gm IV q12h; if over 100 kg, 1.5 gm IV q12h.	**Linezolid** 600 mg po/IV[NFDA-I] bid	Sternal debridement for cultures & removal of necrotic bone. For S. aureus options: Hem.Osteo. Specific Therapy, Table 1(1).
Contiguous Osteomyelitis With Vascular Insufficiency. Ref.: CID S115–22, 2004				
Most pts are **diabetics** with peripheral neuropathy & infected skin ulcers (see Diabetic foot, page 15)	Polymicrobic [Gm+ cocci (to include MRSA) (aerobic & anaerobic) and Gm-neg. bacilli (aerobic & anaerobic)]	Debride overlying ulcer & submit bone for histology & culture. Select antibiotic based on culture results & treat for 6 weeks. **No empiric therapy unless acutely ill.** If acutely ill, see suggestions, Diabetic foot, page 15. Revascularize if possible. Full contact cast.		**Diagnosis of osteo:** Culture bone biopsy (gold standard). Poor concordance of culture results between swab of ulcer and bone – need bone. (CID 42:57, 63, 2006). Osteo more likely if ulcer >2cm², positive probe to bone, ESR >70 & abnormal plain x-ray (JAMA 299:806, 2008). **Treatment:** (1) **Revascularize if possible.** (2) Culture bone. (3) Specific antimicrobial(s). (4) Full contact cast.
Chronic Osteomyelitis: Specific therapy By definition, implies presence of dead bone. **Need valid cultures**	S. aureus, Enterobacteria-ceae, P. aeruginosa	**Empiric rx not indicated.** Base systemic rx on results of culture, sensitivity testing. If acute exacerbation of chronic osteo, rx as acute hematogenous osteo.		Important adjuncts: removal of orthopedic hardware, surgical debridement, vascularized muscle flaps, distraction osteogenesis (Ilizarov) techniques. Antibiotic-impregnated cement & hyperbaric oxygen adjunctive. **NOTE: RIF + (vanco or β-lactam)** effective in animal model and in a clinical trial of S. aureus chronic osteo (SMJ 79:947, 1986).
BREAST: Mastitis—Obtain culture; need to know if MRSA present. Review with definitions: Ob & Gyn Clin No Amer 29:89, 2002				
Postpartum mastitis				
Mastitis without abscess Ref.: JAMA 289:1609, 2003	S. aureus; less often S. pyogenes (Gp A or B), E. coli, bacteroides species, maybe Corynebacterium sp., & selected coagulase-neg. staphylococci (e.g., S. lugdunensis)	**NO MRSA: Outpatient: Dicloxacillin** 500 mg po qid or **cephalexin** 500 mg po qid. **Inpatient: Nafcillin/oxacillin** 2 gm IV q4h	**MRSA Possible: Outpatient: TMP-SMX-DS** tabs 1-2 po bid or, if susceptible, **clinda** 300 mg po qid **Inpatient: Vanco** 1 gm IV q12h; if over 100 kg, 1.5 gm IV q12h.	If no abscess, ↑ freq of nursing may hasten response; no risk to infant. Coryne-bacterium sp. assoc. with chronic granulomatous mastitis (CID 35:1434, 2002). Bartonella henselae infection reported (Ob & Gyn 95:1027, 2000).
Mastitis with abscess				With abscess, d/c nursing, **I&D standard;** needle aspiration reported successful (Am J Surg 182:117, 2001). Resume breast feeding from affected breast as soon as pain allows.
Non-puerperal mastitis with abscess	S. aureus; less often Bacter-oides sp., peptostreptococ-cus, & selected coagulase-neg. staphylococci	Acute: Vanco 1 gm IV q12h; if over 100 kg, 1.5 gm q12h.		**If subareolar & odoriferous**, most likely anaerobes; need to **add metro** 500 mg IV/po tid. If not subareolar, staph. Need pretreatment aerobic/anaerobic cultures. Surgical drainage for abscess.
Breast implant infection	Acute: S. aureus, S. pyogenes. TSS reported. Chronic: Look for rapidly growing Mycobacteria	Acute: Await culture results. See Table 12 for mycobacteria treatment.		Lancet Infect Dis 5:94, 462, 2005

Abbreviations on page 3.   NOTE: All dosage recommendations are for adults (unless otherwise indicated) and assume normal renal function.

TABLE 1A (3)

ANATOMIC SITE/DIAGNOSIS/ MODIFYING CIRCUMSTANCES	ETIOLOGIES (usual)	SUGGESTED REGIMENS*		ADJUNCT DIAGNOSTIC OR THERAPEUTIC MEASURES AND COMMENTS
		PRIMARY	ALTERNATIVE§	
CENTRAL NERVOUS SYSTEM				
Brain abscess				
Primary or contiguous source Ref.: *CID 25:763, 1997*	Streptococci (60–70%), bacteroides (20–40%), Enterobacteriaceae (25–33%), S. aureus (10–15%), S. milleri. Rare: Nocardia (*below*) Listeria (*CID 40:907, 2005*)	**P Ceph 3 ([cefotaxime** 2 gm IV q4h or **ceftriaxone** 2 gm IV q12h) + (**metro** 7.5 mg/kg q6h or 15 mg/kg IV q12h)]	**Pen G** 3-4 million units IV q4h + **metro** 7.5 mg/kg q6h or 15 mg/kg IV q12h	If CT scan suggests cerebritis or abscesses <2.5 cm and pt neurologically stable and conscious, start antibiotics and observe. Otherwise, surgical drainage necessary. Experience with Pen G (HD) + metro without ceftriaxone or nafcillin/oxacillin has been good. We use ceftriaxone because of frequency of isolation of Enterobacteriaceae. **S. aureus rare without positive blood culture; if S. aureus, include vanco until susceptibility known.** Strep. milleri group esp. prone to produce abscess.
		Duration of rx unclear; treat until response by neuroimaging (CT/MRI)		
Post-surgical, post-traumatic	S. aureus, Enterobacteriaceae	For MSSA: (**Nafcillin or oxacillin**) 2 gm IV q4h + (**ceftriaxone or cefotaxime**)	For MRSA: **Vanco** 1 gm IV q12h + (**ceftriaxone or cefotaxime**)	
HIV-1 infected (AIDS)	Toxoplasma gondii	See Table 13A, page 129		
Nocardia: Haematogenous abscess *Can Med J 171:1063, 2004*	N. asteroides & B. basiliensis	**TMP-SMX:** 15 mg/kg/day of TMP & 75 mg/kg/day of SMX, IV/po div in 2-4 doses + **ceftriaxone** 2 gm IV q12h. If multiorgan involvement some add **amikacin** 7.5 mg/kg q12h. After 3-6 wks of IV therapy, switch to po therapy. Immunocompetent pts: **TMP-SMX, minocycline** or **AM-CL** x 3 months. Immunocompromised pts: Treat with 2 drugs for at least one year.	**TMP-SMX + amikacin** as in primary and add **IMP** 500 mg IV q6h.	Measure peak sulfonamide levels: target 100-150 mcg/mL 2 hrs post dose. **Linezolid** 600 mg po bid reported effective (*Ann Pharmacother 41:1694, 2007*). For in vitro susceptibility testing: Wallace (+) 903-877-7680 or U.S. CDC (+1) 404-639-3158. If sulfanomide resistant or sulfa-allergic, **amikacin** plus one of: **IMP, MER, ceftriaxone** or **cefotaxime.**
Subdural empyema: In adult 60-90% are extension of sinusitis or otitis media. Rx same as primary brain abscess. Surgical emergency: must drain (*CID 20:372, 1995*).				
Encephalitis/encephalopathy *IDSA Guideline: CID 47:303, 2008.* (*For Herpes see Table 14A,page 141, and for rabies, page 191*)	Herpes simplex, arboviruses, rabies, West Nile virus. Rarely: listeria, cat-scratch disease, amebic	Start IV **acyclovir** while awaiting results of CSF PCR for H. simplex. For amebic encephalitis see *Table 13A.*		Newly recognized strain of bat rabies. May not require a break in the skin to infect. Eastern equine encephalitis causes focal MRI changes in basal ganglia and thalamus (*NEJM 336:867, 1997*). Cat-scratch ref.: *PIDJ 23:1161, 2004*). Ref. on West Nile & related viruses: *NEJM 351:370, 2004.*
Meningitis, "Aseptic": Pleocytosis of 100s of cells, CSF glucose normal, neg. culture for bacteria (*see Table 14A, page 137*) Ref.: *CID 47:783, 2008*	Enteroviruses, HSV-2, LCM, HIV, other viruses, drugs (NSAIDs, metronidazole, carbamazepine, TMP-SMX, IVIG), rarely leptospirosis	For all but leptospirosis, IV fluids and analgesics. D/C drugs that may be etiologic. For lepto (**doxy** 100 mg IV/po q12h) or (**AMP** 0.5–1 gm IV q6h). Repeat LP if suspect partially-treated bacterial meningitis.		If available, PCR of CSF for enterovirus. HSV-2 unusual without concomitant genital herpes. Drug-induced aseptic meningitis: *AnIM 159:1185, 1999.* For lepto, positive epidemiologic history and concomitant hepatitis, conjunctivitis, dermatitis, nephritis. For complete list of implicated drugs: *Inf Med 25:331, 2008.*
Meningitis, Bacterial, Acute: Goal is empiric therapy, then CSF exam within 30 min. If focal neurologic deficit, give empiric therapy, then head CT, then LP. (*NEJM 354:44,2006; Ln ID 7:191, 2007*) NOTE: In children, treatment caused CSF cultures to turn neg. in 2 hrs with meningococci & partial response with pneumococci in 4 hrs (*Peds 108:1169, 2001*)				
Empiric Therapy—CSF Gram stain is negative—immunocompetent				
Age: Preterm to <1 mo *Ln 361:2139, 2003*	Group B strep 49%, E. coli 18%, listeria 7%, misc. Gm-neg. 10%, misc. Gm-pos. 10%	**AMP + cefotaxime** Intraventricular treatment not recommended. Repeat CSF exam/culture 24-36 hr after start of therapy	**AMP + gentamicin**	Primary & alternative reg active vs Group B strep, most coliforms, & listeria. If premature infant with long nursery stay, S. aureus, enterococci, and resistant coliforms potential pathogens. Optional empiric regimens: [nafcillin + (ceftazidime or cefotaxime)]. **If high risk of MRSA,** use vanco + cefotaxime. Alter regimen after culture/sensitivity data available.
		For dosage, see Table 16		

Abbreviations on page 3.   NOTE: All dosage recommendations are for adults (unless otherwise indicated) and assume normal renal function.

TABLE 1A (4)

ANATOMIC SITE/DIAGNOSIS/ MODIFYING CIRCUMSTANCES	ETIOLOGIES (usual)	SUGGESTED REGIMENS*		ADJUNCT DIAGNOSTIC OR THERAPEUTIC MEASURES AND COMMENTS
		PRIMARY	ALTERNATIVE[5]	
CENTRAL NERVOUS SYSTEM/Meningitis, Bacterial, Acute/Empiric Therapy *(continued)*				
Age: 1 mo– 50 yrs See **footnote**[2] for empiric treatment rationale. For meningococcal immunization, see *Table 20A, page 187.*	S. pneumo, meningococci, H. influenzae now very rare, **listeria unlikely if young & immuno-competent** (add **ampicillin** if suspect listeria 2 gm IV q4h)	Adult dosage: [[Cefotax-ime 2 gm IV q4–6h OR ceftriaxone 2 gm IV q12h]] + **vanco** (see footnote[3]) Peds: see footnote[4]	[[MER 2 gm IV q8h] (Peds: 40 mg/kg IV q8h)] + IV dexamethasone + vanco (see footnote[3]) Peds: see footnote[4]	**For pts with severe pen. allergy: Chloro** 12.5 mg/kg IV q6h (max. 4 gm/day) (for meningococcus) + **TMP-SMX** 5 mg/kg q6–8h (for listeria if immunocom-promised) + **vanco**. Rare meningococcal isolates chloro-resistant (*NEJM 339:868, 1998*). High chloro failure rate in pts with resistant S. pneumo (*Ln 339: 405, 1992; Ln 342:240, 1993*). **So far, no vanco-resistant S. pneumo.** Value of dexamethasone documented in children with H. influenzae and in adults with S. pneumo (*NEJM 347:1549 & 1613, 2002; NEJM 357:2431 & 2441, 2007; LnID 4:139, 2004*). **Give 1st dose 15–20min. prior to or con-comitant with 1st dose of antibiotic. Dose: 0.15 mg/kg IV q6h x 2–4 days.**
		Dexamethasone: 0.15 mg/kg IV q6h x 2–4 days. **Give with or just before 1st dose of antibiotic to block TNF production** (See Comment). See footnote[4] for rest of ped. dosage		
Age: >50 yrs or alcoholism or other debilitating assoc diseases or impaired cellular immunity	S. pneumo, listeria, Gm-neg. bacilli. Note absence of meningo-coccus.	(AMP 2 gm IV q4h) + (ceftriaxone 2 gm IV q12h or cefotaxime 2 gm IV q6h) + vanco + IV dexamethasone For vanco dose, see footnote[3]. Dexamethasone: 0.15 mg/kg IV q6h x 2–4 days; 1st dose before or concomitant with 1st dose of antibiotic.	MER 2 gm IV q8h + vanco + IV dexamethasone **For severe pen. Allergy, see Comment**	**Severe penicillin allergy: Vanco** 500–750 mg IV q6h + **TMP-SMX** 5 mg/kg q6–8h pending culture results. Chloro has failed vs resistant S. pneumo (*Ln 342:240, 1993*).
Post-neurosurgery, post-head trauma, or post-cochlear implant (*NEJM 349:435, 2003*)	S. pneumoniae most common, esp. if CSF leak. Other: S. aureus, coliforms, P. aeruginosa	**Vanco** (until known not MRSA) 500–750 mg IV q6h[2] + **cefepime** or **ceftaz-idime** 2 gm IV q8h)(see Comment	MER 2 gm IV q8h + **vanco** 1 gm IV q6–12h	**Vanco** alone not optimal for S. pneumo. If/when suscept. S. pneumo identified, quickly switch to **ceftriaxone** or **cefotaxime**. If coliform or pseudomonas meningitis, some add intrathecal gentamicin (4 mg q12h into lateral ventricles). Cure of acinetobacter meningitis with intraventricular or intrathecal colistin (*JAC 53:290, 2004; JAC 58:1078, 2006*).
Ventriculitis/meningitis due to infected ventriculo-peritoneal (atrial) shunt	S. epidermidis, S. aureus, coliforms, diphtheroids (rare), P. acnes	**Vanco** 500–750 mg IV q6h + (**cefepime** or **ceftazi-dime** 2 gm IV q8h) If unable to remove shunt, consider intraventricular therapy; for dosages, see footnote[5]	**Vanco** 500–750 mg IV q6h + **MER** 2 gm IV q8h	Usual care: 1st remove infected shunt & culture; external ventricular catheter for drainage/pressure control; antimicrobic for 14 days. For timing of new shunt, see *CID 39:1267, 2004.*
Empiric Therapy—Positive CSF Gram stain				
Gram-positive diplococci	S. pneumoniae	Either (**ceftriaxone** 2 gm IV q12h or **cefotaxime** 2 gm IV q4–6h) + **vanco** 500–750 mg IV q6h + timed **dexametha-sone** 0.15 mg/kg q6h IV x 2–4 days.	**Dexamethasone** 0.15 mg/kg IV q8h or **Moxi** 400 mg IV q24h. **Dexamethasone** does not block penetration of vanco into CSF (*CID 44:250, 2007*).	**Alternatives: MER** 2 gm IV q8h or **Moxi** 400 mg IV q24h or **AMP** 2 gm q4h or **Moxi** 400 mg IV q24h. **In adults**, max dose of 2-3 gm/day is suggested: **500–750 mg IV q6h.**
Gram-negative diplococci	N. meningitidis	(**Cefotaxime** 2 gm IV q4–6h or **ceftriaxone** 2 gm IV q12h)		**Alternatives: Pen G** 4 mill. units IV q4h or **AMP** 2 gm q4h or **chloro** 1 gm IV q6h

---

2 **Rationale:** Hard to get adequate CSF concentrations of anti-infectives, hence MIC criteria for in vitro susceptibility are lower for CSF isolates (*ArIM 161:2538, 2001*).
3 Low & erratic penetration of **vanco** into the CSF (*PIDJ 16:895, 1997*). **children's dosage** 15 mg/kg IV q6h (2x standard adult dose). **In adults**, max dose of 2-3 gm/day is suggested: **500–750 mg IV q6h.**
4 **Dosage of drugs used to treat children ≥1 mo of age:** Cefotaxime 200 mg/kg per day IV div. q6–8h; ceftriaxone 100 mg/kg per day IV div. q12h; vanco 15 mg/kg IV q6h.
5 Dosages for intraventricular therapy. The following are daily adult doses in mg: amikacin 30, gentamicin 4–8, polymyxin E (Colistin) 10, tobramycin 5–20, vanco 10–20. Ref.: *CID 39:1267, 2004.*

Abbreviations on page 3.   NOTE: *All dosage recommendations are for adults (unless otherwise indicated) and assume normal renal function.*

TABLE 1A (5)

ANATOMIC SITE/DIAGNOSIS/ MODIFYING CIRCUMSTANCES	ETIOLOGIES (usual)	SUGGESTED REGIMENS* PRIMARY	ALTERNATIVE§	ADJUNCT DIAGNOSTIC OR THERAPEUTIC MEASURES AND COMMENTS
CENTRAL NERVOUS SYSTEM/Meningitis, Bacterial, Acute/Empiric Therapy (continued)				
Gram-positive bacilli or coccobacilli	Listeria monocytogenes	AMP 2 gm IV q4h ± **gentamicin** 2 mg/kg loading dose then 1.7 mg/kg q8h		If pen-allergic, use TMP-SMX 5 mg/kg q6–8h or **MER 2 gm IV q8h**
Gram-negative bacilli	H. influenzae, coliforms, P. aeruginosa	(**Ceftazidime** or **cefepime** 2 gm IV q8h) + **gentamicin** 2 mg/kg 1st dose then 1.7 mg/kg q8h		Alternatives: **CIP** 400 mg IV q8–12h; **MER** 2 gm IV q8h
Specific Therapy—Positive culture of CSF with in vitro susceptibility results available. Interest in monitoring/reducing intracranial pressure: CID 38:384, 2004				
H. influenzae	β-lactamase positive	Ceftriaxone (peds): 50 mg/kg IV q12h		Pen. allergic: **Chloro** 12.5 mg/kg IV q6h (max. 4 gm/day.)
Listeria monocytogenes (CID 43:1233, 2006)		AMP 2 gm IV q4h ± **gentamicin** 2 mg/kg loading dose, then 1.7 mg/kg q8h		Pen. allergic: **TMP-SMX** 20 mg/kg per day div. q6–12h. One report of greater efficacy of AMP + TMP-SMX as compared to AMP + gentamicin (JID 33:79, 1996). Alternative: **MER 2 gm IV q8h**. Success reported with **linezolid + RIF** (CID 40:908, 2005).
N. meningitidis	MIC 0.1–1 mcg per mL	**Ceftriaxone** 2 gm IV q12h x 7 days (see Comment); if pen. allergic, **chloro** 12.5 mg/kg (up to 1 gm) IV q6h		Rare isolates chloro-resistant (NEJM 339:368 & 917, 1998). Alternatives: **MER** 2 gm IV q8h or **Moxi** 400 mg q24h.
S. pneumoniae NOTES:	Pen G MIC <0.1 mcg/mL	Pen G 4 million units IV q4h or **AMP** 2 gm IV q4h		Alternatives: **Ceftriaxone** 2 gm IV q12h, **chloro** 1 gm IV q6h
1. Assumes dexamethasone just prior to 1st dose & x 4 days.	0.1–1 mcg/mL	**Ceftriaxone** 2 gm IV q12h or **cefotaxime** 2 gm IV q4–6h		Alternatives: **Cefepime** 2 gm IV q8h or **MER** 2 gm IV q8h
2. If MIC ≥1, repeat CSF exam after 24–48h.	≥2 mcg/mL	**Vanco** 500–750 mg IV q6h + (**ceftriaxone** or **cefotaxime** as above)		Alternatives: **Moxi** 400 mg IV q24h
3. Treat for 10–14 days	Ceftriaxone MIC ≥1 mcg/mL	**Vanco** 500–750 mg IV q6h + (**ceftriaxone** or **cefotaxime** as above)		Alternatives: **Moxi** 400 mg IV q24h If MIC to ceftriaxone >2 mcg/mL, add **RIF** 600 mg 1x/day.
E. coli, other coliforms, or P. aeruginosa	Consultation advised— need susceptibility results	(**Ceftazidime** or **cefepime** 2 gm IV q8h) ± **gentamicin**		Alternatives: **CIP** 400 mg IV q8–12h; **MER** 2 gm IV q8h. For discussion of intraventricular therapy: CID 39:1267, 2004
Prophylaxis for H. influenzae and N. meningitides				
Haemophilus influenzae type b Household and/or day care contact: residing with index case or ≥4 hrs. Day care contact: same day care as index case for 5–7 days before onset		**Children: RIF** 20 mg/kg po (not to exceed 600 mg) q24h x 4 doses. **Adults: RIF** 600 mg q24h x 4 days		**Household:** If there is one unvaccinated contact ≤4 yr in the household, give RIF to all household contacts except pregnant women. **Child Care Facilities:** With 1 case, if attended by unvaccinated children ≤2 yr, consider prophylaxis + vaccinate susceptibles. If all contacts >2 yr: no prophylaxis. If ≥2 cases in 60 days & unvaccinated children attend, prophylaxis recommended for children & personnel (Am Acad Ped Red Book 2006, page 313).
Prophylaxis for Neisseria meningitidis exposure (close contact) NOTE: CDC reports CIP-resistant gp B meningococcus from selected counties in N. Dakota & Minnesota. Use ceftriaxone, RIF, or single 500 mg dose of azithro (MMWR 57:173, 2008).		[**CIP** (adults) 500 mg po single dose] OR [**Ceftriaxone** 250 mg IM x 1 dose (child <15 yr 125 mg IM x 1)] OR [**RIF** 600 mg po q12h x 4 doses. (Children >1 mo 10 mg/kg po q12h x 4 doses, <1 mo 5 mg/kg q12h x 4 doses)] OR **Spiramycin**NUS 500 mg po q6h x 5 days. Children 10 mg/kg po q6h x 5 days.		Spread by respiratory droplets, not aerosols, hence close contact req. ↑ risk if close contact for at least 4hrs during wk before illness onset (e.g., housemates, day care contacts, cellmates) or exposure to pt's nasopharyngeal secretions (e.g., kissing, mouth-to-mouth resuscitation, intubation, nasotracheal suction-ing). Since RIF-resistant N. meningitidis documented, post-prophylaxis (EID 11:977, 2005) with CIP or ceftriaxone preferred. Primary prophylactic regimen in many European countries.
Meningitis, chronic Defined as symptoms + CSF pleocytosis for ≥4 wks	M. tbc 40%, cryptococcosis 7%, neoplastic 8%, Lyme, syphilis, Whipple's disease	Treatment depends on etiology. No urgent need for empiric therapy.		Long list of possibilities: bacteria, parasites, fungi, viruses, neoplasms, vasculitis, and other miscellaneous etiologies—see chapter on chronic meningitis in latest edition of Harrison's Textbook of Internal Medicine. Whipple's: JID 188:797 & 801, 2003.

Abbreviations on page 3.   NOTE: All dosage recommendations are for adults (unless otherwise indicated) and assume normal renal function.

TABLE 1A (6)

ANATOMIC SITE/DIAGNOSIS/ MODIFYING CIRCUMSTANCES	ETIOLOGIES (usual)	SUGGESTED REGIMENS* PRIMARY	SUGGESTED REGIMENS* ALTERNATIVE§	ADJUNCT DIAGNOSTIC OR THERAPEUTIC MEASURES AND COMMENTS
CENTRAL NERVOUS SYSTEM (continued)				
Meningitis, eosinophilic *LnID 8:621, 2008*	Angiostrongyliasis, gnathostomiasis, baylisascaris	Corticosteroids	Not sure antihelminthic therapy works	1/3 lack peripheral eosinophilia. Need serology to confirm diagnosis. Steroid ref.: *CID 31:660, 2001; LnID 6:621, 2008*.
Meningitis, HIV-1 infected (AIDS) See *Table 11, Sanford Guide to HIV/AIDS Therapy*	As in adults, >50 yr: also consider cryptococci, M. tuberculosis, syphilis, HIV aseptic meningitis, Listeria monocytogenes	If etiology not identified: treat as adult >50 yr + obtain CSF/serum cryptococcal antigen (see *Comments*)	For crypto rx, see *Table 11A, page 102*	C. neoformans most common etiology in AIDS patients. H. influenzae, pneumococci, Tbc, syphilis, viral, histoplasma & coccidioides also need to be considered. Obtain blood cultures. L. monocytogenes risk >60x ↑, ¾ present as meningitis (*CID 17:224, 1993*).
EAR				
External otitis				
Chronic	Usually 2° to seborrhea	Eardrops: [(**polymyxin B + neomycin + hydrocortisone** qid) + **selenium sulfide shampoo**]		Control seborrhea with dandruff shampoo containing selenium sulfide (Selsun) or [(ketoconazole shampoo) + (medium potency steroid solution, triamcinolone 0.1%)].
Fungal	Candida species	Fluconazole 200 mg po x 1 dose & then 100 mg po x 3-5 days.		
"Malignant otitis externa" Risk groups: Diabetes mellitus, AIDS, chemotherapy. Ref: *Oto Clinics N Amer 41:537, 2008*	Pseudomonas aeruginosa in >90%	(**IMP** 0.5 gm IV q6h) or (**MER** 1 gm IV q8h) or [**CIP** 400 mg IV q12h (or 750 mg po q12h)] or (**ceftaz** 2 gm IV q8h) or (**CFP** 2 gm q12h) or (**PIP** 4–6 gm IV q4–6h + **tobra**) or (**TC** 3 gm IV q4h + **tobra** dose Table 10D)		CIP po for treatment of early disease. Debridement usually required. R/O osteomyelitis: CT or MRI scan. If bone involved: treat for 4–6 wks. PIP without Tazo may be hard to find: extended infusion of PIP-TZ (4 hr infusion of 3.375 gm every 8h) may improve efficacy (*CID 44:357, 2007*).
"Swimmer's ear" *PIDJ 22:299, 2003*	Pseudomonas sp., Enterobacteriaceae, Proteus sp. (Fungi rare.) Acute infection usually 2° S. aureus	Eardrops: **Oflox 0.3% soln bid** or [(**polymyxin B + neomycin + hydrocortisone**) qid] or (**CIP + hydrocortisone bid**) --active vs gm-neg bacilli. For acute disease: **dicloxacillin** 500 mg po 4x/day.		Rx includes gentle cleaning. Recurrences prevented (or decreased) by drying with alcohol drops (1/3 white vinegar, 2/3 rubbing alcohol) after swimming, then antibiotic drops or 2% acetic acid solution. Ointments should not be used in ear. Do not use neomycin drops if tympanic membrane punctured.

Otitis media—infants, children, adults

Acute (*NEJM 347:1169, 2002; Peds 113:1451, 2004*). For correlation of bacterial eradication from middle ear & clinical outcome, see *LnID 2:593, 2002.*

Initial empiric therapy of acute otitis media (AOM) **NOTE:** Pending new data, **treat children <2 yr old**. If >2 yr old, afebrile, no ear pain, neg./questionable exam—consider analgesic treatment without antimicrobials. Favorable results in mostly afebrile pts with waiting 48hrs before deciding on antibiotic use (*JAMA 296:1235, 1290, 2006*)	Overall detection in middle ear fluid: No pathogen 4% Virus 70% Bact. + virus 66% Bacteria only 92% Bacterial pathogens from middle ear: S. pneumo 49%, H. influenzae 29%, M. catarrhalis 28%. Ref.: *CID 43:1417 & 1423, 2006.* Children 6 mo-3 yrs. 2 episodes AOM/yr & 63% are virus positive (*CID 46:815 & 824, 2008*).	**If NO antibiotics in prior month:** **Amox** po HD[6] For dosage, see footnotes[7] and[8] on next page **All doses are pediatric** **Duration of rx:** <2 yr old x 10 days; ≥2 yr x 5-7 days. Approp. duration unclear. 5 days may be inadequate for severe disease (*NEJM 347:1169, 2002*) **For adult dosages, see Sinusitis, pages 46–47, and Table 10**	**Received antibiotics in prior month:** **Amox** HD[6] or **AM-CL** extra-strength[6] or **cefdinir** or **cefpodoxime** or **cefprozil** or **cefuroxime axetil**	**If allergic to β-lactam drugs?** If history unclear or rash, effective oral ceph OK; avoid ceph if IgE-mediated allergy, e.g., anaphylaxis. High failure rate with **TMP-SMX** if etiology is DRSP or H. influenzae (*PIDJ 20:260, 2001*); **azithro x 5 days or clarithro x 10 days** (both have ↓ activity vs DRSP). **Up to 50% S. pneumo resistant to macrolides**. Rationale & data for single dose azithro, 30 mg per kg: *PIDJ 23:S102 & S108, 2004.* **Spontaneous resolution occurred in:** 90% pts infected with M. catarrhalis, 50% with H. influenzae, 10% with S. pneumoniae; overall 80% resolve within 2-14 days (*Ln 363:465, 2004*). Risk of DRSP ↑ if age <2 yr, antibiotics last 3 mo, &/or daycare attendance. Selection of drug based on (1) effectiveness against β-lactamase producing H. influenzae & M. catarrhalis & (2) effectiveness against S. pneumo, inc. DRSP. **Cefaclor, loracarbef, & ceftibuten less active vs resistant S. pneumo.** Other than these other agents listed. Variable acceptance of drug taste/smell by children 4–8 yrs old. [*PIDJ 19 (Suppl.2):S174, 2000*].

Abbreviations: **Amoxicillin UD or HD** = amoxicillin usual dose or high dose; **AM-CL HD** = amoxicillin-clavulanate high dose. **Dosages in footnote[8] on next page.** Data supporting amoxicillin HD: *PIDJ 22:405, 2003.*

[6] **Amoxicillin UD or HD** = amoxicillin usual dose or high dose; **AM-CL HD** = amoxicillin-clavulanate high dose. **Dosages in footnote[8] on next page.** Data supporting amoxicillin HD: *PIDJ 22:405, 2003.*

Abbreviations on page 3.   NOTE: *All dosage recommendations are for adults (unless otherwise indicated) and assume normal renal function.*

TABLE 1A (7)

ANATOMIC SITE/DIAGNOSIS/ MODIFYING CIRCUMSTANCES	ETIOLOGIES (usual)	SUGGESTED REGIMENS*		ADJUNCT DIAGNOSTIC OR THERAPEUTIC MEASURES AND COMMENTS
		PRIMARY	ALTERNATIVE§	
EAR/Otitis media—infants, children, adults (*continued*)				
Treatment for clinical failure after 3 days	Drug-resistant S. pneumoniae main concern	**NO antibiotics in month prior to last 3 days:** **AM-CL** high dose or **cefdinir** or **cefpodoxime** or **cefprozil** or **cefuroxime axetil** or IM **ceftriaxone** x 3 days. For dosage, see *footnotes[7] and[8]* **All doses are pediatric** Duration of rx as above	**Antibiotics in month prior to last 3 days:** [(IM **ceftriaxone**) or (**clindamycin**) and/or tympanocentesis] See *clindamycin Comments*	**Clindamycin** not active vs H. influenzae or M. catarrhalis. S. pneumo resistant to macrolides are usually also resistant to clindamycin. Definition of failure: no change in ear pain, fever, bulging TM or otorrhea after 3 days of therapy. Tympanocentesis will allow culture. **Newer FQs active vs drug-resistant S. pneumo (DRSP), but not approved for use in children** (*PIDJ 23:390, 2004*). **Vanco is active vs DRSP.** Ceftriaxone IM x 3 days superior to 1-day treatment vs DRSP (*PIDJ 19:1040, 2000*). AM-CL HD reported successful for pen-resistant S. pneumo AOM (*PIDJ 20:829, 2001*).
After >48hrs of nasotracheal intubation	Pseudomonas sp., klebsiella, enterobacter	**Ceftazidime** or **CFP** or **IMP** or **MER** or (**Pip-Tz**) or **TC-CL** or **CIP**. (*For dosages, see Ear, Malignant otitis externa, page 10*)		With nasotracheal intubation >48 hrs, about ½ pts will have otitis media with effusion.
Prophylaxis: acute otitis media *PIDJ 22:10, 2003*	Pneumococci, H. influenzae, M. catarrhalis, Staph. aureus, Group A strep (*see Comments*)	**Sulfisoxazole** 50 mg/kg po at bedtime or **amoxicillin** 20 mg/kg q24h	**Use of antibiotics to prevent otitis media is a major contributor to emergence of antibiotic-resistant S. pneumo!** Pneumococcal protein conjugate vaccine decreases freq. AOM & due to vaccine serotypes. Adenoidectomy at time of tympanostomy tubes ↓ need for future hospitalization for AOM (*NEJM 344:1188, 2001*).	
Mastoiditis				
Acute Outpatient	Strep. pneumoniae 22%, S. pyogenes 16%, **Staph. aureus** 7%, H. influenzae 4%, P. aeruginosa 4%; others <1%	Empirically, same as Acute otitis media, above; need **vanco** or **nafcillin/oxacillin** if culture + for S. aureus.		Has become a rare entity, presumably as result of the aggressive treatment of acute otitis media. Small ↑ in incidence in Netherlands where use of antibiotics limited to children with complicated course or high risk (*PIDJ 20:140, 2001*).
Hospitalized		**Cefotaxime** 1–2 gm IV q4–8h (depends on severity) or (**ceftriaxone** 1 gm IV q24h)		
Chronic	Often polymicrobic: anaerobes, S. aureus, Enterobacteriaceae, P. aeruginosa	Treatment for acute exacerbations or perioperatively. No treatment until surgical cultures obtained. Empiric regimens: **IMP** 0.5 gm IV q6h, **TC-CL** 3.1 gm IV q6h, **PIP-TZ** 3.375 gm IV q4–6h or 4.5 gm q8h, or 4 hr infusion of 3.375 gm q8h, **MER** 1 gm IV Q8h.		May or may not be associated with chronic otitis media with drainage via ruptured tympanic membrane. Antimicrobials given in association with surgery. Mastoidectomy indications: chronic drainage and evidence of osteomyelitis by MRI or CT, evidence of spread to CNS (epidural abscess, suppurative phlebitis, brain abscess).

[7] **Amoxicillin UD or HD** = amoxicillin usual dose or high dose: **AM-CL HD** = amoxicillin-clavulanate high dose: *PIDJ 22:405, 2003.*

[8] **Drugs & peds dosage (all po unless specified) for acute otitis media: Amoxicillin UD** = 40 mg/kg per day div q12h or q8h. **Amoxicillin HD** = 90 mg/kg per day div q12h or q8h. **AM-CL HD** = 90 mg/kg per day of amox component. **Extra-strength AM-CL oral suspension** (Augmentin ES-600) available with 600 mg AM & 42.9 mg CL / 5 mL—dose: 90/6.4 mg/kg per day div bid. **Cefuroxime axetil** 30 mg/kg per day div q12h. **Ceftriaxone** 50 mg/kg IM x 3 days. **Clindamycin** 20–30 mg/kg per day div qid (may be effective vs DRSP but no activity vs H. influenzae). **Other drugs suitable for drug (e.g., penicillin)-sensitive S. pneumo: TMP-SMX** 4 mg/kg of TMP q12h. **Erythro-sulfisoxazole** 50 mg/kg per day of erythro div q6–8h. **Clarithro** 15 mg/kg per day q12h; **azithro** 10 mg/kg per day x 1 & then 5 mg/kg q24h on days 2–5. Other FDA-approved regimens: 10 mg/kg q24h x 3 days & 30 mg/kg x 1. **Cefprozil** 15 mg/kg q12h; **cefpodoxime proxetil** 10 mg/kg per day as single dose; **cefaclor** 40 mg/kg per day div q8h; **loracarbef** 15 mg/kg per day div q8h. **Cefdinir** 7 mg/kg q12h or 14 mg/kg q24h.

Abbreviations on page 3.   *NOTE: All dosage recommendations are for adults (unless otherwise indicated) and assume normal renal function.*

TABLE 1A (8)

ANATOMIC SITE/DIAGNOSIS/ MODIFYING CIRCUMSTANCES	ETIOLOGIES (usual)	SUGGESTED REGIMENS* PRIMARY	ALTERNATIVE§	ADJUNCT DIAGNOSTIC OR THERAPEUTIC MEASURES AND COMMENTS
EYE—General Reviews: *CID 21:479, 1995; IDCP 7:447, 1998*				
Eyelid: Little reported experience with CA-MRSA (*Ophtha 113:455, 2006*)				
Blepharitis	Etiol. unclear. Factors include Staph. aureus & Staph. epidermidis, seborrhea, rosacea. & dry eye	Lid margin care with baby shampoo & warm compresses q24h. Artificial tears if assoc. dry eye (see *Comment*).		Usually topical ointments of no benefit. If associated rosacea, add doxy 100 mg po bid for 2 wk and then q24h.
Hordeolum (Stye)				
External (eyelash follicle)	Staph. aureus	Hot packs only. Will drain spontaneously		Infection of superficial sebaceous gland.
Internal (Meibomian glands): Can be acute, subacute or chronic.	Staph. aureus, MSSA	Oral **dicloxacillin** + hot packs		Also called acute meibomianitis. Rarely drain spontaneously; may need I&D and culture. Role of fluoroquinolone eye drops is unclear: MRSA often resistant to lower conc.; may be susceptible to higher concentration of FQ in ophthalmologic solutions of gati, levo or moxi.
	Staph. aureus, MRSA-CA	**TMP/SMX-DS**, tabs ii po bid		
	Staph. aureus, MRSA-HA	**Linezolid** 600 mg po bid possible therapy if multi-drug resistant.		
Conjunctiva: *NEJM 343:345, 2000*				
Conjunctivitis of the newborn (ophthalmia neonatorum): by day of onset post-delivery—all doses pediatric				
Onset 1st day	Chemical due to silver nitrate prophylaxis	None		Usual prophylaxis is erythro ointment; hence, silver nitrate irritation rare.
Onset 2–4 days	N. gonorrhoeae	**Ceftriaxone** 25–50 mg/kg IV x 1 dose (see *Comment*), not to exceed 125 mg		Treat mother and her sexual partners. Hyperpurulent. Topical rx inadequate. **Treat neonate for concomitant Chlamydia trachomatis.**
Onset 3–10 days	Chlamydia trachomatis	**Erythro base or ethylsuccinate syrup** 12.5 mg/kg q6h x 14 days). No topical rx needed.		Diagnosis by antigen detection. Alternative: **Azithro suspension** 20 mg/kg po q24h x 3 days. Treat mother & sexual partner.
Onset 2–16 days	Herpes simplex types 1, 2	See *keratitis on page 13*		Consider IV acyclovir if concomitant systemic disease.
Ophthalmia neonatorum prophylaxis: **Silver nitrate** 1% x 1 or **erythro** 0.5% ointment x 1 or **tetra** 1% ointment x 1 application				
Pink eye (viral conjunctivitis) Usually unilateral	Adenovirus (types 3 & 7 in children, 8, 11 & 19 in adults)	No treatment. If symptomatic, cold artificial tears may help.		Highly contagious. Onset of ocular pain and photophobia in an adult suggests associated keratitis—rare.
Inclusion conjunctivitis (**adult**) Usually unilateral	Chlamydia trachomatis	**Doxy** 100 mg bid po x 1–3 wk	**Erythro** 250 mg po qid x 1–3 wk	Oculogenital disease. Diagnosis by culture or antigen detection or PCR—availability varies by region and institution. Treat sexual partner.
Trachoma --a chronic bacterial keratoconjunctivitis linked to poverty	Chlamydia trachomatis	**Azithro** 20 mg/kg po single dose—78% effective in children; Adults: 1 gm po.	**Doxy** 100 mg po bid x minimum of 21 days or **tetracycline** 250 mg po qid x 14 days.	Starts in childhood and can persist for years with subsequent damage to cornea. Topical therapy of marginal benefit. Avoid doxy/tetracycline in young children. Mass treatment works (*NEJM 358:1777 & 1870, 2008; JAMA 299:778, 2008*).
Suppurative conjunctivitis: Children and Adults				
Non-gonococcal; non-chlamydial *Med Lett 46:25, 2004; Med Lett 50:11, 2008*	Staph. aureus, S. pneumoniae, H. influenzae, et al. Outbreak due to atypical S. pneumo. *NEJM 348:1112, 2003*	Ophthalmic solution: **Gati** 0.3%, **Levo** 0.5%, or **Moxi** 0.5%. All 1–2 gtts q2h while awake 1st 2 days, then q4–8h up to 7 days.	**Polymyxin B + trimethoprim** solution 1–2 gtts q3–6h x 7–10 days. **Azithro** 1%, 1 gtt bid x 2 days, then 1 gtt daily x 5 days.	**FQs** best spectrum for empiric therapy but expensive: $40–50 for 5 mL. High concentrations ↑ likelihood of activity vs S. aureus—even MRSA. **TMP** spectrum may include MRSA. Polymyxin B spectrum only Gm-neg. bacilli but no ophthal. prep of only TMP. Most S. pneumo resistant to **gent** & tobra. **Azithro** active vs common gm+ pathogens.
Gonococcal (peds/adults)	N. gonorrhoeae	**Ceftriaxone** 25–50 mg/kg IV/IM (not to exceed 125 mg) as one dose in children; 1 gm IM/IV as one dose in adults		

Abbreviations on page 3.   NOTE: *All dosage recommendations are for adults (unless otherwise indicated) and assume normal renal function.*

TABLE 1A (9)

ANATOMIC SITE/DIAGNOSIS/ MODIFYING CIRCUMSTANCES	ETIOLOGIES (usual)	SUGGESTED REGIMENS*		ADJUNCT DIAGNOSTIC OR THERAPEUTIC MEASURES AND COMMENTS
		PRIMARY	ALTERNATIVE§	
EYE (continued)				
Cornea (keratitis): Usually serious and often sight-threatening. Prompt ophthalmologic consultation essential! Herpes simplex most common etiology in developed countries; bacterial and fungal infections more common in underdeveloped countries.				
Viral				
H. simplex	H. simplex, types 1 & 2	**Trifluridine**, one drop qh, 9x/day for up to 21 days	**Vidarabine** ointment— useful in children. Use 5x/day for up to 21 days.	Fluorescein staining shows topical dendritic figures. 30–50% rate of recurrence within 2 years. 400 mg acyclovir po bid ↓ recurrences, p 0.005 (NEJM 339:300, 1998). If child fails vidarabine, try trifluridine.
Varicella-zoster ophthalmicus	Varicella-zoster virus	**Famciclovir** 500 mg po tid or **valacyclovir** 1 gm po tid x 10 days	**Acyclovir** 800 mg po 5x/day x 10 days	Clinical diagnosis most common: dendritic figures with fluorescein staining in patient with varicella-zoster of ophthalmic branch of trigeminal nerve.
Bacterial (Med Lett 46:25, 2004) Acute: No comorbidity	S. aureus, S. pneumo, S. pyogenes, Haemophilus sp.	**All rx listed for bacterial, fungal, & protozoan is topical**		
		Moxi: eye gtts. 1 gtt tid x 7 days	**Gati:** eye gtts. 1-2 gtts q2h while awake x 2 days, then q4h x 3-7 days.	Prefer Moxi due to enhanced lipophilicity & penetration into aqueous humor. Survey of Ophthal 50 (suppl 1) 1, 2005. **Note:** despite high conc. may fail vs MRSA.
Contact lens users	P. aeruginosa	**Tobra** or **gentamicin** (14 mg/mL) + **piperacillin** or **ticarcillin** eye drops (6–12 mg/mL) q15–60 min around clock x 24–72 hrs, then slow reduction	**CIP** 0.3% or **Levo** 0.5% drops q15–60 min around clock x 24–72 hrs	Pain, photophobia, impaired vision. Recommend alginate swab for culture and sensitivity testing.
Dry cornea, diabetes, immunosuppression	Staph. aureus, S. epidermidis, S. pneumoniae, S. pyogenes, Enterobacteriaceae, listeria	**Cefazolin** (50 mg/mL) + **gentamicin** or **tobra** (14 mg/mL) q15–60 min around clock x 24–72 hrs, then slow reduction	**Vanco** (50 mg/mL) + **ceftazidime** (50 mg/mL) q15–60 min around clock x 24–72 hrs, then slow reduction. See Comment	Specific therapy guided by results of alginate swab culture and sensitivity. CIP 0.3% found clinically equivalent to cefazolin + tobra; only concern was efficacy of CIP vs S. pneumoniae (Ophthalmology 163:1854, 1996).
Fungal	Aspergillus, fusarium, candida. No empiric therapy—see Comment	**Natamycin** (5%) drops q3–4 hrs with subsequent slow reduction	**Ampho B** (0.05–0.15%) q3–4 hrs with subsequent slow reduction	No empiric therapy. Wait for results of Gram stain or culture in Sabouraud's medium.
Mycobacteria: Post-Lasik	Mycobcterium chelonae	**Moxi** eye gtts. 1 gtt qid	**Gati** eye gtts. 1 gtt qid	Ref: Ophthalmology 113:950, 2006
Protozoan Soft contact lens users. Ref: CID 35:434, 2002.	Acanthamoeba, sp.	No primary/alternative; just one suggested regimen: Topical 0.02%, chlorohexidine & 0.02% polyhexamethylene biguinide (PHMB), alone or in combination. Often combined with either propamidine isothionate or hexanide (see Comment). Eyedrops q waking hour for 1 wk, then slow taper		Uncommon. Trauma and soft contact lenses are risk factors. To obtain suggested drops: Leiter's Park Ave Pharmacy (800-292-6773; www.leiterrx.com). Cleaning solution outbreak: MMWR 56: (Dispatch), 2007.
Lacrimal apparatus				
Canaliculitis	Actinomyces most common. Rarely, Arachnia, fusobacterium, nocardia, candida	Remove granules & irrigate with **pen G** (100,000 mcg/mL)	If fungi, irrigate with **nystatin** approx. 5 mcg/mL: 1 gtt tid	Digital pressure produces exudate at punctum; Gram stain confirms diagnosis. Hot packs to punctal area qid.
		Child: AM-CL or **cefprozil** or **cefuroxime** (Dose—Table 16)		

NOTE: All dosage recommendations are for adults (unless otherwise indicated) and assume normal renal function.

TABLE 1A (10)

ANATOMIC SITE/DIAGNOSIS/ MODIFYING CIRCUMSTANCES	ETIOLOGIES (usual)	SUGGESTED REGIMENS* PRIMARY	ALTERNATIVE§	ADJUNCT DIAGNOSTIC OR THERAPEUTIC MEASURES AND COMMENTS
EYE/ Lacrimal apparatus *(continued)*				
Dacryocystitis (lacrimal sac)	S. pneumo, S. aureus, H. influenzae, S. pyogenes, P. aeruginosa	Often consequence of obstruction of lacrimal duct. Empiric therapy based on Gram stain of aspirate—*see Comment.*		Need ophthalmologic consultation. Can be acute or chronic. Culture to detect MRSA.
Endophthalmitis: For post-op endophthalmitis, see *CID 38:542, 2004*				
Bacterial: Haziness of vitreous key to diagnosis. Needle aspirate of both vitreous and aqueous humor for culture prior to therapy. Intravitreal administration of antimicrobials essential.				
Postocular surgery (cataracts) Early, acute onset (incidence 0.05%)	S. epidermidis 60%, Staph. aureus, streptococci, & enterococci each 5–10%, Gm-neg. bacilli 6%	**Immediate ophthal. consult.** If only light perception or worse, immediate vitrectomy + intravitreal vanco 1 mg & intravitreal ceftazidime 2.25 mg. No clear data on intravitreal steroid. May need to repeat intravitreal antibiotics in 2–3 days. Can usually leave lens in.		
Low grade, chronic	Propionibacterium acnes. S. epidermidis, S. aureus (rare)	May require removal of lens material. Intraocular **vanco** ± vitrectomy.		
Post filtering blebs for glaucoma	Strep. species (viridans & others), H. influenzae	Intravitreal and topical agent and consider systemic **AM-CL, AM-SB** or **cefprozil or cefuroxime**		
Post-penetrating trauma	Bacillus sp., S. epiderm.	Intravitreal agent as above + systemic **clinda** or **vanco**		Use topical antibiotics post-surgery (tobra & cefazolin drops).
None, suspect hematogenous	S. pneumoniae, N. meningitidis, Staph. aureus	**(cefotaxime** 2 gm IV q4h or **ceftriaxone** 2 gm IV q24h) + **vanco** 1 gm IV q12h pending cultures. Intravitreal antibiotics as with early post-operative.		
IV heroin abuse	Bacillus cereus, Candida sp.	Intravitreal agent + (systemic **clinda** or **vanco)**		
Mycotic (fungal) Broad-spectrum antibiotics, often corticosteroids, indwelling venous catheters	Candida sp., Aspergillus sp.	Intravitreal **ampho B** 0.005–0.01 mg in 0.1 mL. *Also see Table 11A, page 100 for concomitant systemic therapy. See Comment.*		With moderate/marked vitritis, options include systemic rx + vitrectomy ± intravitreal ampho B *(CID 27:1130 & 1134, 1998).* Report of failure of ampho B lipid complex *(CID 28:1177, 1999).*
Retinitis				
Acute retinal necrosis	Varicella zoster, Herpes simplex	IV **acyclovir** 10–12 mg/kg IV q8h x 5–7 days, then 800 mg po 5x/day x 6 wk		Strong association of VZ virus with atypical necrotizing herpetic retinopathy *(CID 24:603, 1997).*
HIV+ (AIDS) CD4 usually <100/mm[3]	Cytomegalovirus	See *Table 14, page 140*		Occurs in 5–10% of AIDS patients
Orbital cellulitis *(see page 50 for erysipelas, facial)*	S. pneumoniae, H. influenzae, M. catarrhalis, S. aureus, anaerobes, group A strep, occ. Gm-neg. bacilli post-trauma	**Nafcillin** 2 gm IV q4h (or if **MRSA-vanco** 1 gm IV q12h) + **ceftriaxone** 2 gm IV q24h + **metro** 1 gm IV q12h		**If penicillin/ceph allergy: Vanco + levo** 750 mg IV once daily + **metro** IV. Problem is frequent inability to make microbiologic diagnosis. Image orbit (CT or MRI). Risk of cavernous sinus thrombosis. If vanco intolerant, another option for s. aureus is dapto 6 mg/kg IV q24h.

Abbreviations on page 3.   NOTE: *All dosage recommendations are for adults (unless otherwise indicated) and assume normal renal function.*

TABLE 1A (11)

ANATOMIC SITE/DIAGNOSIS/ MODIFYING CIRCUMSTANCES	ETIOLOGIES (usual)	SUGGESTED REGIMENS*		ADJUNCT DIAGNOSTIC OR THERAPEUTIC MEASURES AND COMMENTS
		PRIMARY	ALTERNATIVE§	
FOOT				
"Diabetic"—Two thirds of patients have triad of neuropathy, deformity and pressure-induced trauma. Refs:: *Ln 366:1725, 2005; NEJM 351:48, 2004.*				
Ulcer without inflammation	Colonizing skin flora	No antibacterial therapy		**General:** 1. Glucose control, eliminate pressure on ulcer 2. **Assess for peripheral vascular disease**—very common (*CID 39:437, 2004*).
Ulcer with <2 cm of superficial inflammation	S. aureus (assume MRSA), S. agalactiae (Gp B), S. pyogenes predominate	**Oral therapy: (TMP-SMX-DS or minocycline)** plus **(Pen VK** or selected **O Ceph 2, 3,** or **FQ)**[9] *Dosages in footnote[9]*		**Principles of empiric antibacterial therapy:** 1. Include drug predictably active vs MRSA. If outpatient, can assume community-associated MRSA (CA-MRSA) until culture results available.
Ulcer with >2 cm of inflammation with extension to fascia. **Osteomyelitis** *See Comment.*	As above, plus coliforms possible	**Oral therapy: (AM-CL-ER** plus **TMP-SMX-DS)** or [(**CIP** or **Moxi)** plus **linezolid]** *Dosages in footnote[10]*		2. As culture results dominated by S. aureus & Streptococcus species, empiric drug regimens should include strep & staph. Role of enterococci uncertain. 3. Severe limb and/or life-threatening infections require initial parenteral therapy
Extensive local inflammation plus systemic toxicity. Treatment modalities of limited efficacy & expensive: Neg pressure (wound vac) (*Ln 366:1704, 2005*); growth factor (becaplermin); and hyperbaric oxygen (*CID 43:188, 193, 2006*)	As above, plus anaerobic bacteria. Role of enterococci unclear.	**Parenteral therapy: (Vanco** plus **β-lactam/β-lactamase inhibitor)** or (**vanco** plus **carbapenem).** Other alternatives: 1. **Dapto** or **linezolid** for vanco 2. (**CIP** or **Levo** or **Moxi** or **aztreonam)** plus **metronidazole** for β-lactam/β-lactamase inhibitor 3. **Ceftobiprole** (investigational) *Dosages in footnote[11]* **Assess for arterial insufficiency!**		with predictable activity vs Gm-positive cocci, coliforms & other aerobic Gm-neg, rods, & anaerobic Gm-neg. bacilli. 4. **NOTE:** The regimens listed are suggestions consistent with above principles. Other alternatives exist & may be appropriate for individual patients. 5. Is there an associated osteomyelitis? Risk increased if ulcer area >2 cm², positive probe to bone, ESR >70 and abnormal plain x-ray. Negative MRI reduces likelihood of osteomyelitis (*JAMA 299:806, 2008*). MRI is best imaging modality (*CID 47:519 & 528, 2008*).
Onychomycosis: See Table 11, page 104, *fungal infections*				
Puncture wound: Nail/Toothpick	P. aeruginosa	Cleanse. Tetanus booster. Observe.		*See page 5. 1–2% evolve to osteomyelitis. After toothpick injury (PIDJ 23:80, 2004)*: S. aureus, Strep sp, and mixed flora.
GALLBLADDER Cholecystitis, cholangitis, biliary sepsis, or common duct obstruction (partial: 2ⁿᵈ to tumor, stones, stricture). Cholecystitis Ref: *NEJM 358:2804, 2008.*	Enterobacteriaceae 68%, enterococci 14%, bacteroides 10%, Clostridium sp. 7%, rarely candida	**PIP-TZ** or **AM-SB** or **TC-CL** or **ERTA** If life-threatening: **IMP** or **MER** or **Dori** *Dosages in footnote[11]*	**P Ceph 3** + **metro** OR **Aztreonam** + **metro** OR **CIP** + **metro** OR **Moxi**	In severely ill pts, antibiotic therapy complements adequate biliary drainage. 15–30% pts will require decompression: surgical, percutaneous or ERCP-placed stent. Whether empirical therapy should always cover pseudomonas & anaerobes is uncertain. Ceftriaxone associated with biliary sludge of drug (by ultrasound 50%, symptomatic 9%, *NEJM 322:1821, 1990*); clinical relevance still unclear but has led to surgery (*MMWR 42:39, 1993*).

[9] **TMP-SMX-DS** 1-2 tabs po bid, **minocycline** 100 mg po bid, **Pen VK** 500 mg po qid, (**O Ceph 2, 3:** **cefprozil** 500 mg po q24h, (**O Ceph 2,** 3: **cefprozil** 500 mg po q24h, **cefuroxime axetil** 500 mg po q12h, **cefdinir** 300 mg po q12h or 600 mg po q24h, **cefpodoxime** 200 mg po q12h) **CIP** 750 mg po bid. **Levo** 750 mg po q24h.

[10] **AM-CL-ER** 2000/125 mg po bid. **TMP-SMX-DS** 1-2 tabs po bid, **CIP** 750 mg po bid, **Levo** 750 mg po q24h, **Moxi** 400 mg po q24h, **linezolid** 600 mg po bid.

[11] **Vanco** 1 gm IV q12h, (**parenteral β-lactam/β-lactamase inhibitors: AM-SB** 3 gm IV q6h, **PIP-TZ** 3.375 gm IV q8h or 4.5 gm IV q8h or 4 hr infusion of 3.375 gm;TC-CL 3.1 gm IV q6h); **carbapenems: Doripenem** 500 mg (1-hr infusion) q8h, **ERTA** 1 gm IV q24h, **IMP** 0.5 gm IV q6h, **MER** 1 gm IV q8h, **daptomycin** 6 mg per kg IV q24h, **linezoid** 600 mg IV q12h, **aztreonam** 2 gm IV q8h, **linezoid** 600 mg IV q12h, **aztreonam** 2 gm IV q8h. **CIP** 400 mg IV q12h, **Levo** 750 mg IV q24h, **Moxi** 400 mg IV q24h, **metro** 1 gm IV loading dose & then 0.5 gm IV q6h or 1 gm IV q12h; **ceftobiprole** 500 mg (2-hr infusion) q8h.

Abbreviations on page 3.   NOTE: All dosage recommendations are for adults (unless otherwise indicated) and assume normal renal function.

TABLE 1A (12)

ANATOMIC SITE/DIAGNOSIS/ MODIFYING CIRCUMSTANCES	ETIOLOGIES (usual)	SUGGESTED REGIMENS*		ADJUNCT DIAGNOSTIC OR THERAPEUTIC MEASURES AND COMMENTS
		PRIMARY	ALTERNATIVE§	
GASTROINTESTINAL				
Gastroenteritis—Empiric Therapy (laboratory studies not performed or culture, microscopy, toxin results NOT AVAILABLE) (Ref.: *NEJM 350:38, 2004*)				
Premature infant with necrotizing enterocolitis	Associated with intestinal flora	Treatment and rationale as for diverticulitis/peritonitis, *page 20. See Table 16, page 178 for pediatric dosages.*		Pneumatosis intestinalis on x-ray confirms diagnosis. Bacteremia-peritonitis in 30–50%. If Staph. epidermidis isolated, add vanco (IV).
Mild diarrhea (≤3 unformed stools/day, minimal associated symptomatology)	Bacterial. (See *Severe,* below), viral (norovirus), parasitic. Viral usually causes mild to moderate disease. For traveler's diarrhea, *see page 18*	Fluids only + lactose-free diet, avoid caffeine		**Rehydration: For po fluid replacement, see Cholera, page 18.** **Antimotility:** Loperamide (Imodium) 4 mg po, then 2 mg after each loose stool to max. of 16 mg per day. Bismuth subsalicylate (Pepto-Bismol) 2 tablets
Moderate diarrhea (≥4 unformed stools/day &/or systemic symptoms)		Antimotility agents *(see Comments)* + fluids		(262 mg) po qid. Do not use if suspect hemolytic uremic syndrome. **Hemolytic uremic syndrome (HUS):** Risk in **children** infected with E. coli 0157:H7 is 8–10%. Early treatment with TMP-SMX or FQs ↑ risk of HUS *(NEJM 342:1930 & 1990, 2000).* Controversial meta-analysis: *JAMA 288:996 & 3111, 2002.*
Severe diarrhea (≥6 unformed stools/day, &/or temp ≥101°F, tenesmus, blood, or fecal leukocytes)	Shigella, salmonella, C. jejuni, E. coli 0157:H7, toxin-positive C. difficile, Klebsiella oxytoca, E. histolytica. *For typhoid fever, see page 56*	**FQ (CIP** 500 mg po q12h or **Levo** 500 mg q24h) times 3–5 days	**TMP-SMX-DS** po bid times 3–5 days. Campylobacter resistance to TMP-SMX common in tropics.	**Norovirus:** Etiology of over 90% of non-bacterial diarrhea (± nausea/vomiting). Lasts 12–60 hrs. Hydrate. No effective antiviral. **Other potential etiologies:** Cryptosporidia—no treatment in immuno-competent host *(see Table 13A & JID 170:272, 1994)*. Cyclospora—usually
NOTE: Severe afebrile bloody diarrhea should ↑ suspicion of E. coli 0157:H7 infection— causes only 1–3% all causes diarrhea in US—but causes up to 36% cases of bloody diarrhea *(CID 32:573, 2001)*		*If recent antibiotic therapy (C. difficile toxin colitis possible)* **add:** **Metro** 500 mg po tid times 10–14 days	**Vanco** 125 mg po qid times 10–14 days	chronic diarrhea, responds to TMP-SMX *(see Table 12A & AIM 123:409, 1995).* Klebsiella oxytoca identified as cause of antibiotic-associated hemorrhagic colitis (cytotoxin positive): *NEJM 355:2418, 2006.*
Gastroenteritis—Specific Therapy (results of culture, microscopy, toxin assay AVAILABLE) (Ref.: *NEJM 350:38, 2004*)				
If culture negative, probably **Norovirus (Norwalk)** or rarely (in adults) **Rotavirus**—see *Norovirus, page 145*	Aeromonas/Plesiomonas	**CIP** 500 mg po bid times 3 days.	**TMP-SMX-DS** po bid times 3 days	Although no absolute proof, increasing evidence as cause of diarrheal illness.
	Amebiasis (Entamoeba histolytica, Cyclospora, Cryptosporidia and Giardia), see Table 13A			
NOTE: In 60 hospital pts with unexplained WBCs ≥15,000, 35% had C. difficile toxin present *(AJM 115:543, 2003; CID 34:1585, 2002)*	**Campylobacter jejuni** H/O[12] fever in 53–83%. Self-limited diarrhea in normal host.	**Azithro** 500 mg po q24h x 3 days.	**Erythro stearate** 500 mg po qid x 5 days or **CIP** 500 mg po bid (CP resistance increasing).	**Post-Campylobacter Guillain-Barré;** assoc. 15% of cases *(Ln 366:1653, 2005)*. Assoc. with small bowel lymphoproliferative disease: may respond to antimicrobials *(NEJM 350:239, 2003)*. **Reactive arthritis** another potential sequelae. See *Traveler's diarrhea, page 18.*
	Campylobacter fetus Diarrhea uncommon. More systemic disease in debilitated hosts	**Gentamicin** *(see Table 10D)*	**AMP** 100 mg/kg IV div q6h or **IMP** 500 mg IV q6h	Draw blood cultures. Do not use erythro for C. fetus. In bacteremic pts, 32% resistant to FQs and 8% resistant to erythromycin *(CID 47:790, 2008).*

[12] **H/O** = history of

Abbreviations on page 3.

NOTE: All dosage recommendations are for adults (unless otherwise indicated) and assume normal renal function.

TABLE 1A (13)

ANATOMIC SITE/DIAGNOSIS/ MODIFYING CIRCUMSTANCES	ETIOLOGIES (usual)	SUGGESTED REGIMENS*		ADJUNCT DIAGNOSTIC OR THERAPEUTIC MEASURES AND COMMENTS
		PRIMARY	ALTERNATIVE§	
GASTROINTESTINAL/Gastroenteritis—Specific Therapy (continued)				
Differential diagnosis of toxin-producing diarrhea: • C. difficile • Klebsiella oxytoca • S. aureus Shiga toxin producing E. coli (STEC) • Entero toxigenic B. fragilis (CID 47:797, 2008) More on C. difficile: 1. Ref: NEJM 359:1932, 2008. 2. Prolonged po vanco taper for relapses is expensive. Anecdotal reports of using generic injectable vanco: use 7 vials (1 gm/vial), each reconstituted with 20 mL sterile water = 140 mL. 2.5 mL = 125 mg dose of vanco.	**C. difficile** toxin positive antibiotic-associated colitis. **Probiotics'** (lactobacillus or saccharomyces) inconsistent in prevention of C. difficile (NEJM 359:1932, 2008).			
	po meds okay: WBC <15,000; no increase in serum creatinine.	Metro 500 mg po tid or 250 mg qid x 10-14 days	Vanco 125 mg po qid x 10-14 days Teicoplanin^NUS 400 mg po bid x 10 days	**D/C antibiotic if possible: avoid antimotility agents, hydration, enteric isolation.** Relapse in 10-20% **Nitazoxanide** 500 mg po bid for 7-10 days equivalent to **Metro** po in phase 3 study^NFDA (CID 43:421, 2006).
	po meds okay; Sicker; WBC >15,000; ≥ 50% increase in baseline creatinine	Vanco 125 mg po qid x 10-14 days. To use IV vanco po. see Table 10C, page 91	Metro 500 mg po tid x 10 days	Vanco superior to metro in sicker pts. Relapse in 10-20% (not due to resistance: JAC 56:988, 2005)
	Post-treatment relapse	**1st relapse** Metro 500 mg po tid x 10 days	**2nd relapse** Vanco as above + rif 300 mg po bid **3rd relapse:** See Comment	**3rd relapse: Vanco** taper (all doses 125 mg po): week 1 – qid; week 2 – bid; week 3 – q24h; week 4 – qod; wks 5&6 – q 3 days. Last resort: stool transplant (CID 36:580, 2003). Other options: 1) After initial vanco, **rifaximin**^NFDA 400-800 mg daily divided bid po tid x 2 wks (CID 44:846, 2007, rifaximin-resistant C. diff. reported); 2) **nitazoxanide**^NFDA 500 mg bid x 10d (JAC 59:705, 2007).
	Post-op ileus; severe disease with toxic megacolon	Metro 500 mg IV q6h + vanco via nasogastric tube (or naso-small bowel tube) ± retrograde catheter in cecum. See comment for dosage.		For vanco instillation into bowel, add 500 mg vanco to 1 liter of saline and perfuse at 1-3 mL/min to maximum of 2 gm in 24 hrs (CID 690.2002). **Note: IV vanco not effective. IVIG:** Reports of benefit of 400 mg/kg x 1-3 doses (JAC 53:882, 2004) and lack of benefit (Am J Inf Cont 35:131, 2007).
	E. coli 0157:H7 H/O[13] bloody stools 63% shiga toxin producing E. Coli (STEC)	**NO TREATMENT** with antimicrobials or anti-motility drugs, may enhance toxin release and ↑risk of hemolytic uremic syndrome (HUS) (NEJM 342:1930 & 1990, 2000). Hydration important (Ln 365:1073, 2005).		NOTE: 5–10% of pts develop HUS (approx. 10% with HUS die or have permanent renal failure; 50% HUS pts have some degree of renal impairment (CID 38:1298, 2004). Non O157:H7 STEC emerging as cause of bloody diarrhea and/or HUS; EIA for shiga toxin available (CID 43:1587, 2006).
	Klebsiella oxytoca— antibiotic-associated	Responds to stopping antibiotic		Suggested that stopping NSAIDs helps. Ref.: NEJM 355:2418, 2006.
	Listeria monocytogenes	AMP 50 mg/kg IV q6h	TMP-SMX 20 mg/kg per day IV div. q6-8h	Recently recognized cause of food poisoning, manifest as febrile gastroenteritis. Percentage with complicating bacteremia/meningitis unknown. Not detected in standard stool culture (NEJM 336:100 & 130, 1997.
	Salmonella, non-typhi— For typhoid (enteric) fever, see page 56 Fever in 71–91%, H/O[13] bloody stools in 34%	If pt asymptomatic or illness mild, antimicrobial therapy not indicated. **Treat if** <1 yr old or >50 yr old, if immunocompromised, if vascular grafts or prosthetic joints, bacteremic, hemoglobinopathy, or hospitalized with fever and severe diarrhea (see typhoid fever, page 56). CIP 500 mg po bid or levo 500 mg once daily x 5–7 days.	Azithro 1 gm po once, then 500 mg q24h x 6 days (AAC 43:1441, 1999)	↑resistance to TMP-SMX and chloro. Ceftriaxone, cefotaxime usually active (see footnote, page 23, for dosage); ceftriaxone & FQ resistance in SE Asia (CID 40:315, 2005; Ln 363:1285, 2004). **Primary treatment of enteritis is fluid and electrolyte replacement.** No adverse effects from FQs in children (Ln 348:547, 1996). If immunocompromised, treat 14 days.
	Shigella Fever in 58%, H/O[13] bloody stools 51%	FQs po: (CIP 500 mg bid or (Levo 500 mg q24h)— x 3 days.	(TMP-SMX-DS po bid x 3 days) or (azithro 500 mg po x 1, then 250 mg q24h x 4 days) See Comment for peds rx per dose	**Peds doses:** TMP-SMX 5/25 mg/kg po x 3 days. For severe disease, ceftriaxone 50-75 mg/kg per day x 2-5 days. CIP suspension 10 mg/kg bid x 5 days. CIP superior to ceftriaxone in children (LnID 3:537, 2003). **Immunocompromised children & adults: Treat for 7-10 days.** Azithro superior to cefixime in trial in children (PIDJ 22:374, 2003).

[13] **H/O** = history of

Abbreviations on page 3.

NOTE: All dosage recommendations are for adults (unless otherwise indicated) and assume normal renal function.

TABLE 1A (14)

ANATOMIC SITE/DIAGNOSIS/ MODIFYING CIRCUMSTANCES	ETIOLOGIES (usual)	SUGGESTED REGIMENS*		ADJUNCT DIAGNOSTIC OR THERAPEUTIC MEASURES AND COMMENTS
		PRIMARY	ALTERNATIVE§	
GASTROINTESTINAL/Gastroenteritis—Specific Therapy *(continued)*				
(continued from above)	**Staphylococcus aureus** See Comment	**Vanco** 1 gm IV q12h + 125 mg po qid reasonable		Case reports of toxin-mediated pseudomembranous enteritis/colitis (pseudomembranes in small bowel) (CID 39:747, 2004). **Clinda** to stop toxin production reasonable if organism susceptible.
	Spirochetosis (Brachyspira pilosicoli)	Benefit of treatment unclear. Susceptible to **metro**, **ceftriaxone**, and **Moxi** (AAC 47:2354, 2003).		Anaerobic intestinal spirochete that colonizes colon of domestic & wild animals plus humans. Case reports of diarrhea with large numbers of the organism present. (AAC 39:347, 2001; Am J Clin Path 120:828, 2003).
	Vibrio cholerae Treatment decreases duration of disease, volume losses, & duration of excretion (CID 37:272, 2003; Ln 363:223, 2004)	**Primary rx is hydration** (see Comment) **Azithromycin** 1 gm po once. (NEJM 354:2452, 2500, 2006.) Increasing number of failures.	**Primary Rx is hydration. CIP** 1 gm po once but high failure rate. Peds dosage in Comments	Primary rx is fluid. **IV** use (per liter): 4 gm NaCl, 1 gm KCl, 5.4 gm Na lactate, 8 gm glucose. **PO** use (per liter potable water): 1 level teaspoon table salt + 4 heaping teaspoons sugar (JTMH 84:73, 1981). Add orange juice or 2 bananas for K+. Volume given = fluid loss. Mild dehydration. Give 5% body weight; for moderate, 7% body weight. (Refs.: CID 20:1485, 1995; TRSM 89:103, 1995). Peds azithro: 20 mg/kg (to 1 gm max.) x 1 (Ln 360:1722, 2002); CIP 20 mg/kg (Ln 366:1085, 2005)
	Vibrio parahaemolyticus Vibrio vulnificus	Antimicrobial rx does not shorten course. Hydration. Usual presentation is skin lesions & bacteremia, life-threatening, treat early. **ceftaz** + **doxy**—see page 51; levo (AAC 46:3580, 2002).		Shellfish exposure common. Treat severe disease: **FQ, doxy, P Ceph 3**
	Yersinia enterocolitica Fever in 68%, bloody stools in 26%	No treatment unless severe. If severe, combine **doxy** 100 mg IV bid + **(tobra** or **gent** 5 mg/kg per day once q24h). **TMP-SMX** or **FQs** are alternatives.		Mesenteric adenitis pain can mimic acute appendicitis. Lab diagnosis difficult: requires "cold enrichment" and/or yersinia selective agar. Desferrioxamine therapy increases severity, discontinue if pt on it. Iron overload states predispose to yersinia (CID 27:1362 & 1367, 1998).
Gastroenteritis—Specific Risk Groups—Empiric Therapy				
Anoreceptive intercourse Proctitis (distal 15 cm only)	Herpes viruses, gonococci, chlamydia, syphilis. See Genital Tract, page 20			
Colitis	Shigella, salmonella, campylobacter, E. histolytica (see Table 13A)			**FQ** (e.g., **CIP** 500 mg po) q12h x 3 days for Shigella, Salmonella, Campylobacter.
HIV-1 infected (AIDS): >10 days diarrhea	G. lamblia			See Table 13A
Acid-fast organisms:	Cryptosporidium parvum, Cyclospora cayetanensis			See Table 13A
Other:	Isospora belli, microsporidia (Enterocytozoon bieneusi, Septata intestinalis)			See Table 13A
Neutropenic enterocolitis or "typhlitis" (CID 27:695 & 700, 1998)	Mucosal invasion by **Clostridium septicum**. Occasionally caused by C. sordelli or P. aeruginosa	As for perirectal abscess: diverticulitis, pg 20. Ensure empiric regimen includes drug active vs Clostridia species; e.g., **pen G, AMP** or **clinda** (see Comment re: resistance). Empiric regimen should have predictive activity vs P. aeruginosa also.		Tender right lower quadrant. Surgical resection controversial but may be necessary. **NOTE:** Resistance of clostridia to clindamycin reported.
Traveler's diarrhea, self-medication. Patient usually afebrile (CID 44:338 & 347, 2007)	**Acute**: 60% due to diarrheogenic E. coli; shigella, salmonella, or campylobacter. C. difficile, amebiasis (see Table 13). If **chronic**: cyclospora, cryptosporidia, giardia, isospora	**For Latin America & Africa: Levo** 500 mg po x 1 dose or **other FQ** bid x 3 days (see footnote[14]) OR **rifaximin** 200 mg po tid x 3 days Add **Imodium**: 4 mg po x 1, then 2 mg after each loose stool to max.16 mg/day.	**For S.E. Asia and elsewhere: Azithro** 1 gm po x 1 dose or 500 mg once daily x 3 days OR (**Levo, Moxi** or **CIP**) po daily x 3 days (dose in footnote[14])	Geographic variability in likely etiology. Increasing resistance of campylobacter to CIP but perhaps less resistance to levo and moxi. Single dose azithro + Imodium as effective as levo + Imodium (CID 45:294 & 301, 2007). Peds & pregnancy: Avoid FQs. Azithro peds dose: 5–10 mg/kg x 1 dose. Rifaximin approved for age 12 or older. Adverse effects similar to placebo. No loperamide if fever or blood in stool. **CIP and rifaximin** equivalent efficacy vs non-invasive pathogens (AJTMH 74:1060, 2006)

[14] **FQ** dosage po for self-rx traveler's diarrhea—mild disease: **CIP** 750 mg x 1; severe 500 mg bid x 3 days. **CIP-XR** 1000 mg once daily x 1-3 days; **Oflox** 300 mg po daily x 1-3 days; **Levo** 500 mg once daily x 1-3 days: **Moxi**, 400 mg probably would work but not FDA-approved indication.

Abbreviations on page 3.   NOTE: All dosage recommendations are for adults (unless otherwise indicated) and assume normal renal function.

TABLE 1A (15)

ANATOMIC SITE/DIAGNOSIS/ MODIFYING CIRCUMSTANCES	ETIOLOGIES (usual)	SUGGESTED REGIMENS*		ADJUNCT DIAGNOSTIC OR THERAPEUTIC MEASURES AND COMMENTS
		PRIMARY	ALTERNATIVE[§]	
GASTROINTESTINAL/Gastroenteritis—Specific Risk Groups–Empiric Therapy *(continued)*				
Prevention of Traveler's diarrhea	Not routinely indicated. Current recommendation is to take **FQ + Imodium** with 1st loose stool.		Alternative during 1st 3 wk & only if activities are essential: **Rifaximin** 200 mg po bid *(AnIM 142:805 & 861, 2005)*.	
Gastrointestinal Infections by Anatomic Site: Esophagus to Rectum				
Esophagitis	Candida albicans, HSV, CMV	*See SANFORD GUIDE TO HIV/AIDS THERAPY and Table 11A, page 100.*		
Duodenal/Gastric ulcer; gastric cancer, MALT lymphomas (not 2° NSAIDs) *(AnIM 148:923 & 962, 2008; Nature Clin Practice G-I; Hepatology 5:321, 2008; JAMA 300:1346, 2008).*	**Helicobacter pylori** See *Comment* Prevalence of pre-treatment resistance increasing	**Treatment:** Due to 10-15% rate of clarithro resistance, failure of previously suggested triple therapy (PPI + clarithro + amox) is unacceptable 20%. Cure rate with sequential therapy is 90%. **Sequential therapy:** (**Rabeprazole** 20 mg + **amox** 1 gm) bid x 5 days, then (**rabeprazole** 20 mg + **clarithro** 500 mg + **tinidazole** 500 mg) bid for another 5 days. See *footnote*[15]	**Rx po for 14 days: Bismuth** (see *footnote*[16]), bismuth subsalicylate 2 tabs qid + **tetracycline** 500 mg qid + **metro** 500 mg tid + **omeprazole** 20 mg bid.	**Dx: Stool antigen**—Monoclonal EIA >90% sens. & 92% specific. *(Amer.J.Gastro. 101:921, 2006)* Other tests: Urea breath test; if endoscoped, rapid urease &/or histology &/or culture. **Test of cure:** Repeat stool antigen and/or urea breath test >8 wks post-treatment. **Treatment:** Failure rate of triple therapy 20% due to clarithro resistance. Cure rate with sequential therapy 90%.
Small intestine: Whipple's disease *(NEJM 356:55, 2007; LnID 8:179, 2008)*	Tropheryma whipplei	**Initial 10–14 days** (**Pen G** 2 million units IV q4h + **streptomycin** 1 gm IM/IV q24h) OR **ceftriaxone** 2 gm IV q24h **Then, for approx. 1 year** **TMP-SMX-DS** 1 tab po bid	**TMP-SMX-DS** 1 tab po bid if allergic to penicillin & cephalosporins. If sulfa-allergic: **Doxy** 100 mg po bid + hydroxychloroquine 200 mg po tid.	Therapy based on empiricism and retrospective analyses. TMP-SMX: CNS relapses during TMP-SMX rx reported. Cultivated from CSF in pts with intestinal disease and no neurologic findings *(JID 188:797 & 801, 2003).* Early experience with combination of doxy 100 mg bid plus hydroxychloroquine 200 mg tid in patients without neurologic disease *(NEJM 356:55, 2007).*
See Infective endocarditis, culture-negative, page 28				
Inflammatory bowel disease: Ulcerative colitis, Crohn's disease Mild to moderate Ref.: *Ln 359:331, 2002*	Unknown	**Sulfasalazine** 1 gm po q6h or **mesalamine (5ASA)** 1 gm po q6h	**Coated mesalamine** (Asacol) 800 mg bid or qid equally effective. Corticosteroid enemas	Check stool for **E. histolytica.** Try aminosalicylates 1st in mild/mod. disease. See review article for more aggressive therapy. If recent antimicrobial exposure, check for C. difficile toxin.
	In randomized controlled trial, CIP + metro had no benefit *(Gastro 123:33, 2002).*			
Severe Crohn's Ref: *CID 44:256, 2007*	Unknown	**Etanercept**	**Infliximab/adalimumab**	Screen for latent TBc before blocking TNF *(MMWR 53:683, 2004).* If possible, delay anti-TNF drugs until TBc prophylaxis complete. For other anti-TNF risks: *LnID 8:601, 2008.*

[15] Can substitute other proton pump inhibitors for omeprazole or rabeprazole--all bid: esomeprazole 20 mg (FDA-approved), lansoprazole 30 mg (FDA-approved), pantoprazole 40 mg (not FDA-approved for this indication).

[16] **3 bismuth preparations:** (1) In U.S., **bismuth subsalicylate (Pepto-Bismol)** 262 mg tabs; adult dose for helicobacter is 2 tabs (524 mg) qid. (2) Outside U.S., colloidal bismuth subcitrate (De-Nol) 120 mg chewable tablets; dose is 1 tablet qid. (3) Another treatment option: Ranitidine bismuth citrate 400 mg; give with metro 500 mg and clarithro 500 mg—all bid times 7 days. Worked despite metro/clarithro resistance *(Gastro 114:A323, 1998).*

Abbreviations on page 3. NOTE: *All dosage recommendations are for adults (unless otherwise indicated) and assume normal renal function.*

TABLE 1A (16)

ANATOMIC SITE/DIAGNOSIS/MODIFYING CIRCUMSTANCES	ETIOLOGIES (usual)	SUGGESTED REGIMENS*		ADJUNCT DIAGNOSTIC OR THERAPEUTIC MEASURES AND COMMENTS
		PRIMARY	ALTERNATIVE§	
GASTROINTESTINAL/Gastrointestinal Infections by Anatomic Site: Esophagus to Rectum (continued)				
Diverticulitis, perirectal abscess, peritonitis Also see Peritonitis, page 44 CID 37:997, 2003	Enterobacteriaceae, occasionally P. aeruginosa, Bacteroides sp., enterococci	**Outpatient rx—mild diverticulitis, drained perirectal abscess:** [(**TMP-SMX-DS** bid) or (**CIP** 750 mg bid or **Levo** 750 mg q24h)] + **metro** 500 mg q6h. All po x 7–10 days.	**AM-CL-ER** 1000/62.5 mg 2 tabs po bid x 7–10 days **OR Moxi** 400 mg po qid x 7–10 days	Must "cover" both Gm-neg. aerobic & Gm-neg. anaerobic bacteria. **Drugs active only vs anaerobic Gm-neg. bacilli:** clinda, metro. **Drugs active only vs aerobic Gm-neg. bacilli:** APAG[7], P Ceph 2/3/4 (see Table 10C, page 88), aztreonam, AP Pen, CIP, Levo. **Drugs active vs both aerobic/anaerobic Gm-neg. bacteria:** cefoxitin, cefotetan, TC-CL, PIP-TZ, AM-SB, ERTA, Dori, IMP, MER, Moxi, & tigecycline.
		Mild-moderate disease—Inpatient—Parenteral Rx: (e.g., focal peri-appendiceal peritonitis, peri-diverticular abscess, endomyometritis) **PIP-TZ** 3.375 gm IV q6h or 4.5 gm IV q8h **or AM-SB** 3 gm IV q6h, or **TC-CL** 3.1 gm IV q6h or **ERTA** 1 gm IV q24h **or MOXI** 400 mg IV q24h	[(**CIP** 400 mg IV q12h) or (**Levo** 750 mg IV q24h)] + (**metro** 500 mg IV q6h) **OR tigecycline** 100 mg IV 1st dose & then 50 mg IV q12h **OR Moxi** 400 mg IV q24h	**Increasing resistance of Bacteroides species** (AAC 51:1649, 2007):
					% Resistant:	Cefoxitin	Cefotetan	Clindamycin
				5–30	17–87	19–35
		Severe life-threatening disease, ICU patient: **IMP** 500 mg IV q6h or **MER** 1 gm IV q8h or **Dori** 500 mg q8h (1-hr infusion).	**AMP** + **metro** + (**CIP** 400 mg IV q12h or **Levo** 750 mg IV q24h) OR [**AMP** 2 gm IV q6h + **metro** 500 mg IV q6h + **aminoglycoside**[17] (see Table 10D, page 96]	Resistance to metro, PIP-TZ rare. Few case reports of metro resistance (CID 40:e67, 2005; J Clin Micro 42:4127, 2004). If prior FQ exposure, increasing moxi resistance in Bacteroides sp. on rectal swabs (Abst 2008 ICAAC). **Ertapenem** less active vs P. aeruginosa/Acinetobacter sp. than IMP, MER or Dori. **Concomitant surgical management important**, esp. with moderate-severe disease. **Role of enterococci remains debatable.** Probably pathogenic in infections of biliary tract. Probably need drugs active vs enterococci in pts with valvular heart disease. **Severe penicillin/cephalosporin allergy:** (aztreonam 2 gm IV q6h) + [metro (500 mg IV q6h) or (1 gm IV q12h)] OR [(**CIP** 400 mg IV q12h) or (**Levo** 750 mg IV q24h) + **metro**].

GENITAL TRACT: Mixture of empiric & specific treatment. Divided by sex of the patient. For sexual assault (rape), see Table 15A, page 168. See Guidelines for Dx of Sexually Transmitted Diseases, MMWR 55 (RR-11), 2006 and focused commentary in CID 44 (Suppl 3), 2007.

Both Women & Men: Chancroid	H. ducreyi	**Ceftriaxone** 250 mg IM single dose OR **azithro** 1 gm po single dose	**CIP** 500 mg bid po x 3 days OR **erythro base** 500 mg qid po x7 days.	In HIV+ pts, failures reported with single dose azithro (CID 21:409, 1995). Evaluate after 7 days, ulcer should objectively improve.
Chlamydia, et al. non-gonococcal or post-gonococcal urethritis, cervicitis NOTE: Assume concomitant **N. gonorrhoeae** Chlamydia conjunctivitis, see page 12	Chlamydia 50%, Mycoplasma hominis. Other unknown etiologies (10–15%): trichomonas, herpes simplex virus, Mycoplasma genitalium. Ref: JID 193:333, 336, 2006.	(**Doxy** 100 mg po x 7 days) or (**azithro** 1 gm po as single dose). Evaluate & treat sex partner. **In pregnancy: erythro base** 500 mg po qid x 7 days OR **amox** 500 mg po tid x 7 days.	(**Erythro base** 500 mg po qid po x 7 days) or (**Oflox** 300 mg q12h po x 7 days) or (**Levo** 500 mg q24h x 7 days) **In pregnancy: azithro** 1 gm po x 1. **Doxy & Oflox contraindicated**	**Diagnosis:** Nucleic acid amplification tests for C. trachomatis & N. gonorrhoeae on urine samples equivalent to cervix or urethra specimens (AnIM 142:914, 2005). **For recurrent or persistent disease:** either metro 2 gm po x 1 + either erythro base 500 mg po qid x 7 days or erythro ethylsuccinate 800 mg po qid x 7 days. **Evaluate & treat sex partners.**
Recurrent/persistent urethritis	Occult trichomonas, tetra-resistant U. urealyticum	**Metro** 2 gm po x 1 + **erythro base** 500 mg po qid x 7 days	**Erythro ethylsuccinate** 800 mg po qid x 7 days	In men with NGU, 20% infected with trichomonas (JID 188:465, 2003). Another option: (metro or tinidazole 2 gm po x 1 dose) plus azithro 1 gm po x 1 dose.

[17] **Aminoglycoside** = antipseudomonal aminoglycosidic aminoglycoside, e.g., amikacin, gentamicin, tobramycin

Abbreviations on page 3.   NOTE: All dosage recommendations are for adults (unless otherwise indicated) and assume normal renal function.

TABLE 1A (17)

ANATOMIC SITE/DIAGNOSIS/ MODIFYING CIRCUMSTANCES	ETIOLOGIES (usual)	SUGGESTED REGIMENS* PRIMARY	ALTERNATIVE§	ADJUNCT DIAGNOSTIC OR THERAPEUTIC MEASURES AND COMMENTS
GENITAL TRACT/ Both Women & Men *(continued)*				
Gonorrhea [*MMWR 55 (RR-11), 2006*]. **FQs no longer recommended for treatment of gonococcal infections (***MMWR* **56:332, 2007).**				
Conjunctivitis (adult)	N. gonorrhoeae	**Ceftriaxone** 1 gm IM or IV times one dose		Consider saline lavage of eye times 1
Disseminated gonococcal infection (DGI, dermatitis-arthritis syndrome)	N. gonorrhoeae	**(Ceftriaxone** 1 gm IV q24h) or **(cefotaxime** 1 gm q8h IV) or **(ceftizoxime** 1 gm q8h IV)—*see Comment*	**Spectinomycin**[NUS] 2 gm IM q12h—*see Comment*	Continue IM or IV regimen for 24hr after symptoms ↓; reliable pts may be discharged 24hr after sx resolve to complete 7 days rx with **cefixime**[18] **400 mg po bid**. R/O meningitis/ endocarditis. **Treat presumptively for concomitant C. trachomatis.**
Endocarditis	N. gonorrhoeae	**Ceftriaxone** 1–2 gm IV q24h x 4 wk		Ref: JID 157:1281, 1988
Pharyngitis	N. gonorrhoeae	**Ceftriaxone** 125 mg IM x 1		If chlamydia not ruled out: **Azithro** 1 gm po x 1 or **doxy** 100 mg po bid x 7 days. Some suggest test of cure culture after 1 wk. **Spectinomycin, cefixime, cefpodoxime & cefuroxime not effective**
Urethritis, cervicitis, proctitis (uncomplicated) For prostatitis, *see page 25.* **Diagnosis:** Nucleic acid amplification test (NAAT) on urine or urethral swab—see *AnIM 142:914, 2005.* **NO FQs:** *MMWR* **56:332, 2007.**	N. gonorrhoeae (50% of pts with urethritis, cervicitis have concomitant C. trachomatis —**treat for both unless NAAT indicates single pathogen**).	[(**Ceftriaxone** 125 mg IM x 1) or (**cefpodoxime** 400 mg po x 1)] **PLUS – if chlamydia infection not ruled out:** [(**Azithro** 2 gm po x 1) or (**doxy** 100 mg po q12h x 7 days)] Severe pen/ceph allergy? Maybe **azithro**—see comment. Understanding risk of FQ-resistance, could try FQ therapy with close follow-up. *See footnote[18]*.	[(**Ceftriaxone** 125 mg IM x 1) or (**cefixime**[18] 400 mg po x 1)]	**Treat for both GC and C. trachomatis unless single pathogen by NAAT.** Screen for syphilis. Other alternatives for **GC:** **Spectinomycin**[NUS] 2 gm IM x 1 Other single-dose cephalosporins: ceftizoxime 500 mg IM, cefotaxime 500 mg IM, cefoxitin 2 gm IM + probenecid 1 gm po. **Azithro** 1 gm po x 1 effective for chlamydia but need 2 gm po for GC: not recommended for GC due to GI side-effects, expense & rapid emergence of resistance.
Granuloma inguinale (Donovanosis)	Klebsiella (formerly Calymmatobacterium) granulomatis	**Doxy** 100 mg po bid x 3–4 wks OR **TMP-SMX-DS** q12h x 3 wk	**Erythro** 500 mg po qid x 3 wks OR **CIP** 750 mg po x 3 wks OR **azithro** 1 gm po q wk x 3 wks	Clinical response usually seen in 1 wk. Rx until all lesions healed, may take 4 wk. Treatment failures & recurrence seen with doxy & TMP-SMX. Report of efficacy with FQ and chloro. Ref.: *CID 25:24, 1997.* If improvement not evidence in first few days, some experts add gentamicin 1 mg/kg IV q8h.
Herpes simplex virus	*See Table 14A, page 141*			
Human papilloma virus (HPV)	*See Table 14A, page 146*			
Lymphogranuloma venereum	Chlamydia trachomatis, serovars. L1, L2, L3	**Doxy** 100 mg po bid x 21 days	**Erythro** 0.5 gm po qid x 21 days	Dx based on serology; biopsy contraindicated because sinus tracts develop. Nucleic acid ampli tests for *C. trachomatis* will be positive. In MSM, presents as fever, rectal ulcer, anal discharge (*CID 39:996, 2004*).
Phthirus pubis (**pubic lice, "crabs"**) & scabies	Phthirus pubis & Sarcoptes scabiei		*See Table 13, page 133*	

[18] Cefixime tablets now available as oral suspension, 200 mg/5 mL and 400 mg tablets (Lupine Pharmaceuticals, (+1) 866-587-4617) (*MMWR 57:435, 2008*).

Abbreviations on page 3.   *NOTE: All dosage recommendations are for adults (unless otherwise indicated) and assume normal renal function.*

TABLE 1A (18)

ANATOMIC SITE/DIAGNOSIS/ MODIFYING CIRCUMSTANCES	ETIOLOGIES (usual)	SUGGESTED REGIMENS*		ADJUNCT DIAGNOSTIC OR THERAPEUTIC MEASURES AND COMMENTS
		PRIMARY	ALTERNATIVE§	
GENITAL TRACT/Both Women & Men (continued)				
Syphilis (JAMA 290:1510, 2003); **Syphilis & HIV:** LnID 4:456, 2004; MMWR 53:RR-15, 2004 and 55 :RR-11, 2006				
Early: primary, secondary, or latent <1 yr	T. pallidum NOTE: Test all pts with syphilis for HIV; test all HIV patients for latent syphilis.	**Benzathine pen G (Bicillin L-A)** 2.4 million units IM x 1 NOTE: **Azithro** 2 gm po x 1 dose but use is problematic due to **emerging azithro resistance** (See Comment)	**(Doxy** 100 mg po bid x 14 days) or **(tetracycline** 500 mg po qid x 14 days) or **(ceftriaxone** 1 gm IM/IV q24h x 8–10 days). Follow-up mandatory.	If early or congenital syphilis, **quantitative VDRL at 0, 3, 6, 12 & 24 mo** after rx. If 1° or 2° syphilis, VDRL should ↓ 2 tubes at 6 mo, 3 tubes 12 mo, & 4 tubes 24 mo. Early latent: 2 tubes ↓ at 12 mo. With 1°, 50% will be RPR seronegative at 12 mo, 24% neg. FTA/ABS at 2–3 yrs (AnIM 114:1005, 1991). If titers fail to fall, examine CSF; if CSF (+), treat as neurosyphilis; if CSF is negative, retreat with benzathine Pen G 2.4 m.u. IM x 3 wks. **Azithro-resistant syphilis** documented in California, Ireland, & elsewhere (CID 44:S130, 2007). NOTE: Use of **benzathine procaine penicillin** is inappropriate!!
More than 1 yr's duration (latent of indeterminate duration, cardiovascular, late benign gumma) For penicillin desensitization method, see Table 7, pg. 76 And MMWR 55 (RR-11),33-35, 2006.		**Benzathine pen G (Bicillin L-A)** 2.4 million units IM q week x 3 = 7.2 million units total	**Doxy** 100 mg po bid x 28 days or **tetracycline** 500 mg po qid x 28 days	No published data on efficacy of alternatives. The value of routine lumbar puncture in asymptomatic late syphilis is being questioned in the U.S., i.e.: no LP, rx all patients as primary recommendation. **Indications for LP (CDC): neurologic symptoms, treatment failure, serum non-treponemal antibody titer ≥1:32, other evidence of active syphilis (aortitis, gumma, iritis), non-penicillin rx, + HIV test.**
Neurosyphilis—Very difficult to treat. Includes ocular (retrobulbar neuritis) syphilis **All need CSF exam.**		**Pen G** 3–4 million units IV q4h x 10–14 days.	**(Procaine pen G** 2.4 million units IM q24h + **probenecid** 0.5 gm po qid) both x 10–14 days—See Comment	**Ceftriaxone** 2 gm (IV or IM) q24h x 14 days. 23% failure rate reported (AJM 93:481, 1992). For penicillin allergy: either desensitize to penicillin or obtain infectious diseases consultation. **Serologic criteria for response to rx: 4-fold or greater ↓ in VDRL titer over 6–12 mo.** [CID 28 (Suppl. 1):S21, 1999].
HIV infection (AIDS) CID 44:S130, 2007.		Treatment same as HIV uninfected with closer follow-up. LP on all HIV-infected pts with late syphilis and serum RPR ≥1:32. Recommend CSF exam of all HIV+ pts regardless of stage of syphilis. Treat early neurosyphilis for 10-14 days regardless of CD4 count: MMWR 56:625, 2007.		HIV+ plus RPR ≥1:32 plus CD4 count ≤350/mcL increases risk of neurosyphilis nearly 19-fold—examine CSF (JID 189:369, 2004); also, CSF changes less likely to normalize (CID 38:1001, 2004). Reviews of syphilis & HIV: LnID 4:456, 2004; MMWR 53:RR-15, 2004.
Pregnancy and syphilis		Same as for non-pregnant, some recommend 2nd dose (2.4 million units) **benzathine pen G** 1 wk after initial dose esp. in 3rd trimester or with 2° syphilis	Skin test for penicillin allergy. Desensitize if necessary, as parenteral pen G is only therapy with documented efficacy!	Monthly quantitative VDRL or equivalent. If 4-fold ↑, re-treat. Doxy, tetracycline contraindicated. Erythro not recommended because of high risk of failure to cure fetus.
Congenital syphilis	T. pallidum	**Aqueous crystalline pen G** 50,000 units/kg per dose IV q12h x 7 days, then q8h for 10 day total.	**Procaine pen G** 50,000 units/kg IM q24h for 10 days	Another alternative: Ceftriaxone ≤30 days old, 75 mg/kg IV/IM q24h or >30 days old 100 mg/kg IV/IM q24h. Treat 10-14 days. If symptomatic, ophthalmologic exam indicated. If more than 1 day of rx missed, restart entire course. **Need serologic follow-up!**
Warts, anogenital	See Table 14, page 146			

Abbreviations on page 3.   NOTE: All dosage recommendations are for adults (unless otherwise indicated) and assume normal renal function.

TABLE 1A (19)

ANATOMIC SITE/DIAGNOSIS/ MODIFYING CIRCUMSTANCES	ETIOLOGIES (usual)	SUGGESTED REGIMENS*		ADJUNCT DIAGNOSTIC OR THERAPEUTIC MEASURES AND COMMENTS
		PRIMARY	ALTERNATIVE[§]	
GENITAL TRACT (continued)				
Women: **Amnionitis, septic abortion**	Bacteroides, esp. Prevotella bivius; Group B, A streptococci; Enterobacteriaceae; C. trachomatis	[(**Cefoxitin** or **TC-CL** or **Dori**[NFDA-I] or **IMP** or **MER** or **AM-SB** or **ERTA** or **PIP-TZ**) + **doxy**] **OR** [**Clinda** + (**aminoglycoside** or **ceftriaxone**)] *Dosage: see footnote*[19]		D&C of uterus. **In septic abortion**, Clostridium perfringens may cause fulminant intravascular hemolysis. **In postpartum patients** with enigmatic fever and/or pulmonary emboli, **consider septic pelvic vein thrombophlebitis** (*see Vascular, septic pelvic vein thrombophlebitis, page 60*). After discharge: doxy or continue clinda. **NOTE:** IV clinda effective for C. trachomatis, no data on po clinda (*CID 19:720, 1994*).
Cervicitis, mucopurulent Treatment based on results of nucleic acid amplification test	N. gonorrhoeae Chlamydia trachomatis	Treat for Gonorrhea, *page 21* Treat for non-gonococcal urethritis, *page 20*		Criteria for dx: yellow or green pus on cervical swab, >10 WBC/oil field. Gram stain for GC, if negative rx for C. trachomatis. If in doubt, send swab or urine for culture, EIA or nucleic acid amplification test and rx for both.
Endomyometritis/septic pelvic phlebitis Early postpartum (1st 48 hrs) (usually after C-section)	Bacteroides, esp. Prevotella bivius; Group B, A streptococci; Enterobacteriaceae; C. trachomatis	[(**Cefoxitin** or **TC-CL** or **ERTA** or **IMP** or **MER** or **AM-SB** or **PIP-TZ**) + **doxy**] **OR** [**Clinda** + (**aminoglycoside** or **ceftriaxone**)] *Dosage: see footnote*[19]		*See Comments under Amnionitis, septic abortion, above*
Late postpartum (48 hrs to 6 wks) (usually after vaginal delivery)	Chlamydia trachomatis, M. hominis	**Doxy** 100 mg IV or po q12h times 14 days		Tetracyclines not recommended in nursing mothers; discontinue nursing. M. hominis sensitive to tetra, clinda, not erythro (*CCTID 17:5200, 1993*).
Fitzhugh-Curtis syndrome	C. trachomatis, N. gonorrhoeae	Treat as for pelvic inflammatory disease immediately below.		Perihepatitis (violin-string adhesions)
Pelvic actinomycosis; usually tubo-ovarian abscess	A. Israeli most common	**AMP** 50 mg/kg/day IV div 3-4 doses x 4-6 wks, then **Pen VK** 2-4 gm/day po x 3-6 mos.	**Doxy** or **ceftriaxone** or **clinda** or **erythro**	Complication of intrauterine device (IUD). Remove IUD. Can use **Pen G** 10-20 million units/day IV instead of **AMP** x 4-6 wks.
Pelvic Inflammatory Disease (PID), salpingitis, tubo-ovarian abscess Outpatient rx: limit to pts with temp <38°C, WBC <11,000 per mm[3], minimal evidence of peritonitis, active bowel sounds & able to tolerate oral nourishment *CID 44:953 & 961, 2007; MMWR 55(RR-11), 2006 & www.cdc.gov/std/treatment*	N. gonorrhoeae, chlamydia, bacteroides, Enterobacteriaceae, streptococci	**Outpatient rx:** [(**ceftriaxone** 250 mg IM or IV x 1) (± **metro** 500 mg po bid x 14 days) + (**doxy** 100 mg po bid x 14 days)]. **OR** (**cefoxitin** 2 gm IM with **probenecid** 1 gm po both as single dose) plus (**doxy** 100 mg po bid with **metro** 500 mg bid—both times 14 days) **Inpatient regimens:** [(**Cefotetan** 2 gm IV q12h or **cefoxitin** 2 gm IV q6h) + (**doxy** 100 mg IV/po q12h)] ----- (**Clinda** 900 mg IV q8h) + (**gentamicin** 2 mg/kg loading dose, then 1.5 mg/kg q8h or 4.5 mg/kg once per day), then **doxy** 100 mg po bid x 14 days		Another alternative parenteral regimen: **AM-SB** 3 gm IV q6h + **doxy** 100 mg IV/po q12h Remember: Evaluate and treat sex partner. FQs not recommended due to increasing resistance (*MMWR 56:332, 2007 & www.cdc.gov/std/treatment*)

[19] **P Ceph 2** (**cefoxitin** 2 gm IV q6-8h, **cefotetan** 2 gm IV q12h, **cefuroxime** 750 mg IV q8h); **TC-CL** 3.1 gm IV q4-6h; **AM-SB** 3 gm IV q6h; **PIP-TZ** 3.375 gm q6h or for nosocomial pneumonia: 4.5 gm IV q6h or 4-hr infusion of 3.375 gm q8h; **doxy** 100 mg IV/po q12h; **clinda** 450-900 mg IV q8h; **aminoglycoside** (**gentamicin**, see *Table 10D, page 96*); **P Ceph 3** (**cefotaxime** 2 gm IV q8h, **ceftriaxone** 2 gm IV q24h); **doripenem** 500 mg IV q8h (1-hr infusión), **ertapenem** 1 gm IV q24h; **IMP** 0.5 gm IV q6h; **MER** 1 gm IV q8h; **azithro** 500 mg IV q24h; **linezolid** 600 mg IV/po q12h; **vanco** 1 gm IV q12h

Abbreviations on page 3.   NOTE: All dosage recommendations are for adults (unless otherwise indicated) and assume normal renal function.

TABLE 1A (20)

ANATOMIC SITE/DIAGNOSIS/ MODIFYING CIRCUMSTANCES	ETIOLOGIES (usual)	SUGGESTED REGIMENS* PRIMARY	ALTERNATIVE$	ADJUNCT DIAGNOSTIC OR THERAPEUTIC MEASURES AND COMMENTS
GENITAL TRACT/Women (continued)				
Vaginitis—*MMWR 51(RR-6), 2002* or *CID 35 (Suppl.2):S135, 2002*				
Candidiasis Pruritus, thick cheesy discharge, pH <4.5 *See Table 11A, page 101*	Candida albicans 80–90%. C. glabrata, C. tropicalis may be increasing—they are less susceptible to azoles	**Oral azoles: Fluconazole** 150 mg po x 1; **itraconazole** 200 mg po bid x 1 day	**Intravaginal azoles:** variety of strengths—from 1 dose to 7–14 days. Drugs available (all end in -azole): butocon, clotrim, micon, tiocon, tercon (*doses: Table 11A, footnote page 101*)	Nystatin vag. tabs times 14 days less effective. Other rx for azole-resistant strains: gentian violet, boric acid. If recurrent candidiasis (4 or more episodes per yr): 6 mos. suppression with: fluconazole 150 mg q week or itraconazole 100 mg po q24h or clotrimazole vag. suppositories 500 mg q week.
Trichomoniasis Copious foamy discharge, pH >4.5 Treat sexual partners—see *Comment*	Trichomonas vaginalis	**Metro** 2 gm as single dose or 500 mg po bid x 7 days OR **Tinidazole** 2 gm po single dose **Pregnancy:** *See Comment*	**For rx failure:** Re-treat with metro 500 mg po bid x 7 days; if 2nd failure: metro 2 gm po q24h x 3–5 days. If still failure, suggest ID consultation and/or contact CDC: 770-488-4115 or www.cdc.gov/std.	**Treat male sexual partners (2 gm metronidazole as single dose).** Nearly 20% men with NGU are infected with trichomonas (*JID 188:465, 2003*). Another option if metro-resistant: **Tinidazole** 500 mg po bid x 14 days. Ref.: *CID 33:1341, 2001*. **Pregnancy:** No data indicating metro teratogenic or mutagenic [*MMWR 51(RR-6), 2002*].
Bacterial vaginosis Malodorous vaginal discharge, pH >4.5 Data on recurrence & review: *JID 193:1475,2006*	Etiology unclear: associated with Gardnerella vaginalis, mobiluncus., Mycoplasma hominis, Prevotella sp., & Atopobium vaginae et al.	**Metro** 0.5 gm po bid x 7 days or **metro vaginal gel[20]** (1 applicator intra-vaginally) 1x/day x 5 days OR **Tinidazole** (2 gm po once daily x 2 days or 1 gm po once daily x 5 days)	**Clinda** 0.3 gm bid po x 7 days or 2% **clinda vaginal cream** 5 gm intravaginally at bedtime x 7 days or **clinda ovules** 100 mg intravag-inally at bedtime x 3 days.	Reported 50% ↑ in cure rate if abstain from sex or use condoms: *CID 44:213 & 220, 2007*. Treatment of male sex partner **not** indicated unless balanitis present. Metro extended release tabs 750 mg po q24h x 7 days available: no published data. **Pregnancy:** Treat same as non-pregnancy, except avoid clindamycin cream (↑ risk premature birth). Atopobium resistant to metro in vitro; suscept. To clinda (*BMC Inf Dis 6:51, 2006*); importance unclear.
Men:				
Balanitis	Candida 40%, Group B strep, gardnerella	Oral **azoles** as for vaginitis		Occurs in 1/4 of male sex partners of women infected with candida. Exclude circinate balanitis (Reiter's syndrome). Plasma cell balanitis (non-infectious) responds to hydrocortisone cream.
Epididymo-orchitis Age <35 years	N. gonorrhoeae, Chlamydia trachomatis	**Ceftriaxone** 250 mg IM x 1 + **doxy** 100 mg po bid x 10 days		Also: bedrest, scrotal elevation, and analgesics.
Age >35 years or homosexual men (insertive partners in anal intercourse)	Enterobacteriaceae (coli-forms)	**FQ: CIP-ER** 500 mg po 1x/day or **CIP** 400 mg IV bid or **Levo** 750 mg IV/po 1x/day) x 10–14 days	**AM-SB, P Ceph 3, TC-CL, PIP-TZ** (*Dosage: see footnote page 23*)	Midstream pyuria and scrotal pain and edema. Also: bedrest, scrotal elevation, and analgesics. NOTE: Do urine NAAT (nucleic acid amplification test) to ensure absence of N. gonorrhoeae with concomitant risk of FQ-resistant gonorrhoeae.
Non-gonococcal urethritis	See *Chlamydia et al, Non-gonococcal urethritis, Table 1A(17), page 20*			

[20] 1 applicator contains 5 gm of gel with 37.5 mg metronidazole

Abbreviations on page 3. NOTE: *All dosage recommendations are for adults (unless otherwise indicated) and assume normal renal function.*

TABLE 1A (21)

ANATOMIC SITE/DIAGNOSIS/ MODIFYING CIRCUMSTANCES	ETIOLOGIES (usual)	SUGGESTED REGIMENS* PRIMARY	ALTERNATIVE§	ADJUNCT DIAGNOSTIC OR THERAPEUTIC MEASURES AND COMMENTS
GENITAL TRACT/Men (continued)				
Prostatitis—Review: AJM 106:327, 1999				
Acute				
≤35 years of age	N. gonorrhoeae, C. trachomatis	**ceftriaxone** 250 mg IM x 1 then **doxy** 100 mg bid x 10 days.		FQs no longer recommended for gonococcal infections. In AIDS pts, prostate may be focus of Cryptococcus neoformans.
≥35 years of age	Enterobacteriaceae (coliforms)	FQ (dosage: see Epididymo-orchitis, >35 yrs, above) or **TMP-SMX** 1 DS tablet (160 mg TMP) po bid x 10–14 days		Treat as acute urinary infection. 14 days (not single dose regimen). Some authorities recommend 3–4 wk therapy. If uncertain, do urine test for C. trachomatis and of N. gonorrhoeae.
Chronic bacterial	Enterobacteriaceae 80%, enterococci 15%, P. aeruginosa	FQ (**CIP** 500 mg po bid x 4 wk, **Levo** 750 mg po q24h x 4 wk—see Comment)	**TMP-SMX-DS** 1 tab po bid x 1–3 mo	With treatment failures consider infected prostatic calculi. FDA approved dose of levo is 500 mg; editors prefer higher dose.
Chronic prostatitis/chronic pain syndrome (New NIH classification, JAMA 282:236, 1999)	The most common prostatitis syndrome. Etiology is unknown; molecular probe data suggest infectious etiology (Clin Micro Rev 11: 604, 1998).	**α-adrenergic blocking agents are controversial** (AnIM 133:367, 2000).		Pt has sx of prostatitis but negative cultures and no cells in prostatic secretions. Rev.: JAC 46:157, 2000. In randomized double-blind study, CIP and an alpha-blocker of no benefit (AnIM 141:581 & 639, 2004).
HAND (Bites: See Skin)				
Paronychia				
Nail biting, manicuring	Staph. aureus (maybe MRSA)	Incision & drainage; do culture	**TMP-SMX-DS** 1-2 tabs po bid while waiting for culture result.	See Table 6 for alternatives
Contact with oral mucosa—dentists, anesthesiologists, wrestlers	Herpes simplex (Whitlow)	**Acyclovir** 400 mg tid po x 10 days	**Famciclovir** or **valacyclovir** should work, see Comment	Gram stain and routine culture negative. Famciclovir/valacyclovir doses used for primary genital herpes should work; see Table 14, page 141
Dishwasher (prolonged water immersion)	Candida sp.	**Clotrimazole** (topical)		Avoid immersion of hands in water as much as possible.
HEART				
Infective endocarditis—Native valve—empirical rx awaiting cultures—No IV illicit drugs	**NOTE: Diagnostic criteria** include evidence of continuous bacteremia (multiple positive blood cultures), new murmur (worsening of old murmur) of valvular insufficiency, definite emboli, and echocardiographic (transthoracic or transesophageal) evidence of valvular vegetations. Refs.: Circulation 111:3167, 2005; Ln 363:139, 2004. For antimicrobial prophylaxis, see Table 15A, pg 168			
Valvular or congenital heart disease but no modifying circumstances See Table 15C, page 172 for prophylaxis	Viridans strep 30–40%. "other" strep 15–25%, enterococci 5–18%, staphylococci 20–35% (including coag-neg staphylococci--CID 46:232, 2008).	[**Pen G** 20 million units IV q24h, continuous or div. q4h) or (**AMP** 12 gm IV q24h, continuous or div. q4h) + (**nafcillin** or **oxacillin** 2 gm IV q4h) + **gentamicin** 1 mg/kg IM or IV q8h (see Comment)]	(**Vanco** 15 mg/kg[21] IV q12h (not to exceed 2 gm q24h unless serum levels monitored) + **gentamicin** 1 mg/kg[21] IM or IV q8h) **OR** **dapto** 6 mg/kg IV q24h	If patient not acutely ill and not in heart failure, we prefer to wait for blood culture results. If initial 3 blood cultures neg. after 24–48 hrs, obtain 2–3 more blood cultures before empiric therapy started. **Nafcillin/oxacillin + gentamicin** may not cover enterococci, hence addition of penicillin G pending cultures. When blood cultures +, modify regimen to specific therapy for organism. **Gentamicin** used for synergy; peak levels need not exceed 4 mcg per mL. **Surgery indications:** heart failure, paravalvular infection, resistant organism (JACC 48.e1, 2006); in selected pts, emboli, esp if after week of therapy (AHJ 154:1086, 2007) and large mobile vegetation.
Infective endocarditis—Native valve—IV illicit drug use ± evidence rt-sided endocarditis—empiric therapy	S. aureus(MSSA & MRSA). All others rare	**Vanco** 1 gm IV q12h; over 100 kg: 1.5 gm IV q12h	**Dapto** 6 mg/kg IV q24h Approved for right-sided endocarditis.	**Quinupristin-dalfopristin** cidal vs S. aureus if both constituents active. In controlled clinical trial, **dapto** equivalent to vanco plus 4 days of gentamicin for right-sided endocarditis (NEJM 355:653, 2006).

[21] Assumes estimated creatinine clearance ≥80 mL per min., see Table 17.

Abbreviations on page 3.   NOTE: All dosage recommendations are for adults (unless otherwise indicated) and assume normal renal function.

TABLE 1A (22)

ANATOMIC SITE/DIAGNOSIS/ MODIFYING CIRCUMSTANCES	ETIOLOGIES (usual)	SUGGESTED REGIMENS*		ADJUNCT DIAGNOSTIC OR THERAPEUTIC MEASURES AND COMMENTS
		PRIMARY	ALTERNATIVE§	
HEART (continued) **Infective endocarditis—Native valve—culture positive (NEJM 345:1318, 2001; CID 36:615, 2003; JAC 54:971, 2004[22])**				
Viridans strep, S. bovis (S. gallolyticus) with **penicillin G MIC ≤0.1 mcg/mL** **Note:** New name for S. bovis, biotype 1 is S. gallolyticus subsp. gallolyticus (JCM 46:2966, 2008).	Viridans strep, S. bovis	[(**Pen G** 12–18 million units/day IV, divided q4h **x 4 wk)** PLUS **gentamicin** 1 mg/kg/h q8h IV x 2 wks)] **OR** (**Pen G** 12–18 million units/day IV, divided - q4h **x 4 wk) OR (ceftriaxone** 2 gm IV q24h x 4 wk)	[(**Ceftriaxone** 2 gm IV q24h + **gentamicin** 1 mg per kg IV q8h both **x 2 wks**)] If allergy pen G or ceftriax, use **vanco** 15 mg/kg IV q12h to 2 gm/day max unless serum levels measured **x 4 wks**	Target **gent levels:** peak 3 mcg/mL, trough <1 mcg/mL. If very obese pt, recommend consultation for dosage adjustment. Infuse vanco over ≥1 hr to avoid "red man" syndrome. **S. bovis suggests occult bowel pathology (new name: S. gallolyticus).** Since relapse rate may be greater in pts ill for >3 mos. prior to start of rx, the penicillin-gentamicin synergism theoretically may be advantageous in this group. **NOTE: Dropped option of continuous infusion of Pen G due to instability of penicillin in acidic IV fluids, rapid renal clearance and rising MICs (JAC 53:675, 2004).**
Viridans strep, S. bovis (S. gallolyticus) with **penicillin G MIC >0.1 to <0.5 mcg/mL**	Viridans strep, S. bovis, nutritionally variant streptococci, (e.g. S. abiotrophia) tolerant strep[23]	**Pen G** 18 million units/day IV (divided q4h) **x 4 wks** PLUS **gentamicin** 1 mg/kg IV q8h **x 2 wks** **NOTE: Low dose of gentamicin**	**Vanco** 15 mg/kg IV q12h to max. 2 gm/day unless serum levels documented **x 4 wks**	Can use cefazolin for pen G in pt with allergy that is not IgE-mediated (e.g., anaphylaxis). Alternatively, can use vanco. (See Comment above on gent and vanco) **NOTE: If necessary to remove infected valve & valve culture neg., 2 weeks antibiotic treatment post-op sufficient (CID 41:187, 2005).**
For viridans strep or S. bovis with **pen G MIC ≥0.5** and enterococci susceptible to AMP/pen G, vanco, gentamicin NOTE: Inf. Dis. consultation suggested	"Susceptible" enterococci, viridans strep, S. bovis, nutritionally variant streptococci (new names are: Abiotrophia sp. & Granulicatella sp.)	[(**Pen G** 18–30 million units per 24h IV, divided q4h **x 4–6 wks**) PLUS (**gentamicin** 1–1.5 mg/kg q8h IV x 4– 6 wks)] OR (**AMP** 12 gm/day IV, divided q4h + **gent** as above x 4–6 wks)	**Vanco** 15 mg/kg IV q12h to max of 2 gm/day unless serum levels measured **PLUS gentamicin** 1–1.5 mg/kg q8h IV x 4–6 wks **NOTE: Low dose of gent**	**4 wks of rx if symptoms <3 mos.; 6 wks of rx if symptoms >3 mos.** Vanco for pen non-allergic pts; do not use cephalosporins. Do **not** give gent once-q24h for enterococcal endocarditis. Target gent levels: peak 3 mcg/mL, trough <1 mcg/mL. Vanco target serum levels: peak 20– 50 mcg/mL, trough 5–12 mcg/mL. **NOTE:** Because of ↑ frequency of resistance (see below), all enterococci causing endocarditis should be tested in vitro for susceptibility to penicillin, gentamicin and vancomycin plus β lactamase production.
Enterococci: MIC streptomycin >2000 mcg/mL; MIC gentamicin >500– 2000 mcg/mL; no resistance to penicillin	Enterococci, high-level aminoglycoside resistance	**Pen G** or **AMP** IV as above **x 8–12 wks** (approx. 50% cure)	If prolonged pen G or AMP fails, consider surgical removal of infected valve. See Comment	10–25% E. faecalis and 45–50% E. faecium resistant to high gent levels. May be sensitive to streptomycin, check MIC. Case report of success with combination of AMP, IMP, and vanco (Scand J Inf Dis 29:628, 1997). **Cure rate of 67% with IV AMP 2 gm q4h plus ceftriaxone 2 gm q12h x 6 wks (AnIM 146:574, 2007).**
Enterococci: β-lactamase production test is **positive** & **no gentamicin** resistance	Enterococci, penicillin resistance	**AM-SB** 3 gm IV q6h PLUS **gentamicin** 1–1.5 mg/kg q8h IV x 4–6 wks. **Low dose of gent**	**AM-SB** 3 gm IV q6h PLUS **vanco** 15 mg/kg IV q12h (check levels if >2 gm) **x 4–6 wks**	β-lactamase **not** detected by MIC tests with standard inocula. Detection requires testing with the chromogenic cephalosporin nitrocefin. **Once-q24h gentamicin rx not** efficacious in animal model of E. faecalis endocarditis (JAC 49:437, 2002)—hence give gent q8h.
Enterococci: β-lactamase test neg.; pen G MIC >16 mcg/mL; no gentamicin resistance	Enterococci, intrinsic pen G/AMP resistance	**Vanco** 15 mg/kg IV q12h (check levels if >2 gm) PLUS **gent** 1–1.5 mg/kg q8h **x 4–6 wks** (see Comment)		Desired vanco serum levels: peak 20–50 mcg/mL, trough 5–12 mcg/mL. **Gentamicin** used for synergy; peak levels need not exceed 4 mcg/mL.

22 Ref. for Guidelines of British Soc. for Antimicrob. Chemother. Includes drugs not available in U.S.: flucloxacillin IV, teicoplanin IV: JAC 54:971, 2004.
23 Tolerant streptococci = MBC 32-fold greater than MIC

Abbreviations on page 3.   NOTE: All dosage recommendations are for adults (unless otherwise indicated) and assume normal renal function.

TABLE 1A (23)

ANATOMIC SITE/DIAGNOSIS/ MODIFYING CIRCUMSTANCES	ETIOLOGIES (usual)	SUGGESTED REGIMENS*		ADJUNCT DIAGNOSTIC OR THERAPEUTIC MEASURES AND COMMENTS
		PRIMARY	ALTERNATIVE§	
HEART/Infective endocarditis—Native valve—culture positive *(continued)*				
Enterococci: Pen/AMP resistant + high-level gent/strep resistant + vanco resistant: usually VRE **Consultation suggested**	Enterococci, vanco-resistant, usually E. faecium	No reliable effective rx. Can try **quinupristin-dalfopristin** (Synercid) or **linezolid**—see Comment, footnote[24] and Table 5	**Teicoplanin** active against a subset of vanco-resistant enterococci. Teicoplanin is not available in U.S. **Dapto** is an option.	**Synercid** activity limited to E. faecium and is usually bacteriostatic, therefore expect high relapse rate. Dose: 7.5 mg per kg IV (via central line) q8h. **Linezolid** active most enterococci, but bacteriostatic. Dose: 600 mg IV or po q12h. Linezolid failed in pt with E. faecalis endocarditis (CID 37:e29, 2003). **Dapto** is bactericidal in vitro; clinical experience in CID 41:1134, 2005.
Staphylococcal endocarditis Aortic &/or mitral valve infection—MSSA Surgery indications: see Comment page 25.	Staph. aureus, methicillin-sensitive	**Nafcillin (oxacillin)** 2 gm IV q4h **x 4–6 wks PLUS gentamicin** 1 mg/kg IV q8h **x 3–5 days** **Note: Low dose of gentamicin for only 3-5 days**	[(**Cefazolin** 2 gm IV q8h **x 4–6 wk) PLUS (gentamicin** 1 mg/kg IV q8h **x 3–5 days).** **Low dose of gent) OR** **Vanco** 15 mg/kg IV q12h (check levels if > 2 gm per day) **x 4–6 wks**	If IgE-mediated penicillin allergy, 10% cross-reactivity to cephalosporins (AnIM 141:16, 2004). **Cefazolin** failures reported (CID 37:1194, 2003). No definitive data, pro or con, on once-q24h **gentamicin** for S. aureus endocarditis. At present, favor q8h dosing times **no more than 3–5 days.**
Aortic and/or mitral valve—MRSA	Staph. aureus, methicillin-resistant	**Vanco** 1 gm IV q12h **x 4–6 wks**	**Dapto** not FDA-approved for left-sided endocarditis	In clinical trial (NEJM 355:653, 2006), high failure rate with both vanco and dapto in small numbers of pts. For other alternatives, see Table 6, pg 75.
Tricuspid valve infection (usually IVDUs): MSSA	Staph. aureus, methicillin-sensitive	**Nafcillin (oxacillin)** 2 gm IV q4h **PLUS gentamicin** 1 mg/kg IV q8h **x 2 wks.** **NOTE: low dose of gent**	**If penicillin allergy:** **Vanco** 15 mg/kg IV q12h + low-dose **gent** 1 mg/kg IV q8h x 2 wks OR **Dapto** 6 mg/kg IV q24h (avoid if concomitant left-sided endocarditis). 8-12 mg/kg IV q24h used in some cases, but not FDA approved.	**2-week regimen not long enough if metastatic infection (e.g., osteo) or left-sided endocarditis.** **What about concomitant rifampin?** Older study of success with 4 wks of CIP 750 mg po bid + RIF 300 mg bid in tricuspid infections due to mostly MSSA (Ln 2:1071, 1989). In a 1991 report, adding RIF prolonged bacteremia in pts with MSSA, but not MSSA, endocarditis (AnIM 115:674, 1991) Recent mostly right-sided MRSA native valve endocarditis, adding RIF again prolonged bacteremia & was associated with hepatotoxicity, drug-drug interactions & emergence of RIF-resistant S. aureus (AAC 52:2463, 2008). **Daptomycin:** Approved for bacteremia and in **right-sided** endocarditis based on randomized study (NEJM 355:653 & 727, 2006).
Tricuspid valve--MRSA	Staph. aureus, methicillin-resistant	**Vanco** 15 mg/kg IV q12h (check levels if >2 gm/day) **x 4–6 wks**	**Dapto** 6 mg/kg IV q24h x 4-6 wk equiv to **vanco** for rt-sided endocarditis; both vanco & dapto did poorly if lt-sided endocarditis (NEJM 355: 653, 2006). (See Comments & table 6, pg 75)	**Quinupristin-dalfopristin** another option.[24] **Linezolid:** Limited experience (see JAC 58:273, 2006) in patients with few treatment options; 64% cure rate; clear failure in 21%; thrombocytopenia in 31%. **Dapto** dose of 8-12 mg/kg may help in selected cases, but not FDA-approved.
Slow-growing fastidious Gm-neg. bacilli--any valve	HACEK group (see Comments) Change to HABCEK if add Bartonella.	**Ceftriaxone** 2 gm IV q24h **x 4 wks** (Bartonella resistant – see below)	**AMP** 12 gm IV q24h (continuous or div. q4h) **x 4 wks + gentamicin** 1 mg/kg IV/IM q8h **x 4 wks.**	**HACEK (acronym for Haemophilus parainfluenzae, H. (aphrophilus) aggregatibacter, Actinobacillus, Cardiobacterium, Eikenella, Kingella).** H. aphrophilus resistant to vanco, clinda and methicillin. Penicillinase-positive HACEK organisms should be susceptible to AM-SB + gentamicin.
Bartonella species--any valve Circ 111:3167, 2005	B. henselae, B. quintana	[**Ceftriaxone** 2 gm IV q24h x 14 days] + **doxy** 100 mg IV/po bid x 6 wks.	[**Ceftriaxone** 2 gm IV q24h x 6 wks + **gentamicin** 1 mg/kg q8h x 14 days) + **doxy** 100 mg IV/po bid x 6 wks.	**Dx:** Immunofluorescent antibody titer ≥1:800; blood cultures only occ. positive, or PCR of tissue from surgery. **Surgery:** Over ½ pts require valve surgery: relation to cure unclear. B. quintana transmitted by body lice among homeless; asymptomatic colonization of RBCs described (Ln 360:226, 2002).

[24] Three interesting recent reports: (1) Successful rx of vanco-resistant E. faecium prosthetic valve endocarditis with Synercid without change in MIC (CID 25:163, 1997); (2) resistance to Synercid emerged during therapy of E. faecium bacteremia (CID 24:90, 1997); and (3) super-infection with E. faecalis occurred during Synercid rx of E. faecium (CID 24:91, 1997).

Abbreviations on page 3.   *NOTE: All dosage recommendations are for adults (unless otherwise indicated) and assume normal renal function.*

TABLE 1A (24)

ANATOMIC SITE/DIAGNOSIS/ MODIFYING CIRCUMSTANCES	ETIOLOGIES (usual)	SUGGESTED REGIMENS*		ADJUNCT DIAGNOSTIC OR THERAPEUTIC MEASURES AND COMMENTS
		PRIMARY	ALTERNATIVE§	
HEART (continued)				
Infective endocarditis—"culture negative" Fever, valvular disease, and ECHO vegetations ± emboli and neg. cultures. Rev.: *Medicine 84:162, 2005*				Etiology in 348 cases studied by serology, culture, histopath, & molecular detection: C. burnetii 48%, Bartonella sp. 28%, and rarely (Abiotrophia elegans (nutritionally variant strep), Mycoplasma hominis, Legionella pneumophila, Tropheryma whipplei—together 1%), & rest without etiology identified (most on antibiotic). Ref.: *NEJM 356:715, 2007.*
Infective endocarditis—Prosthetic valve—empiric therapy (cultures pending) S. aureus now most common etiology *(JAMA 297:1354, 2007).*				
Early (<2 mo post-op)	S. epidermidis, S. aureus. Rarely, Enterobacteriaceae, diphtheroids, fungi	**Vanco** 15 mg/kg IV q12h + **gentamicin** 1 mg/kg IV q8h + **RIF** 600 mg po q24h		Early surgical consultation advised especially if etiology is S. aureus, evidence of heart failure, presence of diabetes and/or renal failure, or concern for valve ring abscess *(JAMA 297:1354, 2007; CID 44:364, 2007).*
Late (>2 mo post-op)	S. epidermidis, viridans strep, enterococci. S. aureus			
Infective endocarditis— Prosthetic valve— positive blood cultures **Surgical consultation advised:** Indications for surgery: severe heart failure, S. aureus infection, prosthetic dehiscence, resistant organism, emboli due to large vegetation *(JACC 48:e1, 2006).*	Staph. epidermidis	(**Vanco** 15 mg /kg IV q12h + **RIF** 300 mg po q8h) **x 6 wks** + **gentamicin** 1 mg/kg IV q8h **x 14 days.**		If S. epidermidis is susceptible to nafcillin/oxacillin in vitro (not common), then substitute nafcillin (or oxacillin) for vanco.
	Staph. aureus	Methicillin sensitive: (**Nafcillin** 2 gm IV q4h + **RIF** 300 mg po q8h) **times 6 wks** + **gentamicin** 1 mg per kg IV q8h **times 14 days.** Methicillin resistant: (**Vanco** 1 gm IV q12h + **RIF** 300 mg po q8h) **times 6 wks** + **gentamicin** 1 mg per kg IV q8h **times 14 days.**		
	Viridans strep, enterococci	See *infective endocarditis, native valve, culture positive, page 26*		
	Enterobacteriaceae or P. aeruginosa	**Aminoglycoside** (tobra if P. aeruginosa) + (**AP Pen** or **P Ceph 3 AP** or **P Ceph 4**)		In theory, could substitute CIP for APAG, but no clinical data.
	Candida, aspergillus	**Ampho B** ± an azole, e.g., fluconazole *(Table 11, page 99)*		High mortality. Valve replacement plus antifungal therapy standard therapy but some success with antifungal therapy alone *(CID 22:262, 1996).*
Infective endocarditis—Q fever *LnID 3:709, 2003; NEJM 356:715, 2007.*	Coxiella burnetii	**Doxy** 100 mg po bid + **hydroxychloroquine** 600 mg/day x 1.5–3 yrs *(J Infection 45:127, 2002).* *Pregnancy: Need long term* **TMP-SMX** *(see CID 45:548, 2007).*		**Dx:** Complement-fix or ELISA IgG antibody to phase II antigen diagnostic of acute Q fever; IgG antibody of to phase I antigen diagnostic of chronic Q fever *(JCM 43:4238, 2005; 44:2283, 2006).* Want doxy serum conc. >5 mcg/mL *(JID 188:1322, 2003).*
Pacemaker/defibrillator infections	S. aureus, S. epidermidis, rarely others	**Device removal** + **vanco** 1 gm IV q12h + **RIF** 300 mg po bid	**Device removal** + **dapto** 6 mg per kg IV q24h[NFDA] ± **RIF** *(no data)* 300 mg po bid	**Duration of rx after device removal:** For "pocket" or subcutaneous infection, 10–14 days; if lead-assoc. endocarditis, 4–6 wks depending on organism. Refs.: *Circulation 108:2015, 2003; NEJM 350:1422, 2004.*
Pericarditis, purulent— empiric therapy Rev.: *Medicine 82:385, 2003*	Staph. aureus, Strep. pneumoniae, Group A strep, Enterobacteriaceae	**Vanco + CIP** *(Dosage, see footnote[25])*	**Vanco + CFP** *(see footnote[25])*	Drainage required if signs of tamponade. Forced to use empiric vanco due to high prevalence of MRSA.
Rheumatic fever with carditis Ref.: *Ln 366:155, 2005*	Post-infectious sequelae of Group A strep infection (usually pharyngitis)	**ASA,** and usually **prednisone** 2 mg/kg po q24h for symptomatic treatment of fever, arthritis, arthralgia. May not influence carditis.		Clinical features: Carditis, polyarthritis, chorea, subcutaneous nodules, erythema marginatum. *Prophylaxis: see page 56*
Ventricular assist device-related infection Ref.: *LnID 6:426, 2006*	S. aureus, S. epidermidis, aerobic gm-neg bacilli, Candida sp	After culture of blood, wounds, drive line, device pocket and maybe pump: **Vanco** 1 gm IV q12h + (**Cip** 400 mg IV q12h or **levo** 750 mg IV q24h) + **fluconazole** 800 mg IV q24h.		Can substitute **daptomycin** 6 mg/kg/d for **vanco, cefepime** 2 gm IV q12h for FQ, and (**vori, caspo, micafungin or anidulafungin**) for **fluconazole**.

[25] **Aminoglycosides** *(see Table 10D, page 96),* **IMP** 0.5 gm IV q6h, **MER** 1 gm IV q6h, **nafcillin** or **oxacillin** 2 gm IV q8h, **TC-CL** 3.1 gm IV q6h, **PIP-TZ** 3.375 gm IV q6h or 4.5 gm q8h, **AM-SB** 3 gm IV q6h, **P Ceph** 1 (cephalothin 2 gm IV q4h or cefazolin 2 gm IV q8h), **vanco** 1 gm IV q12h, **CIP** 750 mg po bid or 400 mg IV q12h, **RIF** 600 mg po q24h, **aztreonam** 2 gm IV q8h, **CFP** 2 gm IV q12h

Abbreviations on page 3. NOTE: *All dosage recommendations are for adults (unless otherwise indicated) and assume normal renal function.*

TABLE 1A (25)

29

ANATOMIC SITE/DIAGNOSIS/ MODIFYING CIRCUMSTANCES	ETIOLOGIES (usual)	SUGGESTED REGIMENS*		ADJUNCT DIAGNOSTIC OR THERAPEUTIC MEASURES AND COMMENTS
		PRIMARY	ALTERNATIVE§	
JOINT—Also see Lyme Disease, page 54				
Reactive arthritis **Reiter's syndrome** (See *Comment for definition*)	Occurs wks after infection with C. trachomatis, Campylobacter jejuni, Yersinia enterocolitica, Shigella/Salmonella sp.	Only treatment is non-steroidal anti-inflammatory drugs		Definition: Urethritis, conjunctivitis, arthritis, and sometimes uveitis and rash. Arthritis: asymmetrical oligoarthritis of ankles, knees, feet, sacroiliitis. Rash: palms and soles—keratoderma blennorrhagia; circinate balanitis of glans penis. HLA-B27 positive predisposes to Reiter's.
Poststreptococcal reactive arthritis (See *Rheumatic fever, above*)	Immunologic reaction after strep pharyngitis: (1) arthritis onset in <10 days, (2) lasts months, (3) unresponsive to ASA	Treat strep pharyngitis and then NSAIDs (prednisone needed in some pts)		A reactive arthritis after a β-hemolytic strep infection in absence of sufficient Jones criteria for acute rheumatic fever. Ref.: *Mayo Clin Proc 75:144, 2000.*
Septic arthritis: Treatment requires both adequate drainage of purulent joint fluid and appropriate antimicrobial therapy. **There is no need to inject antimicrobials into joints.** Empiric therapy after collection of blood and joint fluid for culture; review Gram stain of joint fluid.				
Infants <3 mo (neonate)	Staph. aureus, Enterobacteriaceae, Group B strep, N. gonorrhoeae	**If MRSA not a concern:** (Nafcillin or oxacillin) + P Ceph 3	**If MRSA a concern: Vanco +** P Ceph 3	Blood cultures frequently positive. Adjacent bone involved in 2/3 pts. Group B strep and gonococci most common community-acquired etiologies.
Children (3 mo–14 yr)	Staph. aureus 27%, S. pyogenes & S. pneumo 14%, H. influenzae 3%, Gm-neg. bacilli 6% other (GC, N. meningitidis) 14%, unknown 36%	**Vanco + P Ceph 3** until culture results available *(Dosage, see Table 16, page 178)* See Table 16 for dosage Steroids—see Comment		Marked ↓ in H. influenzae since use of conjugate vaccine. **NOTE:** Septic arthritis due to salmonella has no association with sickle cell disease, unlike salmonella osteomyelitis. Duration of treatment varies with specific microbial etiology. Short-course steroid: Benefit reported *(PIDJ 22:883, 2003).*
Adults *(review Gram stain):* See page 54 for **Lyme Disease** and page – for gonococcal arthritis				
Acute monoarticular **At risk for sexually-transmitted disease**	**N. gonorrhoeae** *(see page 21),* S. aureus, streptococci, rarely aerobic Gm-neg. bacilli	**Gram stain negative:** **Ceftriaxone** 1 gm IV q24h or **cefotaxime** 1 gm IV q8h or **ceftizoxime** 1 gm IV q8h	**If Gram stain shows Gm+ cocci in clusters: vanco** 1 gm IV q12h; if >100 kg, 1.5 gm IV q12h.	For treatment comments, see *Disseminated GC, page 21*
Not at risk for sexually-transmitted disease	S. aureus, streptococci, Gm-neg. bacilli	**All empiric choices guided by Gram stain** **Vanco + P Ceph 3** *For treatment duration, see Table 3, page 66 For dosage, see footnote page 31*	**Vanco + (CIP or Levo)** See Table 2 & Table 12	Differential includes gout and chondrocalcinosis (pseudogout). **Look for crystals in joint fluid.** **NOTE:** *See Table 6 for MRSA treatment.*
Chronic monoarticular	Brucella, nocardia, mycobacteria, fungi			
Polyarticular, usually acute	**Gonococci,** B. burgdorferi, acute rheumatic fever; viruses, e.g., hepatitis B, rubella vaccine, parvo B19	Gram stain usually negative for GC. If sexually active, culture urethra, cervix, anal canal, throat, blood, joint fluid, and then: **ceftriaxone** 1 gm IV q24h		If GC, usually associated petechiae and/or pustular skin lesions and tenosynovitis. Consider Lyme disease if exposure areas known to harbor infected ticks. See page 54.
Septic arthritis, post intra-articular injection	MSSE/MRSE 40%, MSSA/ MRSA 20%, P. aeruginosa, Propionibacteria, mycobacteria	**NO empiric therapy.** Arthroscopy for culture/sensitivity, crystals, washout		Expanded differential includes gout, pseudogout, reactive arthritis (HLA-B27 pos). Treat based on culture results x 14 days (assumes no foreign body present).

Abbreviations on page 3.   NOTE: *All dosage recommendations are for adults (unless otherwise indicated) and assume normal renal function.*

TABLE 1A (26)

ANATOMIC SITE/DIAGNOSIS/ MODIFYING CIRCUMSTANCES	ETIOLOGIES (usual)	SUGGESTED REGIMENS*		ADJUNCT DIAGNOSTIC OR THERAPEUTIC MEASURES AND COMMENTS
		PRIMARY	ALTERNATIVE§	
JOINT (continued)				
Infected prosthetic joint	Cultures pending	**No empiric therapy.** Need culture & sens. results. Can ↑ yield of culture by sonication (NEJM 357:654, 2007). Surgical options in Comment.		**Surg. options: 1. 2-stage:** Remove infected prosthesis & leave spacer, anti-microbics, then new prosthesis. Highest cure rate (CID 42:216, 2006). **2. 1-stage:** Remove infected prosthesis, debride, new prosthesis, then antibiotics. **3. Extensive debridement & leave prosthesis in place** plus antibiotic therapy; 53% failure rate, esp. if ≥8 days of symptoms (CID 42:471, 2006)
See surgical options in Comments	S. pyogenes: Gps A, B, or G; viridans strep	Debridement & prosthesis retention: (**Pen G** or **ceftriax**) IV x 4 wks. Cured 17/19 pts (CID 36:847, 2003).		Other: Remove prosthesis & treat ± bone fusion of joint. Last option: debridement and chronic antimicrobic suppression.
Drug dosages in footnote[26]	MSSE/MSSA--see surgical options	(**Nafcillin/oxacillin** IV + **RIF** po) x 6 wks	(**Vanco** + **RIF** po) OR (**Dapto** IV + **RIF** po) x 6 wk	**RIF** bactericidal vs surface-adhering, slow-growing, & biofilm-producing bacteria. Never use **RIF** alone due to rapid development of resistance (JAMA 279:1537, 1575, 1998). **RIF + Fusidic acid**[NUS] (dosage in footnote) another option (Ci.Micro.&Inf. 12(53):93, 2006).
For dental prolylaxis, see Table 15B	MRSE/MRSA--see surgical options	(**Vanco** IV + **RIF** po) x 6 wks	[(**CIP** or **Levo**—if suscepti-ble—po) + (**RIF** po)] OR (**linezolid** po) OR (**Dapto** + **RIF**) x 6 wk	Limited linezolid experience is favorable (JAC 55:387, 2005). Watch for toxicity if over 2 wks of therapy, Table 10C, page 92. **Dapto** experience: IDCP 14:144, 2006
Gentamicin often added to bone cement. Efficacy unclear. May reduce mechanical performance of cement. Theoretical source of Gent toxicity. (Acta Ortho 78:774, 2007.)	P. aeruginosa	**Ceftaz** IV + (**CIP** or **Levo** po)		AAC 39:2423, 1995
Rheumatoid arthritis	TNF inhibitors (adalimumab, anakinra, etanercept, infliximab) ↑ risk of TBc, fungal infection and malignancy. (LnID 8:601, 2008; JAMA 295:2275, 2006). Treat latent TBc first (MMWR 53:683, 2004).			
Septic bursitis: Olecranon bursitis; prepatellar bursitis	Staph. aureus >80%, M. tuberculosis (rare), M. marinum (rare)	(**Nafcillin** or **oxacillin** 2 gm IV q4h or **dicloxacillin** 500 mg po qid) if MSSA	(**Vanco** 1 gm IV q12h or **line-zolid** 600 mg po bid) if **MRSA**	**Initially aspirate q24h and treat for a minimum of 2-3 weeks.** Surgical excision of bursa should not be necessary if treated for at least 3 weeks. Ref.: Semin Arth & Rheum 24:391, 1995 (a classic).
		Other doses, see footnote page 31		
KIDNEY, BLADDER AND PROSTATE [For review, see AJM 113(Suppl.1A):1S, 2002 & NEJM 349:259, 2003]				
Acute uncomplicated urinary tract infection (cystitis-urethritis) in females [NOTE: Routine urine culture not necessary; self-rx works (AnIM 135.9, 2001)].				
NOTE: Resistance of E. coli to TMP-SMX approx. 15–20% (CID 36:183, 2003) & correlates with microbiological/ clinical failure (CID 34:1061 & 1165, 2002). **Recent reports of E. coli resistant to FQs as well.** 5-day nitrofurantoin ref: AnIM 167:2207, 2007	Enterobacteriaceae (E. coli), Staph. saprophyticus, enterococci	<20% of Local E. coli resistant to TMP-SMX & no allergy: **TMP-SMX-DS** bid x 3 days; if sulfa allergy, **nitrofurantoin** 100 mg po bid x 5 days or **fosfomycin** 3 gm po x one dose. All plus **Pyridium**	>20% Local E. coli resistant to TMP-SMX or sulfa allergy: then 3 days of **CIP** 250 mg, **CIP-ER** 500 mg q24h, **Levo** 250 mg q24h OR **Moxi** 400 mg q24h OR **Nitrofurantoin** 100 mg bid OR single 3 gm dose of **fosfomycin.** All plus **Pyridium**	7-day rx recommended **in pregnancy** [discontinue or do not use sulfonamides (TMP-SMX) near term (2 weeks before EDC) because of potential ↑ in kernicterus]. If failure on 3-day course, culture and rx 2 weeks. **Fosfomycin** 3 gm po times 1 less effective vs E. coli than multi-dose TMP-SMX or FQ. Fosfo active vs E. faecalis; poor activity vs other coliforms. **Moxifloxacin:** Not approved for UTIs. Moxi equivalent to comparator drugs in unpublished clinical trials (on file with Bayer). **Phenazopyridine (Pyridium)**—non-prescription—may relieve dysuria: 200 mg po tid times 2 days. Hemolysis if G6PD deficient.
Risk factors for STD, Dipstick: positive leukocyte esterase or hemoglobin, neg. Gram stain	C. trachomatis	**Doxy** 100 mg po bid x 7 days	**Azithro** 1 gm po single dose	Pelvic exam for vaginitis & herpes simplex, urine LCR/PCR for GC and C. trachomatis.
Recurrent (3 or more episodes/ year) in young women	Any of the above bacteria	Eradicate infection, then TMP-SMX 1 single-strength tab po q24h long term		A cost-effective alternative to continuous prophylaxis is self-administered single dose rx (TMP-SMX DS, 2 tabs, 320/1600 mg) at symptom onset. Another alternative: 1 DS tablet TMP-SMX post-coitus.
Child: ≤5 yrs old & grade 3–4 reflux	Coliforms	[**TMP-SMX** (2 mg TMP/10 mg SMX) per kg q24h] or (**nitrofurantoin** 2 mg per kg po q24h). **CIP** approved as alternative drug ages 1–17 yrs.		**CIP** approved as alternative drug ages 1–17 yrs

[26] **Aqueous Pen G** 2 million units IV q4h; **cefazolin** 1 gm IV q4h; **ceftriaxone** 2 gm IV q8h; **ceftriaxone** 2 gm IV q24h; **nafcillin** or **oxacillin** 2 gm IV q4h; **vancomycin** 1 gm IV q12h; **Daptomycin** 6 mg/kg IV q24h; **RIF** 300 mg/po q24h; **CIP** 750 mg IV/po bid; **Levo** 750 mg IV/po bid; **ceftazidime** 2 gm IV q8h; **Fusidic Acid**[NUS] 500 mg po/IV tid.

Abbreviations on page 3.   NOTE: All dosage recommendations are for adults (unless otherwise indicated) and assume normal renal function.

TABLE 1A (27)

ANATOMIC SITE/DIAGNOSIS/ MODIFYING CIRCUMSTANCES	ETIOLOGIES (usual)	SUGGESTED REGIMENS* PRIMARY	ALTERNATIVE§	ADJUNCT DIAGNOSTIC OR THERAPEUTIC MEASURES AND COMMENTS
KIDNEY, BLADDER AND PROSTATE/Acute uncomplicated urinary tract infection (cystitis-urethritis) in females *(continued)*				
Recurrent UTI in postmenopausal women *See CID 30:152, 2000*	E. coli & other Enterobacteriaceae, enterococci, S. saprophyticus	Treat as for uncomplicated UTI. Evaluate for potentially correctable urologic factors—*see Comment.* **Nitrofurantoin** more effective than vaginal cream in decreasing frequency, but Editors worry about pulmonary fibrosis with long-term NF rx (CID 36:1362, 2003).		Definition: ≥3 culture + symptomatic UTIs in 1 year or 2 UTIs in 6 months. Urologic factors: (1) cystocele, (2) incontinence, (3) ↑ residual urine volume (≥50 mL).
Acute uncomplicated pyelonephritis (usually women 18–40 yrs, temperature >102°F, definite costovertebral tenderness) [NOTE: Culture of urine and blood indicated prior to therapy. Report of hemolytic uremic syndrome as result of toxin-producing E. coli UTI (NEJM 335:635, 1996)]. **If male, look for obstructive uropathy or other complicating pathology.**				
Moderately ill (outpatient) **NOTE:** May need one IV dose due to nausea. Resistance of E. coli to TMP/SMX 13–45% in collaborative ER study (CID 47:1150, 2008).	Enterobacteriaceae (most likely E. coli), enterococci (Gm stain of **uncentrifuged** urine may allow identification of Gm-neg. bacilli vs Gm+ cocci)	FQs po times 5-7 days: **CIP** 500 mg bid or **CIP-ER** 1000 mg q24h, **Levo** 750 mg q24h, **Oflox** 400 mg bid, **Moxi**[NFDA-I] 400 mg q24h possibly ok— see comment.	**AM-CL, O Ceph, or TMP-SMX-DS po.** Treat for 14 days. Dosage in footnote[27]. Beta-lactams not as effective as FQs: JAMA 293:949, 2005	In randomized double-blind trial, bacteriologic and **clinical success higher for 7 days of CIP than for 14 days of TMP-SMX,** failures correlated with TMP-SMX in vitro resistance (JAMA 283:1583, 2000). Since **CIP** worked with 7-day rx, suspect other FQs effective with 7 days of therapy: **Levo** 750 mg FDA-approved for 5 days. **Moxi** urine concentrations high (Internat J Antimicrob Agents 24:168, 2004).
Acute pyelonephritis-- Hospitalized	E. coli most common, enterococci 2nd in frequency	**FQ** (IV) or (**AMP + gentamicin**) or **ceftriaxone** or **PIP-TZ**. Treat for 14 days. *Dosages in footnote[27] page 31* Do not use cephalosporins for suspect or proven enterococcal infection	**TC-CL** or **AM-SB** or **PIP-TZ** or **ERTA** or **DORI**: 500 mg q8h. Treat for 14 days.	Treat IV until pt afebrile 24–48 hrs, then complete 2-wk course with oral drugs (as Moderately ill, above). **DORI** approved for 10 day treatment. **If pt hypotensive, prompt imaging (Echo or CT) is recommended to ensure absence of obstructive uropathy.** **NOTE: Cephalosporins & ertapenem not active vs enterococci.**
Complicated UTI/catheters Obstruction, reflux, azotemia, transplant, **Foley catheter-related, R/O obstruction**	Enterobacteriaceae, P. aeruginosa, enterococci, rarely S. aureus (CID 42:46, 2006)	(**AMP + gent**) or **PIP-TZ** or **TC-CL** or **DORI** or **IMP** or **MER** for up to 2-3 wks Switch to po **FQ** or **TMP-SMX** when possible *For dosages, see footnote[27] page 31*	(IV **FQ: CIP, Gati, Levo**) or **Ceftaz** or **CFP** for up to 2-3 wks	Not all listed drugs predictably active vs enterococci or P. aeruginosa. **CIP** approved in children (1-17 yrs) as alternative. Not 1st choice secondary to increased incidence joint adverse effects. Peds dose: 6-10 mg/kg (400 mg max) **IV** q8h or 10-20 mg/kg (750 mg max) **po** q12h. **Levo:** FDA approved dose of 750 mg IV/po x 5 days. **DORI:** FDA approved duration of 10 days.
Asymptomatic bacteriuria. IDSA Guidelines: CID 40:643, 2005; U.S. Preventive Services Task Force 149:43, 2008.				
Preschool children		Base regimen on C&S, not empirical		Diagnosis requires ≥10⁵ CFU per mL urine of same bacterial species in 2 specimens obtained 3–7 days apart.
Pregnancy	Aerobic Gm-neg. bacilli & Staph. hemolyticus	Screen 1st trimester. If positive, rx 3–7 days with **amox, nitrofurantoin. O Ceph. TMP-SMX,** or **TMP** alone		Screen monthly for recurrence. Some authorities treat continuously until delivery (stop TMP-SMX 2 wks before EDC). ↑ resistance of E. coli to TMP-SMX.
Before and after invasive urologic intervention, e.g., Foley catheter	Aerobic Gm-neg. bacilli	Obtain urine culture and then rx 3 days with **TMP-SMX DS,** bid. For prevention of UTI: Consider removal after 72 hrs (CID 46:243 & 251, 2008).		Clinical benefit of antimicrobial-coated Foley catheters is uncertain (AnIM 144:116, 2006).
Neurogenic bladder – see "spinal cord injury" below		No therapy in asymptomatic patient; intermittent catheterization if possible		Ref.: AJM 113(1A):67S, 2002—Bacteriuria in spinal cord injured patient.

[27] **AM-CL** 875/125 mg po q12h or 500/125 mg po q12h or 1000 /125 mg po bid; Antipseudomonal penicillins: **AM-SB** 3 gm IV q6h; **PIP** 3 gm IV q4-6h; **PIP-TZ** 3.375 gm IV q4-6h (4.5 gm IV q6h for pseudomonas pneumonia); **TC-CL** 3.1 gm IV q6h; Antipseudomonal cephalosporins: **ceftaz** 2 gm IV q8h; **CFP** 2 gm IV q12h; Carbapenems: **DORI** 500 mg IV q8h (1 hr infusion); **ERTA** 1 gm IV q24h; **IMP** 0.5 gm IV q12h (max 4 gm/day); **MER** 1 gm IV q8h; Parenteral cephalosporins: **cefotaxime** 1 gm IV q8h (2 gm IV q4h for severe infection); **cefoxitin** 2 gm IV q8h; **ceftriaxone** 1-2 gm IV q24h; Oral cephalosporins-- see Table 10C, page 90; **FQs: CIP** 400 mg IV q12h; **Gati**[NUS] 400 mg IV q24h; **levo** 750 mg IV q24h; **gentamicin**-- see Table 10D, page 96; **linezolid** 600 mg IV/po q12h; **metro** 500 mg po q6h or 15 mg/kg IV q12h (max 4 gm/day); **nafcillin/oxacillin** 2 gm IV q4h; **TMP-SMX** 2 mg/kg (TMP component) IV q6h; **vanco** 1 gm IV q12h (if over 100 kg, 1.5 gm IV q12h).

Abbreviations on page 3.   NOTE: All dosage recommendations are for adults (unless otherwise indicated) and assume normal renal function.

TABLE 1A (28)

ANATOMIC SITE/DIAGNOSIS/ MODIFYING CIRCUMSTANCES	ETIOLOGIES (usual)	SUGGESTED REGIMENS*		ADJUNCT DIAGNOSTIC OR THERAPEUTIC MEASURES AND COMMENTS
		PRIMARY	ALTERNATIVE§	
KIDNEY, BLADDER AND PROSTATE/Asymptomatic bacteriuria (continued)				
Asymptomatic, advanced age, male or female Ref: *CID 40:643, 2005*		No therapy indicated unless in conjunction with surgery to correct obstructive uropathy; measure residual urine vol. in females; prostate exam/PSA in males. No screening recommended in men and non-pregnant women (*AnIM 149:43, 2008*).		
Malacoplakia	E. coli	**Bethanechol chloride + (CIP** or **TMP-SMX)**		Chronic pyelo with abnormal inflammatory response. *See CID 29:444, 1999*
Perinephric abscess Associated with staphylococcal bacteremia	Staph. aureus	If **MSSA, Nafcillin/ oxacillin** or **cefazolin** (*Dosage, see footnote page 30*)	If **MRSA: Vanco** 1 gm IV q12h **OR dapto** 6 mg/kg IV q24h	Drainage, surgical or image-guided aspiration
Associated with pyelonephritis	Enterobacteriaceae	See *pyelonephritis, complicated UTI, above*		Drainage, surgical or image-guided aspiration
Post Renal Transplant Obstructive Uropathy (*CID 46:825, 2008*)	Corynebacterium urealyticum	**Vanco** or **Teicoplanin**[NUS]		Organism can synthesize struvite stones. Requires 48-72 hr incubation to detect in culture
Prostatitis		See *prostatitis, page 25*		
Spinal cord injury pts with UTI	E. coli, Klebsiella sp., enterococci	**CIP** 250 mg po bid x 14 days		If fever, suspect assoc. pyelonephritis. Microbiologic cure greater after 14 vs 3 days of CIP (*CID 39:658 & 665, 2004*); for asymptomatic bacteriuria see AJM 113(1A):675, 2002.
LIVER (*for spontaneous bacterial peritonitis, see page 44*)				
Cholangitis		See *Gallbladder, page 15*		
Cirrhosis & variceal bleeding	Esophageal flora	(**Norfloxacin** 400 mg po bid **or CIP** 400 mg IV q12h) x max. of 7 days	**Ceftriaxone** 1 gm IV once daily for max. of 7 days	Short term prophylactic antibiotics in cirrhotics with G-I hemorr., with or without ascites, decreases rate of bacterial infection & ↑ survival (*Hepatology 46:922, 2007*).
Hepatic abscess Pyogenic abscess ref.: *CID 39:1654, 2004* Klebsiella liver abscess ref.: *CID 47:642, 2008*	Enterobacteriaceae (esp. Klebsiella sp.), bacteroides, enterococci, Entamoeba histolytica, Yersinia enterocolitica (rare), Fusobacterium necrophorum (*Lemierre's*). For echinococcus, see Table 13, page 132. For cat-scratch disease (CSD), see pages 43 & 53	**Metro** + (**ceftriaxone** or **cefoxitin** or TC-CL or **PIP-TZ** or **AM-SB** or **CIP** or **levo** (*Dosage, see footnote[27] on page 31*) **AMP + aminoglycoside + metro** traditional & effective but AMP-resistant Gm-neg. bacilli ↑and aminoglycoside toxicity an issue.	**Metro** (for amoeba) + either **IMP**, **MER** or **Dori** (*Dosage, see footnote[27] on page 31*)	**Serological tests for amebiasis should be done on all patients;** if neg., surgical drainage or percutaneous aspiration. In pyogenic abscess, ½ have identifiable GI source or underlying biliary tract disease. If amoeba serology positive, treat with **metro** alone without surgery. Empiric **metro** included for both E. histolytica & bacteroides. **Hemochromatosis** associated with Yersinia enterocolitica liver abscess (*CID 18:938, 1994*); regimens listed are effective for yersinia. Klebsiella pneumonia genotype K1 associated ocular & CNS Klebsiella infections (*CID 45:284, 2007*).
Leptospirosis	Leptospirosis, see page 55	See page 53		
Peliosis hepatis in AIDS pts	Bartonella henselae and B. quintana			
Post-transplant infected "biloma" (*CID 39:517, 2004*)	Enterococci (incl. VRE), candida, Gm-neg. bacilli (P. aeruginosa 8%), anaerobes 5%	**Linezolid** 600 mg IV bid + **CIP** 400 mg IV q12h + **fluconazole** 400 mg IV q24h	**Dapto** 6 mg/kg per day + **Levo** 750 mg IV q24h + **fluconazole** 400 mg IV q24h	Suspect if fever & abdominal pain post-transplant. Exclude hepatic artery thrombosis. Presence of candida and/or VRE bad prognosticators.
Viral hepatitis	Hepatitis A, B, C, D, E, G	See *Table 14, page 138*		

NOTE: bid = twice a day; tid = 3 times a day; qid = 4 times a day.

NOTE: All dosage recommendations are for adults (unless otherwise indicated) and assume normal renal function.

TABLE 1A (29)

ANATOMIC SITE/DIAGNOSIS/ MODIFYING CIRCUMSTANCES	ETIOLOGIES (usual)	SUGGESTED REGIMENS*		ADJUNCT DIAGNOSTIC OR THERAPEUTIC MEASURES AND COMMENTS
		PRIMARY	ALTERNATIVE[§]	
LUNG/Bronchi				
Bronchiolitis/wheezy bronchitis (expiratory wheezing)				
Infants/children (≤ age 5) See RSV, *Table 14B page 147* Ref.: *Ln 368:312, 2006*	**Respiratory syncytial virus** (RSV) 50%, parainfluenza 25%, human metapneumovirus	Antibiotics not useful, mainstay of therapy is oxygen. Ribavirin for severe disease: 6 gm vial (20 mg/mL) in serile H₂O by SPAG-2 generator over 18-20 hrs daily times 3-5 days.		RSV most important. Rapid diagnosis with antigen detection methods. For prevention a humanized mouse monoclonal antibody, **palivizumab**. See *Table 14, page 147*. RSV immune globulin is no longer available. Review: *Red Book of Peds 2006, 27th Ed.*
Bronchitis				
Infants/children (≤ age 5)	< Age 2: Adenovirus; age 2–5: Respiratory syncytial virus, parainfluenza 3 virus, human metapneumovirus	Antibiotics indicated only with associated sinusitis or heavy growth on throat culture for S. pneumo., Group A strep, H. influenzae or no improvement in 1 week. Otherwise rx is symptomatic.		
Adolescents and adults with acute tracheobronchitis (Acute bronchitis) Ref.: *NEJM 355:2125, 2006*	Usually viral. M. pneumoniae 5%; C. pneumoniae 5%. See *Persistent cough, below*	**Antibiotics not indicated.** Antitussive ± inhaled bronchodilators		Purulent sputum alone not an indication for antibiotic therapy. Azithro was no better than low-dose vitamin C in a controlled trial (*Ln 359:648, 2002*). Expect cough to last 2 weeks. If fever/rigors, get chest x-ray. M. pneumoniae & C. pneumoniae ref.: *LnID 1:334, 2001*. Rare pt with true C. pneumo infection may require 6 wks of clarithro to clear organism (*J Med Micro 52:265, 2003*).
Persistent cough (>14 days), afebrile during community outbreak: Pertussis (whooping cough) 10–20% adults with cough >14 days have pertussis (*MMWR 54 (RR-14), 2005*). Review: *Chest 130:547, 2006*	Bordetella pertussis & occ. Bordetella parapertussis. Also consider asthma, gastroesophageal reflux, post-nasal drip	**Peds doses: Azithro/ clarithro** OR **erythro estolate**[28] OR **erythro base**[28] OR **TMP/SMX** *(doses in footnote*[27] *page 31)*	**Adult doses: Azithro** po 500 mg day 1, 250 mg q24h days 2–5 OR **erythro estolate** 500 mg po qid times 14 days OR **TMP-SMX-DS** 1 tab po bid times 14 days OR (**clarithro** 500 mg po bid or 1 gm **ER** q24h times 7 days)	**3 stages of illness:** catarrhal (1–2 wks), paroxysmal coughing (2–4 wks), and convalescence (1–2 wks). Treatment may abort or eliminate pertussis in catarrhal stage. but does not shorten paroxysmal stage. **Diagnosis:** PCR on nasopharyngeal secretions or ↑ pertussis-toxin antibody. **Rx aimed at eradication of NP carriage. Azithro** works fastest (*PIDJ 22:847, 2003*). Hypertrophic pyloric stenosis reported in infants under 6 wks of age given erythro (*MMWR 48:1117, 1999*).
Pertussis: Prophylaxis of household contacts		Drugs and doses as per treatment immediately above		Recommended by Am. Acad. Ped. Red Book 2006 for all household or close contacts; community-wide prophylaxis not recommended.
Acute bacterial exacerbation of chronic bronchitis (ABECB), adults (almost always smokers with COPD) Ref: *NEJM 359:2355, 2008.*	Viruses 20–50%, C. pneumoniae 5%, M. pneumoniae <1%; role of S. pneumo, H. influenzae & M. catarrhalis controversial. Tobacco use, air pollution contribute. Non-pathogenic H. haemolyticus may be mistaken for H. influenza (*JID 195:81, 2007*).	**Severe ABECB** = ↑ dyspnea, ↑ sputum viscosity/purulence, ↑ sputum volume. For severe ABECB: (1) consider chest x-ray, esp. if febrile &/or low O₂ sat.; (2) inhaled anticholinergic bronchodilator; (3) oral corticosteroid; taper over 2 wks (*Cochrane Library 3, 2006*); (4) D/C tobacco use; (5) non-invasive positive pressure ventilation. **Role of antimicrobial therapy debated even for severe disease. For mild or moderate disease, no antimicrobial treatment** or maybe amox, doxy, TMP-SMX, or O Ceph. **For severe disease,** AM-CL, azithro/clarithro, or O Ceph or FQs with enhanced activity vs drug-resistant S. pneumo (Gemi, Levo, or Moxi). ***Drugs & doses in footnote. Duration** varies with drug; range 3–10 days. Limit Gemi to 5 days to decrease risk of rash **Placebo-controlled studies:** *Pul Pharm & Therap 14:449, 2001; Ln 358:2020, 2001.*		

[28] **ADULT DOSAGE: AM-CL:** 875/125 mg po bid or 500/125 mg po bid or 2000/125 mg po bid; **azithro** 500 mg po x 1 dose, then 250 mg po q24h x 4 days or 500 mg po q24h x 3 days; *Oral cephalosporins:* **cefaclor** 500 mg po q8h or 500 mg extended release q12h; **cefdinir** 300 mg po q12h or 600 mg po q24h; **cefditoren** 200 mg po q12h; **cefixime** 400 mg po q24h; **cefpodoxime proxetil** 200 mg po q12h; **cefprozil** 500 mg po q12h; **ceftibuten** 400 mg po q24h; **cefuroxime axetil** 250 or 500 mg q12h; **clarithro** extended release 1000 mg po q24h; **doxy** 100 mg po bid; **erythro base** 40 mg/kg/day po div q6h; **erythro estolate** 40 mg/kg/day po on day 1, then 5 mg/kg po q24h x 4 days; **clarithro** 7.5 mg/kg po q12h; **gemi** 320 mg po q24h; **levo** 500 mg po q24h; **moxi** 400 mg po q24h; **TMP-SMX** 1 DS tab po bid.
PEDS DOSAGE: azithro 10 mg/kg/day po on day 1, then 5 mg/kg po q24h x 4 days; **clarithro** 7.5 mg/kg po q12h; **erythro base** 40 mg/kg/day div q6h;
TMP-SMX (>6 mos. of age) 8 mg/kg/day (TMP component) div bid.

Abbreviations on page 3.   *NOTE: All dosage recommendations are for adults (unless otherwise indicated) and assume normal renal function.*

TABLE 1A (30)

ANATOMIC SITE/DIAGNOSIS/ MODIFYING CIRCUMSTANCES	ETIOLOGIES (usual)	SUGGESTED REGIMENS*		ADJUNCT DIAGNOSTIC OR THERAPEUTIC MEASURES AND COMMENTS
		PRIMARY	ALTERNATIVE$	
LUNG/Bronchi (continued)				
Fever, cough, myalgia during influenza season	Influenza A & B	**Oseltamivir** 75 mg po bid x 5 days (see Table 14A for data on resistant virus)		**Complications: Influenza pneumonia, secondary bacterial pneumonia** (S. pneumo., S. aureus, S. pyogenes, H. Influenzae), S. aureus TSS. Ref: LnID 6:296, 2006.
Bronchiectasis. Ref: Chest 134:815, 2008 Acute exacerbation	H. influ., P. aeruginosa, and rarely S. pneumo.	**Gemi, levo,** or **moxi** x 7-10 days. Dosage in footnote[28].		Many potential etiologies: obstruction, ↓ immune globulins, cystic fibrosis, dyskinetic cilia, tobacco, prior severe or recurrent necrotizing bronchitis: e.g. pertussis.
Prevention of exacerbation	Not applicable	One option: **Erythro** 500 mg po bid or **azithro** 250 mg q24h x 8 wks (JAMA 290:1749, 2003; Eur Resp J 13:361, 1999)		
Specific organisms	Aspergillus (see Table 11) MAI (Table 12) and P. aeruginosa (Table 5), MAI (Table 12) and Aspergillus (Table 11).			
Pneumonia **Neonatal: Birth to 1 month**	**Viruses:** CMV, rubella, H. simplex **Bacteria:** Group B strep, listeria, coliforms, S. aureus, P. aeruginosa **Other:** Chlamydia trachomatis, syphilis	**AMP + gentamicin ± cefotaxime.** Add **vanco** if MRSA a concern. For chlamydia therapy, **erythro** 12.5 mg per kg po or IV qid times 14 days.		Blood cultures indicated. Consider C. trachomatis if afebrile pneumonia, staccato cough, IgM >1:8; therapy with erythro or sulfisoxazole. If MRSA documented, **vanco**, **TMP-SMX**, & **linezolid** alternatives. **Linezolid** dosage from birth to age 11 yrs is **10 mg per kg q8h.** Ref.: PIDJ 22(Suppl.):S158, 2003.

CONSIDER TUBERCULOSIS IN ALL PATIENTS: ISOLATE ALL SUSPECT PATIENTS

ANATOMIC SITE/DIAGNOSIS/ MODIFYING CIRCUMSTANCES	ETIOLOGIES (usual)	SUGGESTED REGIMENS*		ADJUNCT DIAGNOSTIC OR THERAPEUTIC MEASURES AND COMMENTS
		PRIMARY	ALTERNATIVE$	
Age 1–3 months (Adapted from NEJM 346:429, 2002) Pneumonitis syndrome. Usually afebrile	C. trachomatis, RSV, parainfluenza virus 3, human metapneumovirus, Bordetella, S. pneumoniae, S. aureus (rare)	**Outpatient: po erythro** 12.5 mg/kg q6h x 14 days or po **azithro** 10 mg/kg x dose, then 5 mg/kg x 4 days. For **RSV**, see Bronchiolitis, page 33	**Inpatient: If afebrile erythro** 10 mg/kg IV q6h or **azithro** 2.5 mg/kg IV q12h (see Comment). **If febrile,** add **cefotaxime** 200 mg/kg per day div q8h	Pneumonitis syndrome: cough, tachypnea, dyspnea, diffuse infiltrates, afebrile. Usually requires hospital care. Reports of hypertrophic pyloric stenosis after erythro under age 6 wks; not sure about azithro; bid azithro dosing theoretically might ↓ risk of hypertrophic pyloric stenosis. If lobar pneumonia, give AMP 200– 300 mg per kg per day for S. pneumoniae. No empiric coverage for S. aureus, as it is rare etiology.

(Continued on next page)

Abbreviations on page 3.   NOTE: All dosage recommendations are for adults (unless otherwise indicated) and assume normal renal function.

TABLE 1A (31)

ANATOMIC SITE/DIAGNOSIS/ MODIFYING CIRCUMSTANCES	ETIOLOGIES (usual)	SUGGESTED REGIMENS*		ADJUNCT DIAGNOSTIC OR THERAPEUTIC MEASURES AND COMMENTS
		PRIMARY	ALTERNATIVE§	
LUNG/Bronchi/Pneumonia (continued)				
Age 4 months–5 years For RSV, see bronchiolitis, page 33, & Table 14	RSV, human metapneumovirus, other resp. viruses, S. pneumo. H. flu, mycoplasma, S. aureus (rare). M. tbc	**Outpatient: Amox** 100 mg/kg/day div q8h. **Inpatient (not ICU): No** antibiotic if viral or IV **AMP** 200 mg/kg per day div q6h	**Inpatient (ICU): Cefotaxime** 200 mg per kg per day IV div q8h plus **azithro** 5 mg/kg (max 500 mg/day) IV q24h plus **vanco** (for CA-MRSA) 40 mg/kg/day div q6h.	Common "other" viruses: rhinovirus, influenza, parainfluenza, adenovirus. Often of mild to moderate severity. S. pneumo, non-type B H. flu in 4–20%. Treat for 10–14 days. Ref: http://www.cincinnatichildrens.org/svc/alpha/h/health-policy/ev-based pneumonia.htm
Age 5 years–15 years, Non-hospitalized, immuno-competent NEJM 346:429, 2002; PIDJ 21:592, 2002; http://www.cincinnatichildrens. org/svc/alpha/h/health-policy/ev-based pneumonia.htm	Mycoplasma, Chlamydophila pneumoniae, S. pneumo-niae, Mycobacterium tuber-culosis Respiratory viruses: mixed, e.g., influenza Bacterial/viral infection in 23% (Peds 113:701, 2004) Legionella: especially in pts with malignancy Ln Inf Dis 6:529, 2006	[(**Amox** 100 mg/kg per day) + (**Clarithro** 500 mg po bid or 1 gm ER q24h; Peds dose: 7.5 mg/kg q12h)] **OR** (**azithro** 0.5 gm po x 1, then 0.25 gm/day; Peds dose: 10 mg/kg per day, max. of 500 mg po. then 5 mg/kg per day, max. 250 mg) **See Comment regarding macrolide resistance**	[(**Amox** 100 mg/kg per day) + [**Doxy** 100 mg po bid (if pt >8 yrs old) or **erythro** 500 mg po qid. (Peds dose: 10 mg/kg po q6h)]	If otherwise healthy and if not concomitant with (or post-) influenza, S. pneumoniae & S. aureus uncommon in this subset; suspect S. pneumo if sudden onset and large amount of purulent sputum. **Macrolide-resistant S. pneumo** an issue. Higher prevalence of macrolide-resistant S. pneumo in pts <5 yrs old (JAMA 286:1857, 2001). Also reports of macrolide-resistant M. pneumoniae. Mycoplasma PCR/viral culture usually not done for outpatients. **Mycoplasma requires 2–3 wks of therapy,** C. pneumoniae up to 6 wks. (LnID 1:334, 2001; J Med Micro 52:265, 2003).: Macrolide-resistant M. pneumo reported (AAC 50:709, 2006) **Linezolid** approved for peds use for pen-susceptible & multi-drug resistant S. pneumo (including bacteremia) & methicillin-sensitive S. aureus.
Children, hospitalized, immunocompetent— 2–18 yrs	S. pneumoniae, viruses, mycoplasma; consider S. aureus if abscesses or necrotizing, esp. during influenza season	**Ceftriaxone** 50 mg per kg per day IV (to max. 2 gm per day) + **azithro** 10 mg per kg per day up to 500 mg IV div q12h. Add anti-staph drug if evidence of lung necrosis: **vanco** 40 mg/kg/day divided q8h.		**Alternatives are a problem in children:** If proven S. pneumo resistant to azithro & ceftriaxone (or severe ceftriaxone allergy): IV vanco, linezolid, or off-label respiratory FQ. No doxy under age 8. Linezolid reported efficacious in children (PIDJ 22:677, 2003). Cefuroxime failures vs drug-resistant S. pneumo (CID 29:462, 1999).

(Continued on next page)

Abbreviations on page 3.   NOTE: All dosage recommendations are for adults (unless otherwise indicated) and assume normal renal function.

TABLE 1A (32)

ANATOMIC SITE/DIAGNOSIS/ MODIFYING CIRCUMSTANCES	ETIOLOGIES (usual)	SUGGESTED REGIMENS*		ADJUNCT DIAGNOSTIC OR THERAPEUTIC MEASURES AND COMMENTS
		PRIMARY	ALTERNATIVE§	
LUNG/Bronchi/Pneumonia (continued)				
Adults (over age 18)— IDSA/ATS Guideline for CAP in adults: *CID 44 (Suppl 2): S27-S72, 2007.*				
Community-acquired, not hospitalized **Prognosis prediction:** **CURB-65** *(AnIM 118:384, 2005).* C: confusion = 1 pt U. BUN >19 mg/dl = 1 pt R. RR >30 min = 1 pt B. BP <90/60 = 1 pt Age ≥65 = 1 pt **If score = 1, ok for outpatient therapy; if >1, hospitalize.** The higher the score, the higher the mortality. Lab diagnosis of invasive pneumococcal disease: *CID 46:926, 2008.*	Varies with clinical setting. **No co-morbidity:** Atypicals—M. pneumoniae, et al [29] S. pneumo, viral **Co-morbidity:** Alcoholism: S. pneumo, anaerobes, coliforms Bronchiectasis: *see Cystic fibrosis, page 41* COPD: H. influenzae, M. catarrhalis, S. pneumo IVDU: Hematogenous S. aureus Post-CVA aspiration: Oral flora, incl. S. pneumo Post-obstruction of bronchi: S. pneumo, anaerobes Post-influenza: S. pneumo. and S. aureus	**No co-morbidity:** **Azithro** 0.5 gm po times 1, then 0.25 gm per day **OR azithro-ER** 2 gm times 1 **OR clarithro** 500 mg po bid or **clarithro-ER** 1 gm po q24h **OR doxy** 100 mg po bid **OR if prior antibiotic within 3 months: (azithro or clarithro) + (amox** 1gm po tid or high dose **AM-CL OR Respiratory FQ** **Duration of rx:** S. pneumo—Not bacteremic: until afebrile 3 days —Bacteremic: 10–14 days reasonable C. pneumoniae—Unclear. Some reports suggest 21 days. Some bronchitis pts required 5–6 wks of clarithro *(J Med Micro 52:265, 2003)* Legionella—10–21 days Necrotizing pneumonia 2° to coliforms, S. aureus, anaerobes: ≥2 weeks **Cautions:** 1. **If local macrolide resistance to S. pneumoniae >25%, use alternative empiric therapy.** 2. **Esp. during influenze season, look for S. aureus.**	**Co-morbidity present:** **Respiratory FQ** (*see footnote[30]*) OR **[(azithro or clarithro) + (high dose amox, high dose AM-CL, cefdinir, cefpodoxime, cefprozil)]** OR **telithromycin—see comment, page 37** *Doses in footnote[31]*	**Azithro/clarithro:** Pro: appropriate spectrum of activity; more in vitro resistance than clinical failure *[CID 34(Suppl.1):S27, 2002]*; q24h dosing; better tolerated than erythro *(Chest 131:1205, 2007).* If pen G resist. S. pneumo, up to 50% + resistance to azithro/clarithro. Influence of prior macrolide use on macrolide resistant S. pneumo *(CID 40:1288, 2005).* Con: Overall S. pneumo resistance in vitro 20–30% and may be increasing **Amoxicillin:** Pro: Active 90–95% S. pneumo at 3–4 gm per day Con: No activity atypicals or β-lactamase + bacteria. Need 3–4 gm per day **AM-CL:** Pro: Spectrum of activity includes β-lactamase + H. influenzae, M. catarrhalis, MSSA, & Bacteroides sp. Con: No activity atypicals **Cephalosporins**—po: Cefditoren, cefpodoxime, cefprozil, cefuroxime & others—*see footnote[31]* Pro: Active 75–85% S. pneumo & H. influenzae. Cefuroxime least active & higher mortality rate when S. pneumo resistant *(CID 37:230, 2003).* Con: Inactive vs atypical pathogens **Doxycycline:** Pro: Active vs S. pneumo *(DMID 49:147, 2004)* but resistance may be increasing. Active vs H. influenzae, atypicals, & bioterrorism agents (anthrax, plague, tularemia). Con: Resistance of S. pneumo 18–20% *(CID 35:633, 2002).* Sparse clinical data *(AnIM 159: 266, 1999; CID 37:870, 2003).*
Community-acquired, hospitalized—NOT in the ICU **Empiric therapy** Treat for minimum of 5 days, afebrile for 48-72 hrs, with stable BP, adequate oral intake, and room air O₂ saturation of >90% *(COID 20:177, 2007).*	Etiology by co-morbidity & risk factors as above. Culture sputum & blood. S. pneumo, urine antigen reported helpful *(CID 40: 1608, 2005)* Legionella urine antigen indicated. In general, the sicker the pt, the more valuable culture data. Look for S. aureus.	**Ceftriaxone** 1 gm IV q24h + **azithro** 500 mg IV q24h OR **Ertapenem** 1 gm q24h plus **azithro** 500 mg IV q24h No rigid time window for first dose; if in ER, first dose in ER. If diagnosis of pneumonia vague, OK for admitting diagnosis of "uncertain." *(Chest 130:16, 2006).*	**Levo** 750 mg IV q24h or **Moxi** 400 mg IV q24h **Gati**[nus] 400 mg IV q24h (gati no longer marketed in US due to hypo- and hyperglycemic reactions)	**FQs—Respiratory FQs:** Moxi, levo & gemi Pro: In vitro & clinically effective vs pen-sensitive & pen-resistant S. pneumo. **NOTE: dose of Levo is 750 mg q24h.** Q24H dosing. Gemi only available po. Con: Geographic pockets of resistance with clinical failure *(NEJM 346:747, 2002).* Important Drug-drug interactions *(see Table 22A, page 193).* Reversible rash in young females given Gemi for >7 days. **Ceftriaxone/cefotaxime:** Pro: Drugs of choice for pen-sens. S. pneumo, active H. influenzae, M. catarrhalis, & MSSA Con: Not active vs atypicals or pneumonia due to bioterrorism pathogens. Add macrolide for atypicals and perhaps their anti-inflammatory activity.

[29] Atypical pathogens: Chlamydophila pneumoniae, C. psittaci, Legionella sp., M. pneumoniae, C. burnetii (Q fever) (Ref.: *LnID 3:709, 2003*)

[30] Respiratory FQs with enhanced activity vs S. pneumo with high-level resistance to penicillin: **Gati**[nus] 400 mg IV/po q24h (no longer marketed in US due to hypo- and hyperglycemic reactions), **Gemi** 320 mg po q24h, **Levo** 750 mg IV/po q24h, **Moxi** 400 mg IV/po q24h. Ketolide: **telithro** 800 mg po q24h (physicians warned about rare instances of hepatotoxicity).

[31] O Ceph dosage: **Cefdinir** 300 mg po q12h, **cefditoren pivoxil** 200 mg po q12h, **cefpodoxime proxetil** 200 mg po q12h, **cefprozil** 500 mg po q12h, **high dose amox** 1 gm po q12h, **high dose amox** 1 gm po tid; **high dose AM-CL**—use **AM-CL-ER** 1000/62.5 mg, 2 tabs po bid. **telithromycin** 800 mg po q24h times 7–10 days.

Abbreviations on page 3.   *NOTE: All dosage recommendations are for adults (unless otherwise indicated) and assume normal renal function.*

TABLE 1A (33)

ANATOMIC SITE/DIAGNOSIS/ MODIFYING CIRCUMSTANCES	ETIOLOGIES (usual)	SUGGESTED REGIMENS*		ADJUNCT DIAGNOSTIC OR THERAPEUTIC MEASURES AND COMMENTS
		PRIMARY	ALTERNATIVE§	
LUNG/Bronchi/Pneumonia/Adults (over age 18) (continued)				
Community-acquired, hospitalized—IN ICU Empiric therapy **NOTE:** Not all ICU admissions meet IDSA/ATS CAP Guideline criteria for severe CAP. Do not believe that all ICU pneumonia patients need 2 drugs with activity vs. gram-negative bacilli. Hence, 4 example clinical settings are outlined: **severe COPD; post-influenza, suspect gm-neg bacilli; risk of pen-resistant S. pneumo**	**Severe COPD** pt with pneumonia: S. pneumoniae, H. influenzae, Moraxella sp. Legionella sp. Rarely S. aureus. Culture sputum, blood and maybe pleural fluid. Look for respiratory virsues. Urine antigen for both Legionella and S. pneumoniae. Sputum PCR for Legionella.	**Levo** 750 mg IV q24h or **Moxi** 400 mg IV q24h **Gati** not available in US due to hypo- and hyperglycemic reactions	[**Ceftriaxone** 1 gm IV q24h + **azithro** 500 mg IV q24h] or **ERTA** 1 gm q24h IV + **azithro** 500 mg IV q24h (see Comment)	**Telithromycin:** Pro: Virtually no resistant S. pneumo. Active vs atypical pathogens. (Anlm 244:415, 2006; NEJM 355:2260, 2006). Con: Concern of severe hepatotoxicity. Transient reversible blurry vision due to paralysis of lens accommodation; avoid in myasthenia gravis pts **(Black Box Warning).** **Various studies** indicate improved outcome when azithro added to a β-lactam (CID 36:389 & 1239, 2003; ArIM 164:1837, 2001 & 159:2562, 1999). Similar results in prospective study of critically ill pts with pneumococcal bacteremia (AJRCCM 170:440, 2004). **Ertapenem** could substitute for ceftriaxone: need azithro for atypical pathogens. Do not use if suspect P. aeruginosa. **Legionella:** Not all Legionella species detected by urine antigen; if suspicious culture or PCR on airway secretions. Value of specific diagnosis: CID 46:1356 & 1365, 2008. In patients with normal sinus rhythm and not receiving beta-blockers, relative bradycardia suggests Legionella, psittacosis, Q-fever, or typhoid fever (Clin Micro Infect 6:633, 2000).
		Addition of a macrolide to beta-lactam empiric regimens lowers mortality for patients with bacteremic pneumococcal pneumonia (CID 36:389, 2003). Benefit NOT found with use of FQ or tetracycline for "atypicals" (Chest 131:466, 2007). Combination therapy benefited patients with concomitant "shock." (CCM 35:1493 & 1617, 2007).		
Community-acquired, hospitalized—IN ICU Empiric therapy	**If concomitant with or post-influenza,** S. aureus and S. pneumoniae possible.	**Vanco** 1 gm IV q12h + (**Levo** 750 mg IV q24h or **moxi** 400 mg IV q24h)	**Linezolid** 600 mg IV bid + (**levo** or **moxi**)	Sputum gram stain may help. S. aureus post-influenza ref: EID 12:894, 2006. Empiric therapy vs MRSA decreases risk of mortality (CCM 34:2069, 2006).
Community-acquired, hospitalized—IN ICU Empiric therapy	**Suspect aerobic gm-neg bacilli:** eg, P. aeruginosa and/or life-threatening infection (see comment). Hypoxic and/or hypotensive "Cover" S. pneumo & Legionella	Anti-pseudomonal beta-lactam[32] + (respiratory **FQ** or aminoglycoside). Add **azithro** if no FQ. Drugs and doses in footnote[32]	If severe IgE-mediated beta-lactam allergy: **aztreonam** + **FQ** or (**aztreonam** + **aminoglycoside** + **azithro**).	At risk for gm-neg rod pneumonia due to: alcoholism with necrotizing pneumonia, underlying chronic bronchiectasis (e.g. cystic fibrosis), chronic trachostomy and/or mechanical ventilation, febrile neutropenia and pulmonary infiltrates, septic shock, underlying malignancy, or organ failure. Microbiologic documentation of pneumonia due to an aerobic gm-neg rod acquired in the community and admitted to the ICU is an uncommon event (AnlM 162:1849, 2002, COID 16:135, 2003; AJRCCM 160:397, 1999).
	Risk of Pen G-resistant S. pneumoniae 2° antibiotic use in last 3 months.	High dose IV **amp** (or **Pen G**) + **azithro** + **respiratory FQ**	Beta-lactam allergy: **vanco + respiratory FQ**	**If Pen G MIC>4 mg/mL, vanco. Very rare event.**
Health care-associated pneumonia (HCAP) Ref: CID 46(54):S295, 2008.	HCAP used to designate large diverse population of pts with many co-morbidities who reside in nursing homes, other long-term care facilities, require home IV therapy or are dialysis pts. Pneumonia in these pts frequently resembles hospital-acquired pneumonia (see next section).			

NOTE: q24h = once q24h; bid = twice q24h; tid = 3 times a day; qid = 4 times a day.

[32] Antipseudomonal beta-lactams: **Aztreonam** 2 gm IV q6h; **piperacillin** 3 gm IV q4h; **piperacillin/tazobactam** 3.375 mg IV q4h or 4.5 gm IV q6h or 4-hr infusion of 3.375 gm q8h(high dose for Pseudomonas); **cefepime** 2 gm IV q12h; **ceftazidime** 2 gm IV q8h; **doripenem** 500 mg IV q8h as 1 or 4 hr infusion; **imipenem/cilastatin** 500 mg IV q6h; **meropenem** 1 gm IV q8h; **gentamicin or tobramycin** (see Table 10D, pg. 96). FQ for P. aeruginosa: **CIP** 400 mg IV q8h or **levo** 750 mg IV once daily. **Respiratory FQs: levofloxacin** 750 mg IV q24h or **moxifloxacin** 400 mg IV q24h; **high-dose ampicillin** 2 gm IV q6h; **azithromycin** 500 mg IV q24h; **vanco** 1 gm IV q12h.

Abbreviations on page 3.   NOTE: *All dosage recommendations are for adults (unless otherwise indicated) and assume normal renal function.*

TABLE 1A (34)

ANATOMIC SITE/DIAGNOSIS/ MODIFYING CIRCUMSTANCES	ETIOLOGIES (usual)	SUGGESTED REGIMENS* PRIMARY	ALTERNATIVE§	ADJUNCT DIAGNOSTIC OR THERAPEUTIC MEASURES AND COMMENTS
LUNG/Bronchi/Pneumonia/Adults (over age 18) *(continued)*				
Hospital-acquired—usually with mechanical ventilation (VAP) (empiric therapy) Refs: *U.S. Guidelines: AJRCCM 171:388, 2005; U.S. Review: JAMA 297:1583, 2007; Canadian Guidelines: Can J Inf Dis Med Micro 19:19, 2008; British Guidelines: JAC 62:5, 2008*	Highly variable depending on clinical setting: S. pneumo, S. aureus, Legionella, coliforms, P. aeruginosa, stenotrophomonas, acinetobacter[33] anaerobes all possible	(**IMP** 0.5 gm IV q6h or **DORI** 500 mg IV q8H (1 or 4-hr infusion) or **MER** 1 gm IV q8h)[33] plus, if suspect legionella or bioterrorism, **respiratory FQ (Levo or Moxi)** **NOTE:** *Regimen not active vs MRSA—see specific rx below* *See Comment regarding diagnosis* **Dosages:** *See footnote[25]* *Duration of therapy, see footnote[35]*	If suspect P. aeruginosa, empirically start 2 anti-P. aer drugs to increase likelihood that at least one will be active, e.g.: (**IMP** or **CFP** or **PIP-TZ**[34]) + (**CIP** or **tobra**). Ref.: *CCM 35:1888, 2007*	**Dx of ventilator-associated pneumonia:** Fever & lung infiltrates often **not** pneumonia *(Chest 106:221, 1994).* Quantitative cultures helpful: bronchoalveolar lavage ($>10^4$ per mL pos.) or protect. spec. brush ($>10^3$ per mL pos.) Ref.: *AJRCCM 165:867, 2002; AnIM 132:621, 2000.* **Microbial etiology:** No empiric regimen covers all possibilities. Regimens listed active majority of **S. pneumo, legionella, & most coliforms.** Regimens **not active vs MRSA, Stenotrophomonas & others;** *see below: Specific therapy when culture results known.* **Ventilator-associated pneumonia—Prevention:** Keep head of bed elevated 30° or more. Remove N-G, endotracheal tubes as soon as possible. If available, continuous subglottic suctioning. Chlorhexidine oral care. Refs.: *Chest 130:251, 2006; AJRCCM 173:1297, 1348, 2006.* **Misc. clarithro** accelerated resolution of VAP *(CID 46:1157, 2008).* Silver-coated endotracheal tubes reported to reduce incidence of VAP. *(JAMA 300:805 & 842, 2008).*
Hospital- or community-acquired, neutropenic pt ($<$500 neutrophils per mm³)	Any of organisms listed under community- & hospital-acquired + fungi (aspergillus). *See Table 11*	*See Hospital-acquired, immediately above.* Vanco not included in initial therapy unless high suspicion of infected IV access or drug-resistant S. pneumo. Ampho not used unless still febrile after 3 days or high clinical likelihood. *See Comment*		See consensus document on management of febrile neutropenic pt: *CID 34:730, 2002.*
Adults—Selected specific therapy after culture results (sputum, blood, pleural fluid, etc.) available. *Also see Table 2, page 63*				
Acinetobacter baumani *(See also Table 5).* Ref: *NEJM 358:1271, 2008*	Patients with VAP	Use **IMP** if susceptible	If IMP resistant: **colistin** (polymyxin E). In U.S.: 2.5–5 mg/kg/day div into 2–4 doses	Sulbactam portion of AM-SB often active; dose: 3 gm IV q6h. Reported more efficacious than colistin. *(JAC 61:1369, 2008 & J Inf 56:432, 2008)* Colistin summary: *LnID 8:403, 2008*
Burkholderia (Pseudo-monas) pseudomallei (etiology of melioidosis) Ref.: *Ln 361:1715, 2003* Can cause primary or secondary skin infection *(CID 47:603, 2008)*	Gram-negative	**Initial parenteral rx: Ceftazidime** 30–50 mg per kg IV q8h or **IMP** 20 mg per kg IV q8h. Rx minimum 10 days & improving, then po therapy → *see Alternative column*	**Post-parenteral po rx: Adults** *(see Comment for children):* **Chloro** 10 mg per kg q6h times 8 wks: **Doxy** 2 mg per kg bid times 20 wks; **TMP-SMX** 5 mg per kg (TMP component) bid times 20 wks	**Children ≤8 yrs old & pregnancy:** For oral regimen, use **AM-CL-ER** 1000/62.5, 2 tabs po bid times 20 wks. Even with compliance, relapse rate is 10%. Max. daily ceftazidime dose: 6 gm. Tigecycline: No clinical data but active in vitro *(AAC 50:1555, 2006)*
Haemophilus influenzae	β-lactamase negative β-lactamase positive	**AMP** IV, **amox** po, **TMP-SMX, azithro/clarithro, doxy** **AM-CL, O Ceph 2/3, P Ceph 3, FQ, azithro/clarithro, telithro**[36] Dosage: *Table 10C*		25–35% strains β-lactamase positive. ↑ resistance to both TMP-SMX and doxy. *See Table 10C, page 88 for dosages.* High % of comensal H. hemolyticus misidentified as H. influenza *(JID 195:81, 2007).*
Klebsiella sp.—ESBL pos. & other coliforms[37]	β-lactamase positive	**Dori, IMP** or **MER**: if resistant, **polymyxin E (colistin)** or **B** Usually several wks of therapy.		**ESBL**[37] inactivates all cephalosporins, β-lactam/β-lactamase inhibitor drug activ. not predictable: co-resistance to all FQs & often aminoglycosides.

33 If Acinetobacter sp., **susceptibility to IMP & MER** may be discordant *(CID 41:758, 2005)*

34 **PIP-TZ** for P. aeruginosa pneumonia : 3.375 gm IV over 4 hrs & repeat q8h *(CID 44:357, 2007)* plus **tobra.**

35 Dogma on duration of therapy not possible with so many variables: ie, certainty of diagnosis, infecting organism, severity of infection and number/severity of co-morbidities. Agree with efforts to de-escalate & shorten course. Treat at least 7-8 days. Need clinical evidence of response: fever resolution, improved oxygenation, falling WBC. Refs: *AJRCCM 171:388, 2005; CID 43:S75, 2006; COID 19:185, 2006.*

36 **Telithro** = telithromycin 800 mg po q24h. Rare severe hepatotoxic reactions reported *(AnIM 144:415, 2006; NEJM 355:2260, 2006).*

37 **ESBL** = Extended spectrum beta-lactamase

Abbreviations on page 3.   NOTE: All dosage recommendations are for adults (unless otherwise indicated) and assume normal renal function.

TABLE 1A (35)

ANATOMIC SITE/DIAGNOSIS/ MODIFYING CIRCUMSTANCES	ETIOLOGIES (usual)	SUGGESTED REGIMENS*		ADJUNCT DIAGNOSTIC OR THERAPEUTIC MEASURES AND COMMENTS
		PRIMARY	ALTERNATIVE§	
LUNG/Pneumonia/Adults— Selected specific therapy after culture results (sputum, blood, pleural fluid, etc.) available *(continued)*				
Legionella species Relative bradycardia common feature	Hospitalized/ immunocompromised	**Azithro IV** or **Levo IV** or **Moxi IV.** *See Table 10C, pages 91 & 93 for dosages.* Treat for 7–14 days *(CID 39:1734, 2004)*		Legionella website: www.legionella.org. Two studies support superiority of **Levo** over macrolides *(CID 40:794 & 800, 2005).*
Moraxella catarrhalis	93% β-lactamase positive	**AM-CL, O Ceph 2/3, P Ceph 2/3, macrolide**[38] **telithro** *(see footnote*[36] *on page 38),* **FQ, TMP-SMX. Doxy** another option. *See Table 10C, page 88 for dosages*		
Pseudomonas aeruginosa	Often ventilator-associated	**(PIP-TZ** 3.375 gm IV q4h or prefer 4-hr infusion of 3.375 gm q8h) + **tobra** 5 mg/kg IV once q24h (see Table 10D, page 96). Could substitute anti-pseudomonal cephalosporin or carbapenem (**DORI, IMP, MER**) for **PIP-TZ** if pt. strain is susceptible.		**NOTE: PIP-TZ** for P. aeruginosa *(CID 44:357, 2007);* other options: **CFP** 2 gm IV q 12h; **CIP** 400 mg IV q8h + **PIP-TZ; IMP** 500 mg IV q6h + **CIP** 400 mg IV q12h; if multi-drug resistant, **polymyxin**—parenteral & perhaps by inhalation, 80 mg IV bid *(CID 41:754, 2005).*
Staphylococcus aureus Duration of treatment: 3 wks if just pneumonia; 4-6 wks if concomitant endocarditis and/or osteomyelitis.	Nafcillin/oxacillin susceptible	**Nafcillin/oxacillin** 2 gm IV q4h	**Vanco** 1 gm IV q12h or **linezolid** 600 mg IV q12h	Retrospective analysis of 2 prospective randomized double-blind studies of hospital-acquired **MRSA** showed enhanced survival with linezolid, p 0.03 *(Chest 124:1632, 2003);* efficacy perhaps related to superb linezolid lung concentrations. Concern of possible misinterpretation of post hoc subgroup analysis *(Chest 126:314, 2004).*
	MRSA	**Vanco** 1 gm IV q12h	**Linezolid** 600 mg IV q12h; if >10–14days check CBC q week	
Stenotrophomonas maltophilia		**TMP-SMX**	**TC-CL** ± aztreonam	Potential synergy: **TMP-SMX + TC-CL.**
Streptococcus pneumoniae Note: Case fatality rate lower with combination therapy that includes azithro. *(AJM 107:345, 1999; CID 42:304, 2006)*	Penicillin-susceptible	**AMP** 2 gm IV q6h, **amox** 1 gm po tid, *page 88 for other dosages.*	**macrolide**[38], **pen G** IV[39], **doxy**, **O Ceph 2, P Ceph 2/3, telithro** 800 mg po q24h. *See Table 10C,* Treat until afebrile. 3-5 days (min. of 5 days).	
	Penicillin-resistant, high level	**FQs** with enhanced activity: , **Gemi, Levo, Moxi; P Ceph 3** (resistance rare); high-dose IV **AMP.** If all options not possible (e.g., allergy), linezolid active: 600 mg IV or po q12h. Treat until afebrile. 3-5 days (min. of 5 days).	**vanco** IV—*see Table 5, page 74 for more data.* **Telithro** 800 mg po q24h. *Dosages Table 10C.*	
Yersinia pestis (Plague)	Aerosol Y. pestis (See Table 1B(2))	**Gentamicin** 5 mg/kg IV q24h	**Doxy** 200 mg IV times 1, then 100 mg IV bid	Refs.: *JAMA 283:2281, 2000; CID 42:614, 2006; JID 19:782, 2007.*

[38] **Macrolide** = azithromycin, clarithromycin and erythromycin.

[39] **IV Pen G dosage:** Blood cultures neg., 1 million units IV q4h; blood cultures pos. & no meningitis, 2 million units IV q4h. Another option is continuous infusion (CI) 3 million units loading dose & then CI of 10–12 million units over 12 hrs *(Chest 112:1657, 1997).* If concomitant meningitis, 4 million units IV q4h.

Abbreviations on page 3. NOTE: *All dosage recommendations are for adults (unless otherwise indicated) and assume normal renal function.*

TABLE 1A (36)

ANATOMIC SITE/DIAGNOSIS/ MODIFYING CIRCUMSTANCES	ETIOLOGIES (usual)	SUGGESTED REGIMENS* PRIMARY	ALTERNATIVE§	ADJUNCT DIAGNOSTIC OR THERAPEUTIC MEASURES AND COMMENTS
LUNG—Other Specific Infections				
Actinomycosis	A. Israeli and rarely others	**AMP** 50 mg/kg/day IV div in 3-4 doses x 4-6 wks, then **Pen VK** 2-4 gm/day po x 3-6 wks	**Doxy** or **ceftriaxone** or **clinda** or **erythro**	Can use **Pen G** instead of AMP: 10-20 million units/day IV x 4-6 wks.
Anthrax Inhalation (applies to oropharyngeal & gastrointestinal forms): **Treatment** (Cutaneous: See page 48) Refs.: *MMWR 50:909, 2001; www.bt.cdc.gov*	*Bacillus anthracis* **To report possible bioterrorism event: 770-488-7100** Plague, tularemia: see *Table 1B, page 62* Chest x-ray: mediastinal widening & pleural effusion	**Adults (including pregnancy):** (**CIP** 400 mg IV q12h) or (**Levo** 500 mg IV q24h) or (**doxy** 100 mg IV q12h) **plus (clindamycin** 900 mg IV q8h &/or **RIF** 300 mg IV q12h). Switch to po when able & lower CIP to 500 mg po bid; clinda to 450 mg po q8h; & RIF 300 mg po bid. Treat times 60 days. Other alternatives: *Table 1B, page 61*	**Children:** (**CIP** 10 mg/kg IV q12h or 15 mg/kg po q12h) or (**Doxy:** >8 y/o & >45 kg: 100 mg IV q12h; >8 y/o & ≤45 kg: 2.2 mg/kg IV q12h; ≤8 y/o: 2.2 mg/kg IV q12h) **plus clindamycin** 7.5 mg/kg IV q6h **and/or RIF** 20 mg/kg (max. 600 mg) IV q24h. Treat times 60 days. *See Table 16, page 178 for oral dosage.*	1. Clinda may block toxin production 2. Rifampin penetrates CSF & intracellular sites. 3. If isolate shown penicillin-susceptible: a. **Adults: Pen G** 4 million units IV q4h b. **Children: Pen G** <12 y/o: 50,000 units per kg IV q6h; >12 y/o: 4 million units IV q4h c. Constitutive & inducible β-lactamases—do not use pen or amp alone. 4. Do not use cephalosporins or TMP-SMX. 5. Erythro, azithro activity borderline; clarithro active. 6. No person-to-person spread. 7. Antitoxins in development 8. Moxi should work, but no clinical data 9. Case report of survival with use of anthrax immunoglobulin (*CID 44:968, 2007*).
Anthrax, prophylaxis	Info: www.bt.cdc.gov	**Adults (including pregnancy) or children >50 kg: (CIP** 500 mg po bid or **Levo** 500 mg po q24h) x 60 days. **Children <50 kg: CIP** 20-30 mg/kg per day div q12h x 60 days or **levo** 8 mg/kg q12h x 60 days	**Adults (including pregnancy): Doxy** 100 mg po bid x 60 days. **Children** (see Comment): **Doxy** >8 y/o & >45kg: 100 mg po bid: >8 y/o & ≤45 kg: 2.2 mg/kg po bid; ≤8 y/o: 2.2 mg/kg po bid. All for 60 days.	1. Once organism shows suscept. to penicillin, switch to amoxicillin 80 mg per kg per day div. q8h (max. 500 mg q8h); pregnant pt to amoxicillin 500 mg po tid. 2. Do **not** use cephalosporins or TMP-SMX. 3. Other FQs (Gati, Moxi) & clarithro should work but no clinical experience.
Aspiration pneumonia ± lung abscess Refs.: *CID 40:915 & 923, 2005*	Transthoracic culture in 90 pts—% of total isolates: anaerobes 34%, Gm-pos. cocci 26%, S. milleri 16%, Klebsiella pneumoniae 25%, nocardia 3%	**PIP-TZ** 3.375 gm IV q6h or 4-hr infusion of 3.375 gm q8h (*CID 44:357, 2007*).	**Ceftriaxone** 1 gm IV q24h plus **metro** 500 mg IV q6h or 1 gm IV q12h	Suggested regimens based on retrospective evaluation of 90 pts with cultures obtained by transthoracic aspiration (*CID 40:915 & 923, 2005*). Surprising frequency of Klebsiella pneumoniae. **Moxi** 400 mg IV/po q24h another option (*CID 41:764, 2005*). Note switch from clinda due to prevalence of Gm-neg bacilli.
Chronic pneumonia with fever, night sweats and weight loss	M. tuberculosis, coccidioidomycosis, histoplasmosis	*See Table 11, Table 12.* For risk associated with TNF inhibitors, see *CID 41(Suppl.3):S187, 2005.*		HIV+, foreign-born, alcoholism, contact with TB, travel into developing countries

Abbreviations on page 3.   *NOTE: All dosage recommendations are for adults (unless otherwise indicated) and assume normal renal function.*

TABLE 1A (37)

ANATOMIC SITE/DIAGNOSIS/ MODIFYING CIRCUMSTANCES	ETIOLOGIES (usual)	SUGGESTED REGIMENS*		ADJUNCT DIAGNOSTIC OR THERAPEUTIC MEASURES AND COMMENTS
		PRIMARY	ALTERNATIVE§	
LUNG—Other Specific Infections *(continued)*				
Cystic fibrosis **Acute exacerbation of pulmonary symptoms** Refs.: *Ln 361:681, 2003; AJRCCM 168:918, 2003; J.Peds&ChildHealth 42:601,2006.*	S. aureus or H. influenzae early in disease; P. aeruginosa later in disease	**For P. aeruginosa:** (Peds doses) **Tobra** 3.3 mg/kg q8h or 12 mg/kg IV q24h. Combine tobra with (**PIP** or **ticarcillin** 100 mg/kg q6h) **or ceftaz** 50 mg/kg IV q8h to max of 6 gm per day. If resistant to above, **CIP/Levo** used if P. aeruginosa susceptible. *See footnote[40] & Comment*	**For S. aureus: (1) MSSA— oxacillin/nafcillin** 2 gm IV q4h *(Peds dose, Table 16)*. **(2) MRSA—vanco** 1 gm q12h & check serum levels. *See Comment*	May be hard to get pieracillin without tazobactam. Older children and adults need high dose PIP-TZ for P. aeruginosa (3.375 gm IV q4h). Extended infusion better: 4-hr infusion of 3.375 gm q8h. For pharmacokinetics of aminoglycosides in CF, *J.Peds&ChildHealth 42:601, 2006* For chronic suppression of P. aeruginosa, **inhaled phenol-free tobra** 300 mg bid x 28 days, then no rx x 28 days, then repeat cycle *(AJRCCM 167:841, 2003).* Inhaled aztreonam lysine in Phase III trials.
	Burkholderia (Pseudomonas) cepacia	**TMP-SMX** 5 mg per kg (TMP) IV q6h	**Chloro** 15–20 mg per kg IV/po q6h	B. cepacia has become a major pathogen. Patients develop progressive respiratory failure, 62% mortality at 1 yr. **Fail to respond to aminoglycosides,** piperacillin, & ceftazidime. Patients with B. cepacia should be isolated from other CF patients.
Empyema Refs.: Pleural effusion review: *NEJM 346:1971, 2002; CID 45:1480, 2007*			*For other alternatives, see Table 2*	
Neonatal	Staph. aureus	*See Pneumonia, neonatal, page 34*		Drainage indicated.
Infants/children (1 month–5 yrs)	Staph. aureus, Strep. pneumoniae, H. influenzae	*See Pneumonia, age 1 month–5 years, page 34*		Drainage indicated.
Child >5 yrs to ADULT—Diagnostic thoracentesis; chest tube for empyemas Acute, usually parapneumonic Strep. pneumoniae, Group A strep For dosage, see Table 10 or footnote page 23 Microbiologic diagnosis: *CID 42:1135, 2006.*		**Cefotaxime** or **ceftriaxone** *(Dosage, see footnote[19] page 23)*	Vanco	In large multicenter double-blind trial, **intrapleural streptokinase** did not improve mortality, reduce the need for surgery or the length of hospitalization *(NEJM 352:865, 2005).* Success using S. pneumoniae urine antigen test on pleural fluid *(Chest 131:1442, 2007).*
	Staph. aureus: Check for MRSA	**Nafcillin** or **oxacillin** if MSSA	Vanco if MRSA	Usually complication of S. aureus pneumonia &/or bacteremia.
	H. influenzae	**Ceftriaxone**		
Subacute/chronic	Anaerobic strep, Strep. milleri, Bacteroides sp., Enterobacteriaceae, M. tuberculosis	**Clinda** 450–900 mg IV q8h + **ceftriaxone**	**TMP-SMX** or **AM-SB** **Cefoxitin** or **IMP** or **TC-CL** or **PIP-TZ** or **AM-SB** *(Dosage, see footnote[19] page 23)*	Pleomorphic Gm-neg. bacilli. ↑ resistance to TMP-SMX. If organisms not seen, treat as subacute. Drainage. R/O tuberculosis or tumor. Pleural biopsy with culture for mycobacteria and histology if TBc suspected.
Human immunodeficiency virus infection (HIV+): See SANFORD GUIDE TO HIV/AIDS THERAPY				
CD4 T-lymphocytes <200 per mm³ or clinical AIDS Dry cough, progressive dyspnea, & diffuse infiltrate **Prednisone first if suspect pneumocystis (see Comment)**	Pneumocystis carinii most likely; also M. tbc, fungi, Kaposi's sarcoma, & lymphoma NOTE: AIDS pts may develop pneumonia due to DRSP or other pathogens—see next box below	Rx listed here is for *severe* pneumocystis; see Table 13, page 128 for po regimens for mild disease. **Prednisone 1st (see Comment),** then: **TMP-SMX** [IV: 15 mg per kg per day div q8h (TMP component) or po: 2 DS tabs q8h], total of 21 days	**(Clinda** 600 mg IV q8h + **primaquine** 30 mg po q24h) or **(pentamidine isethionate** 4 mg per kg per day IV) times 21 days. *See Comment*	**Diagnosis (induced sputum or bronchial wash) for:** histology or monoclonal antibody strains or PCR. Serum beta-glucon (Fungitell) levels under study *(CID 46:1928 & 1930, 2008).* **Prednisone 40 mg bid po times 5 days then 40 mg q24h po times 5 days then 20 mg q24h po times 11 days is indicated with PCP (pO₂ <70 mmHg), should be given at initiation of anti-PCP rx; don't wait until pt's condition deteriorates.** If PCP studies negative, consider bacterial pneumonia, TBc, cocci, histo, crypto, Kaposi's sarcoma or lymphoma. **Pentamidine not active vs bacterial pathogens.** **NOTE: Pneumocystis resistant to TMP-SMX, albeit rare, does exist.**

[40] Other options: (Tobra + aztreonam 50 mg per kg IV q8h); (IMP 15–25 mg per kg IV q6h + tobra); **CIP commonly used in children**, e.g., CIP IV/po + ceftaz IV *(LnID 3:537, 2003).*

Abbreviations on page 3.   *NOTE: All dosage recommendations are for adults (unless otherwise indicated) and assume normal renal function.*

TABLE 1A (38)

ANATOMIC SITE/DIAGNOSIS/ MODIFYING CIRCUMSTANCES	ETIOLOGIES (usual)	SUGGESTED REGIMENS* PRIMARY	ALTERNATIVE§	ADJUNCT DIAGNOSTIC OR THERAPEUTIC MEASURES AND COMMENTS
LUNG—Other Specific Infections/Human immunodeficiency virus infection (HIV+) *(continued)*				
CD4 T-lymphocytes normal Acute onset, purulent sputum & pulmonary infiltrates ± pleuritic pain. **Isolate pt until TBc excluded: Adults**	Strep. pneumoniae, H. influenzae, aerobic Gm-neg. bacilli (including P. aeruginosa), Legionella rare, M. tbc	Ceftriaxone 1 gm IV q24h (over age 65 1 gm IV q24h) + **azithro.** Could use **, Levo,** or **Moxi** IV as alternative *(see Comment)*		If Gram stain of sputum shows Gm-neg. bacilli, options include **P Ceph 3 AP, TC-CL, PIP-TZ, IMP,** or **MER**. **FQs: Levo** 750 mg po/IV q24h; **Moxi** 400 mg po/IV q24h. Gati not available in US due to hypo- & hyperglycemic reactions.
As above: Children	Same as adult with HIV + lymphoid interstitial pneumonia (LIP)	As for HIV+ adults with pneumonia. If diagnosis is LIP, rx with steroids.		In children with AIDS, LIP responsible for 1/3 of pulmonary complications, usually >1 yr of age vs PCP, which is seen at <1 yr of age. Clinically: clubbing, hepatosplenomegaly, salivary glands enlarged (take up gallium), lymphocytosis.
Nocardia pneumonia Expert Help: Wallace Lab (+1) 903-877-7680; CDC (+1) 404-639-3158	N. asteroides, N. brasiliensis	**TMP-SMX** 15 mg/kg/day based on TMP IV/po div in 2-4 doses x 3-4 wks; then reduce dose to 10 mg/kg/ day IV/po div in 2-4 doses x 3-6 mos *(See Comment)*	**IMP** 500 mg IV q6h + **amikacin** 7.5 mg/kg IV q12h x 3-4 wks & then po **TMP-SMX**	**Duration:** 3 mos. if immunocompetent; 6 mos. if immunocompromised. **Measure peak sulfonamide levels:** Target is 100-150 mcg/mL 2 hrs post po dose. **Linezolid** active in vitro *(An Pharmacother 41:1694, 2007).*
Viral (interstitial) pneumonia suspected *(See Table 14, page 137)* Ref: *Chest 133:1221, 2008.*	Consider: Adenovirus, coronavirus (SARS), hantavirus, influenza, metapneumovirus, parainfluenza virus, respiratory syncytial virus	Presently **influenza** treatment complicated by 2008-9 isolates of **influenza A/H1N1** demonstrating near 100% resistance to **oseltamivir**. *See CDC advisory bulletin of 12/9/2008:* www.cdc.gov/flu/professionals/antivirals/recommendations. htm		No known efficacious drugs for adenovirus, coronavirus (SARS), hantavirus, metapneumovirus, parainfluenza or RSV. Need travel (SARS) & exposure (Hanta) history. RSV and human metapneumovirus as serious as influenza in the elderly *(NEJM 352:1749 & 1810, 2005: CID 44:1752 & 1759, 2007).* NOTE: As of 01/01/09, most influenza A/N1N1 resistant to oseltamivir: *see Table 14A, Influenza A.*
LYMPH NODES (approaches below apply to lymphadenitis without an obvious primary source)				
Lymphadenitis, acute **Generalized**	Etiologies: EBV, early HIV infection, syphilis, toxoplasma, tularemia, Lyme disease, sarcoid, lymphoma, systemic lupus erythematosus, and **Kikuchi-Fujimoto** disease *(CID 39:138, 2004).* Complete history and physical examination followed by appropriate serological tests. Treat specific agent (s).			**Kikuchi-Fujimoto** disease causes fever and benign self-limited adenopathy; the etiology is unknown *(CID 39:138, 2004).*
Regional **Cervical—see cat-scratch disease (CSD), below**	CSD (B. henselae), Grp A strep, Staph. aureus, anaerobes, M. TBc (scrofula), M. avium, M. scrofulaceum, M. malmoense, toxo, tularemia			History & physical exam directs evaluation. If nodes fluctuant, aspirate and base rx on Gram & acid-fast stains. *Review of mycobacterial etiology: CID 20:954, 1995.*
Inguinal Sexually transmitted	HSV, chancroid, syphilis, LGV			
Not sexually transmitted	GAS, SA, tularemia, CSD			
Axillary	GAS, SA, CSD, tularemia, Y. pestis, sporotrichosis			
Extremity, with associated nodular lymphangitis	Sporotrichosis, leishmania, Nocardia brasiliensis, Mycobacterium marinum, Mycobacterium chelonae, tularemia	Treatment varies with specific etiology		A distinctive form of lymphangitis characterized by subcutaneous swellings along inflamed lymphatic channels. Primary site of skin invasion usually present; regional adenopathy variable.
Nocardia lymphadenitis & skin abscesses	N. asteroides, N. brasiliensis	**TMP-SMX** 5-10 mg/kg/day based on TMP IV/po div in 2-4 doses	**Sulfisoxazole** 2 gm po qid or **minocycline** 100-200 mg po bid.	**Duration:** 3 mos. if immunocompetent; 6 mos. if immunocompromised. **Linezolid** 600 mg po bid reported effective *(An Pharmacother 41:1694, 2007).*

Abbreviations on page 3.   NOTE: All dosage recommendations are for adults (unless otherwise indicated) and assume normal renal function.

TABLE 1A (39)

ANATOMIC SITE/DIAGNOSIS/ MODIFYING CIRCUMSTANCES	ETIOLOGIES (usual)	SUGGESTED REGIMENS* PRIMARY	ALTERNATIVE§	ADJUNCT DIAGNOSTIC OR THERAPEUTIC MEASURES AND COMMENTS
LYMPH NODES/Lymphadenitis, acute/Regional (continued)				
Cat-scratch disease— immunocompetent patient Axillary/epitrochlear nodes 46%, neck 26%, inguinal 17%	Bartonella henselae Reviews: AAC 48:1921, 2004; PIDJ 23:1161, 2004	**Azithro** dosage—**Adults** (>45.5 kg): 500 mg po x 1, then 250 mg/day x 4 days. **Children** (<45.5 kg): liquid azithro 10 mg/kg x 1, then 5 mg/kg per day x 4 days. Rx is controversial	No therapy; resolves in 2–6 mos. Needle aspiration relieves pain in suppurative nodes. Avoid I&D.	**Clinical**: Approx. 10% nodes suppurate. Atypical presentation in <5% pts, i.e., lung nodules, liver/spleen lesions, Parinaud's oculoglandular syndrome, CNS manifestations in 2% of pts (encephalitis, peripheral neuropathy, retinitis), FUO. **Dx**: Cat exposure. Positive IFA serology. Rarely need biopsy. **Rx**: Only 1 prospective randomized blinded study, used azithro with ↑ rapidity of resolution of enlarged lymph nodes (PIDJ 17:447, 1998). **Note**: In elderly, endocarditis more frequent; lymphadenitis less frequent (CID 41:969, 2005).
MOUTH				
Odontogenic infection, including Ludwig's angina Can result in parapharyngeal space infection (see page 46)	Oral microflora: infection polymicrobial	**Clinda** 300–450 mg po bid or 600 mg IV q6–8h	(**AM-CL** 875/125 mg po bid or 500/125 mg tid or 2000/125 mg bid) or **cefotetan** 2 gm IV q12h	Surgical drainage & removal of necrotic tissue essential. β-lactamase pro-ducing organisms are ↑ in frequency. Other parenteral alternatives: **AM-SB, PIP-TZ, or TC-CL.** For Noma (cancrum oris) see Ln 368:147, 2006.
Buccal cellulitis Children <5 yrs	H. influenzae	**Cefuroxime** or **ceftriaxone**	**AM-CL** or **TMP-SMX**	With Hib immunization, invasive H. influenzae infections have ↓ by 95%. Now occurring in infants prior to immunization.
		Dosage: see Table 16, page 178		
Cervico-facial actinomycosis (lumpy jaw) Review: AJM 117:420, 2004	Actinomyces israeli and rarely others	**AMP** 50 mg/kg/day IV div in 3-4 doses x 4-6 wks, then **Pen VK** 2-4 gm/day po x 3-6 mos.	**Doxy** or **ceftriaxone** or **clinda** or **erythro**	Presents as lumps & sinus tracts after dental/jaw trauma. Can use Pen G IV instead of AMP: 10-20 million units/day x 4-6 wks.
Herpetic stomatitis	Herpes simplex virus 1 & 2	See Table 14		
Aphthous stomatitis, recurrent	Etiology unknown	Topical steroids (Kenalog in Orabase) may ↓ pain and swelling; if AIDS, see SANFORD GUIDE TO HIV/AIDS THERAPY.		
MUSCLE				
"Gas gangrene" Contaminated traumatic wound Can be spontaneous without trauma (CID 28:159, 1999)	Cl. perfringens, other histo-toxic Clostridium sp.	(**Clinda** 900 mg IV q8h) + (**pen G** 24 million units/day div. q4–6h IV)	**Ceftriaxone** 2 gm IV q12h or **erythro** 1 gm q6h IV (not by bolus)	Surgical debridement primary therapy. Hyperbaric oxygen adjunctive: efficacy debated, consider if debridement not complete or possible. Clinda decreases toxin production.
Pyomyositis Review: AJM 117:420, 2004	Staph. aureus, Group A strep, (rarely Gm-neg. bacilli), variety of anaerobic organisms	**Nafcillin** or **oxacillin** 2 gm IV q4h) or [**P Ceph 1** (**cefazolin** 2 gm IV q8h)] if **MSSA**	**Vanco** 1 gm IV q12h if **MRSA**	Common in tropics; rare, but occurs, in temperate zones. Follows exercise or muscle injury, see Necrotizing fasciitis. Now seen in HIV/AIDS. Add **metro** if anaerobes suspected or proven.
PANCREAS: Reviews—Ln 361:1447, 2003; JAMA 291:2865, 2004; NEJM 354:2142, 2006.				
Acute alcoholic (without necrosis) (idiopathic) pancreatitis	Not bacterial	None No necrosis on CT		1–9% become infected but prospective studies show no advantage of prophylactic antimicrobials (Ln 346:652, 1995). Observe for pancreatic abscesses or necrosis which require therapy.
Pancreatic abscess, infected pseudocyst, post-necrotizing pancreatitis	Enterobacteriaceae, entero-cocci, S. aureus, S. epider-midis, anaerobes, candida	Need culture of abscess/infected pseudocyst to direct therapy		Can often get specimen by fine-needle aspiration.
Antimicrobic prophylaxis, necrotizing pancreatitis	As above	Controversial: Cochrane Database 2: CD 002941, 2004 supports prophylaxis. Subsequent, double-blind, randomized, controlled study, showed no benefit (Gastroenterol 126:997, 2004). Consensus conference voted against prophylaxis (CCM 32:2524, 2004).		

Abbreviations on page 3.   NOTE: All dosage recommendations are for adults (unless otherwise indicated) and assume normal renal function.

44

TABLE 1A (40)

ANATOMIC SITE/DIAGNOSIS/ MODIFYING CIRCUMSTANCES	ETIOLOGIES (usual)	SUGGESTED REGIMENS*		ADJUNCT DIAGNOSTIC OR THERAPEUTIC MEASURES AND COMMENTS
		PRIMARY	ALTERNATIVE§	
PAROTID GLAND "Hot" tender parotid swelling	S. aureus, S. pyogenes, oral flora, & aerobic Gm-neg, bacilli (rare), mumps, rarely enteroviruses/influenza: **Natcillin** or **oxacillin** 2 gm IV q4h if MSSA; **vanco** if MRSA			Predisposing factors: stone(s) in Stensen's duct, dehydration. Therapy depends on ID of specific etiologic organism.
"Cold" non-tender parotid swelling	Granulomatous disease (e.g., mycobacteria, fungi, sarcoidosis, Sjögren's syndrome), drugs (iodides, et al.), diabetes, cirrhosis, tumors			History/lab results may narrow differential; may need biopsy for diagnosis
PERITONEUM/PERITONITIS: *Reference—CID 31:997, 2003*				
Primary (spontaneous bacterial peritonitis, SBP) *CDBSR 2001, Issue 3, Article No CD002232*	Enterobacteriaceae 63%, S. pneumo 15% enterococci 6–10%, anaerobes <1%. Extended β-lactamase (ESBL) positive Klebsiella species.	[**Cefotaxime** 2 gm IV q8h (if life-threatening, q4h)] or [**TC-CL** or **PIP-TZ** or **AM-SB**] OR [**ceftriaxone** 2 gm IV q24h] or [**ERTA** 1 gm IV q24h] **If resistant E. coli/Klebsiella species (ESBL+), then:** (**DORI, ERTA, IMP** or **MER**) or (**FQ: CIP, Levo, Moxi**) *(Dosage in footnote[41])*. Check in vitro susceptibility.		One-year **risk of SBP** in pts with ascites and cirrhosis as high as 29% (*Gastro 104:1133, 1993*). 30–40% of pts have neg. cultures of blood and ascitic fluid. % pos. cultures ↑ if 10 mL of pt's ascitic fluid added to blood culture bottles (*JAMA 299:1166, 2008*). **Duration of rx unclear.** Suggest 2 wks if blood culture +. One report suggests repeat paracentesis after 48hrs of cefotaxime. If PMNs <250/mm³ & ascitic fluid sterile, success with 5 days of treatment (*AJM 97:169, 1994*). IV albumin (1.5 gm/kg at dx & 1 gm/kg on day 3) may ↓ frequency of renal impairment (p 0.002) & ↓ hospital mortality (p 0.01) (*NEJM 341:403, 1999*).
Prevention of SBP: Cirrhosis & ascites *For prevention after UGI bleeding, see Liver, page 32*		**TMP-SMX-DS** 1 tab po 5 days/wk or **CIP** 750 mg po q wk	**TMP-SMX** ↓ peritonitis or spontaneous bacteremia from 27% to 3% (*AnIM 122:595, 1995*). Ref. for CIP: *Hepatology 22:1171, 1995*	
Secondary (bowel perforation, ruptured appendix, ruptured diverticula) Refs.: *CID 37:997, 2003*	Enterobacteriaceae, Bacteroides sp., enterococci, P. aeruginosa (3+–15%)	**Mild-moderate disease—Inpatient—parenteral rx:** (e.g., focal periappendiceal peritonitis, peridiverticular abscess, endomyometritis) **PIP-TZ** 3.375 gm IV q6h or 4.5 gm IV q8h or 4-hr infusion of 3.375 gm q8h **AM-SB** 3 gm IV q6h OR TC-CL 3.1 gm IV q6h OR ERTA 1 gm IV q24h OR MOXI 400 mg IV q24h **Severe life-threatening disease—ICU patient:** **IMP** 500 mg IV q6h or **MER** 1 gm IV q8h or **DORI** 500 mg IV q8h (1-hr infusion)	[(**CIP** 400 mg IV q12h or **Levo** 750 mg IV q24h) **+** (**metro** 1 gm IV q12h)] or (**CFP** 2 gm q12h + **metro**) or **tigecycline** 100 mg IV times 1 dose, then 50 mg q12h [**AMP** + **metro** + (**CIP** 400 mg IV q8h or **Levo** 750 mg IV q24h)] OR [**AMP** 2 gm IV q6h + **metro** 500 mg IV q6h + **aminoglycoside** *(see Table 10D, page 96)*	Must "cover" both Gm-neg. aerobic & Gm-neg. anaerobic bacteria. **Drugs active only vs anaerobic Gm-neg. bacilli:** clinda, metro. **Drugs active only vs aerobic Gm-neg. bacilli:** APAG, P Ceph 2/3/4, aztreonam, AP Pen, CIP, Levo. **Drugs active vs both aerobic/anaerobic Gm-neg. bacteria:** cefoxitin, cefotetan, TC-CL, PIP-TZ, AM-SB, Dori, IMP, MER, Gati, Moxi. Increasing resistance (R) of Bacteroides species (AAC 51:1649, 2007):

(cont.)

Cefoxitin — Cefotetan — Clindamycin
% R — 5-30 — 17–87 — 19-35

Essentially no resistance: **metro**. **PIP-TZ**. Case reports of metro resistance: *CID 40:e67, 2005; JCM 42:4127, 2004.* **Ertapenem** not active vs P. aeruginosa/Acinetobacter species.
If absence of ongoing fecal contamination, aerobic/anaerobic culture of peritoneal exudate/abscess of help in guiding specific therapy.
Less need for aminoglycosides. **With severe pen allergy** can "cover" Gm-neg. aerobes with **CIP** or **aztreonam. Remember IMP/MER are β-lactams.**

Concomitant surgical management important.

41 Parenteral **IV therapy** for peritonitis: **TC-CL** 3.1 gm q6h, **PIP-TZ** 3.375 gm q6h or 4.5 gm q8h or 4-hr infusion of 3.375 gm q8h, **AM-SB** 3 gm q6h, **Dori** 500 mg IV q8h (1-hr infusion), **IMP** 0.5 gm q6h, **FQ** [**CIP** 400 mg q12h, **Oflox** 400 mg q12h, **Levo** 750 mg q24h, **Moxi** 400 mg q24h], **AMP** 1 gm q6h, **aminoglycoside** *(see Table 10D, page 96)*, **cefotetan** 2 gm q12h, **cefoxitin** 2 gm q8h, **P Ceph 3** (**cefotaxime** 2 gm q4–8h, **ceftriaxone** 2 gm q4–8h, **ceftizoxime** 1–2 gm q8h, **ceftazidime** 2 gm q8h), **P Ceph 4** (**CFP** 2 gm q12h, **cefpirome**NUS 2 gm q12h), **clinda** 450–900 mg q8h, **metro** 1 gm loading then 0.5 gm q6h or 1 gm q12h, **AP Pen** (**ticarcillin** 4 gm q6h, **PIP** 4 gm q6h, **aztreonam** 2 gm q8h)

Abbreviations on page 3.   NOTE: *All dosage recommendations are for adults (unless otherwise indicated) and assume normal renal function.*

TABLE 1A (41)

ANATOMIC SITE/DIAGNOSIS/ MODIFYING CIRCUMSTANCES	ETIOLOGIES (usual)	SUGGESTED REGIMENS* PRIMARY	SUGGESTED REGIMENS* ALTERNATIVE§	ADJUNCT DIAGNOSTIC OR THERAPEUTIC MEASURES AND COMMENTS
PERITONEUM/PERITONITIS/Secondary *(continued)*				
Abdominal actinomycosis	A. israeli and rarely others	**AMP** 50 mg/kg/day IV div in 3-4 doses x 4-6 wks, then **Pen VK** 2-4 gm/day po x 3-6 mos.	**Doxy** or **clinda** or **erythro**	Presents as mass +/- fistula tract after abdominal surgery, e.g., for ruptured appendix. Can use IV Pen G instead of AMP: 10-20 million units/day IV x 4-6 wks.
Associated with chronic ambulatory peritoneal dialysis (defined as > 100 WBC per mcL, >50% PMNs)	Staph. aureus (most common), Staph. epidermidis, P. aeruginosa 7%, Gm-neg. bacilli 11%, sterile 20%, M. fortuitum (rare)	If of moderate severity, can rx by adding drug to dialysis fluid—see *Table 17 for dosage*. Reasonable empiric combinations: (**vanco** + **ceftazidime**) or (**vanco** + **gent**). If severely ill, rx with same drugs IV (adjust dose for renal failure, *Table 17*) & via addition to dialysis fluid. Excellent ref.: *Perit Dialysis Int 13:14, 1993*		For diagnosis: concentrate several hundred mL of removed dialysis fluid by centrifugation. Gram stain concentrate and then inject into aerobic/anaerobic blood culture bottles. A positive Gram stain will guide initial therapy. If culture shows Staph. epidermidis, good chance of "saving" dialysis catheter; **if multiple Gm-neg. bacilli cultured, consider bowel perforation and catheter removal.**
PHARYNX				
Pharyngitis/Tonsillitis—Reviews: *NEJM 344:205, 2001; AnIM 139:113, 2003.* Guideline for Group A strep: *CID 35:113, 2002* **Exudative or diffuse erythema** *For relationship to acute rheumatic fever, see footnote42* Rheumatic fever ref.: *Ln 366:155, 2005*	Group A, C, G strep, "viral," infectious mononucleosis (*NEJM 329:156, 1993*), C. diphtheriae, A. haemolyticum, Mycoplasma pneumoniae In adults, only 10% pharyngitis due to Group A strep	**Pen V** po x 10 days or if compliance unlikely, **benzathine pen** IM times 1 dose Up to 35% of isolates resistant to erythro, azithro, clarithro, clinda (*AAC 48:473, 2004*) **See footnote43 for adult and pediatric dosages** Acetaminophen effective for pain relief. **If macrolide-resistant & pen-allergy:** Children—**Linezolid** should work; Adults—**FQ**	**O Ceph 2** x 4–6 days (*CID 38:1526 & 1535, 2004*) or **clinda** or **azithro** x 5 days or **clarithro** x 10 days or **erythro** x 10 days	**Dx:** Rapid strep test or culture: (*JAMA 292:167, 2004*). *Rapid strep test valid in adults: An IM 166:640, 2006.* **Pen allergy & macrolide resistance:** No penicillin or cephalosporin-resistant S. pyogenes, but now **macrolide-resist. S. pyogenes** (7% 2000–2003). Culture & susceptibility testing if clinical failure with azithro/clarithro (*CID 41:599, 2005*). **S. pyogenes Groups C & G cause pharyngitis but not a risk for post-strep rheumatic fever.** To prevent rheumatic fever, eradicate Group A strep. Requires 10 days of pen V po; 4–6 days of po O Ceph 2; 5 days of po azithro; 10 days of clarithro. In controlled trial, better eradication rate with 10 days clarithro (91%) than 5 days azithro (82%)(*CID 32: 1798,2001*)
	Gonococci	**Ceftriaxone** 125 mg IM x 1 dose+ (**azithro** or **doxy**) *(see Comment)*	**FQs** no longer recommended due to high prevalence of resistance: *MMWR 56:332, 2007.*	Because of risk of concomitant genital C. trachomatis, add either (azithro 1 gm po times 1 dose) or (doxy 100 mg po q12h times 7 days).
	Group A strep	**No rx required** **Clinda** or **AM-CL** po	Parenteral **benzathine pen G** ± **RIF** *(see Comment)*	Routine post-rx throat culture not advised.
Asymptomatic post-rx carrier Multiple repeated culture-positive episodes (*CID 25:574, 1997*)	Group A strep	*Dosages in footnote43*		Small % of pts have recurrent culture-pos. Group A strep with symptomatic tonsillo-pharyngitis. Hard to tell if true Group A strep infection or active viral infection in carrier of Group A strep. Addition of **RIF** may help: 20 mg per kg per day times 4 days to max. of 300 mg bid.
Whitish plaques, HIV+ (thrush)	Candida albicans (*see Table 11, page 100*)			

42 Primary rationale for therapy is eradication of Group A strep (GAS) and prevention of acute rheumatic fever (ARF). Benzathine penicillin G has been shown in clinical trials to ↓ rate of ARF from 2.8 to 0.2%. This was associated with clearance of GAS on pharyngeal cultures (*CID 19:1110, 1994*). Subsequent studies have been based on cultures, not actual prevention of ARF. Treatment decreases duration of symptoms.

43 Treatment of Group A strep: **All po unless otherwise indicated. PEDIATRIC DOSAGE: Benzathine penicillin** 25,000 units per kg IM to max. 1.2 million units; **Pen V** 25–50 mg per kg per day div. q6h times10 days; **AM-CL** 45 mg per kg per day div. q12h times 10 days; **erythro estolate** 20 mg per kg per day div. bid times 10 days; **succinate** 40 mg per kg per day div. bid times10 days; **cefuroxime axetil** 20 mg per kg per day div. bid for 4–10 days (*PIDJ 14:295, 1995*); **cefpodoxime proxetil** 10 mg per kg per day div. bid times10 days; **cefdinir** 7 mg per kg per day q12h times 5–10 days or 14 mg per kg q24h times 10 days; **cefprozil** 15 mg per kg per day per day div. bid times 10 days; **clarithro** 15 mg per kg per day div. bid times 10 days; **azithro** 12 mg per kg per day times 5 days; **clinda** 20–30 mg per kg per day div. q8h times 10 days. **ADULT DOSAGE: Benzathine penicillin** 1.2 million units IM times 1; **Pen V** 500 mg bid or 250 mg qid times 10 days; **erythro**, dosage varies—with erythro base 500 mg qid times 10 days; **cefditoren** 200 mg bid times 10 days; **cefuroxime axetil** 250 mg bid times 4 days; **cefpodoxime proxetil** 100 mg bid times 4 days; **cefdinir** 300 mg q12h times 5–10 days or 600 mg q24h times 10 days; **cefprozil** 500 mg q24h times 10 days; **NOTE:** All O Ceph 2 drugs approved for 10-day rx of strep. pharyngitis; increasing number of studies show efficacy of 4–6 days; **clarithro** 250 mg bid times 10 days; **azithro** 500 mg times 1 and then 250 mg q24h times 4 days or 500 mg q24h times 3 days.

Abbreviations on page 3. NOTE: *All dosage recommendations are for adults (unless otherwise indicated) and assume normal renal function.*

TABLE 1A (42)

ANATOMIC SITE/DIAGNOSIS/ MODIFYING CIRCUMSTANCES	ETIOLOGIES (usual)	SUGGESTED REGIMENS*		ADJUNCT DIAGNOSTIC OR THERAPEUTIC MEASURES AND COMMENTS
		PRIMARY	ALTERNATIVE§	
PHARYNX/Pharyngitis/Tonsillitis (continued)				
Vesicular, ulcerative	Coxsackie A9, B1-5, ECHO (multiple types), Enterovirus 71, Herpes simplex 1,2	Antibacterial agents not indicated. For HSV-1,2: **acyclovir 400 mg tid po x 10 days.**		
Membranous—Diphtheria or Vincent's angina	C. diphtheriae	[**Antitoxin + erythro** 20–25 mg/kg IV q12h times 7–14 days (*JAC 35:717, 1995*)] or [**benzyl pen G** 50,000 units/kg per day x 5 days, then po **pen VK** 50 mg/kg per day x 5 days]		Diphtheria occurs in immunized individuals. Antibiotics may ↓ toxin production, ↓ spread of organisms. Penicillin superior to erythro in randomized trial (*CID 27:845, 1998*).
	Vincent's angina (anaerobes/spirochetes)	**Pen G** 4 million units IV q4h	**Clinda** 600 mg IV q8h	May be complicated by F. necrophorum bacteremia, *see jugular vein phlebitis* (**Lemierre's syndrome**), *page 46.*
Epiglottitis Children	H. influenzae (rare), S. pyogenes, S. pneumoniae, S. aureus	**Peds dosage: Cefotaxime** 50 mg per kg IV q8h or **ceftriaxone** 50 mg per kg IV q24h	**Peds dosage: AM-SB** 100–200 mg/kg per day div q6h or **TMP-SMX** 8–12 mg TMP component /kg per day div q12h	Have tracheostomy set "at bedside." **Chloro** is effective, but potentially less toxic alternative agents available. Review (adults): *JAMA 272:1358, 1994*).
Adults	Group A strep, H. influenzae (rare)	**Adult dosage: See footnote**[44]		
Parapharyngeal space infection Poor dental hygiene, dental extractions, foreign bodies (e.g., toothpicks, fish bones)	[Spaces include: sublingual, submandibular, submaxillary (Ludwig's angina, used loosely for these), lateral pharyngeal, retropharyngeal, pretracheal] Polymicrobic: Strep sp., anaerobes, Eikenella corrodens	[[**Clinda** 600–900 mg IV q8h) or (**pen G** 24 million units by cont. infusion or div. q4–6h IV] + **metro** 1 gm load and then 0.5 gm IV q6h)	**Cefoxitin** 2 gm IV q8h or **clinda** 600-900 mg IV q8h or **TC-CL** or **PIP-TZ** or **AM-SB** (*Dosage, see footnote*[44])	Close observation of airway, 1/3 require intubation. MRI or CT to identify abscess; if present, surgical drainage. **Metro** may be given 1 gm IV q12h.
Jugular vein septic phlebitis (**Lemierre's disease**) (*PIDJ 22:921, 2003; CID 31:524, 2000*)	Fusobacterium necrophorum in vast majority	**Pen G** 24 million units q24h by cont. infusion or div. q4–6h	**Clinda** 600–900 mg IV q8h	Usual therapy includes external drainage of lateral pharyngeal space. Emboli: pulmonary and systemic common. Erosion into carotid artery can occur.
Laryngitis (hoarseness)/tracheitis	Viral (90%)	Not indicated		
Sinusitis, acute; current terminology: acute rhinosinusitis. **Obstruction of sinus ostia, viral infection, allergens** Refs.: *Otolaryn-Head & Neck Surgery 130:S1, 2004; AnIM 134:495 & 498, 2001.* For rhinovirus infections (common cold), see Table 14, page 147 Pediatric Guidelines: *Peds 108:798, 2001*	Strep. pneumoniae 31%, H. influenzae 21%, M. catarrhalis 2%, Group A strep 2%, anaerobes 6%, viruses 15%, Staph. aureus 4% By CT scans, sinus mucosa inflamed in 87% of viral URIs; only 2% develop bacterial rhinosinusitis	**Reserve antibiotic therapy for pts given decongestants/ analgesics for 7 days who have (1) maxillary/facial pain & (2) purulent nasal discharge; if severe illness (pain, fever), treat sooner—usually requires hospitalization.** **For mild/mod. disease: Ask if antibiotics in prior month.**		**Rx goals:** (1) Resolve infection, (2) prevent bacterial complications, e.g., subdural empyema, epidural abscess, brain abscess, meningitis and cavenous sinus thrombosis (*LnID 7:62, 2007*), (3) avoid chronic sinus disease, (4) avoid unnecessary antibiotic rx. High rate of spontaneous resolution. **For pts with pen/cephalosporin allergy, esp. severe IgE-mediated allergy, e.g., hives, anaphylaxis, treatment options: clarithro, azithro, TMP-SMX, doxy or FQs. Avoid FQs if under age 18. *Dosages in footnote*[43] *page 45.* If allergy just skin rash, po cephalosporin OK.** (*continued on next page*)

[44] **Ceftriaxone** 2 gm IV q24h; **cefotaxime** 2 gm IV q4-8h; **AM-SB** 3 gm IV q4-8h; **AM-SB** 3 gm IV q6h; **PIP-TZ** 3.375 gm IV q6h or 4-hr infusion of 3.375 gm IV q8h; **TC-CL** 3.1 gm IV q4-6h; **TMP-SMX** 8-10 mg per kg per day (based on TMP component) div q6h, q8h, or q12h.

Abbreviations on page 3.   *NOTE: All dosage recommendations are for adults (unless otherwise indicated) and assume normal renal function.*

TABLE 1A (43)

ANATOMIC SITE/DIAGNOSIS/ MODIFYING CIRCUMSTANCES	ETIOLOGIES (usual)	SUGGESTED REGIMENS*		ADJUNCT DIAGNOSTIC OR THERAPEUTIC MEASURES AND COMMENTS
		PRIMARY	ALTERNATIVE§	
PHARYNX/Sinusitis, acute; current terminology: acute rhinosinusitis *(continued)*				
Meta-analysis of 10 double-blind trials found no clinical signs/symptoms that justify treatment--even after 7-10 days of symptoms *(Ln 371:908, 2008).*		**No Recent Antibiotic Use:** Amox-HD or AM-CL-ER or cefdinir or cefpodoxime or cefprozil	**Recent Antibiotic Use:** AM-CL-ER (adults) or resp. FQ (adults). For pen. allergy, see Comments. Use AM-CL susp. in peds.	**Usual rx 10 days. Azithro,** FQs often given for 5 days (see NOTE below). Watch for pts with fever & fascial erythema; ↑ risk of S. aureus infection, requires IV **nafcillin/oxacillin (antistaphylococcal penicillin, penicillinase-resistant for MSSA or vanco for MRSA).** Pts aged 1–18 yrs with **clinical diagnosis** of sinusitis randomized to placebo, amox, or AM-CL for 14 days **No difference** in multiple measures of efficacy *(Peds 107:619, 2001).* Similar study in adults: *AnM 163:1793, 2003.* Hence, without bacteriologic endpoints, data are hard to interpret.
		In general, treat 10 days (see Comment); Adult and pediatric doses, footnote[45] and footnote[8], page 11 (Otitis)		
Clinical failure after 3 days	As above; consider diagnostic tap/aspirate	**Mild/Mod. Disease: AM-CL-ER OR (cefpodoxime, cefprozil, or cefdinir)**	**Severe Disease:** Gati[NUS], Gemi, Levo, Moxi	NOTE: **Levo** 750 mg q24h x 5 days vs **levo** 500 mg q24h x 10 days equivalent microbiologic and clinical efficacy *(Otolaryngol Head Neck Surg 134:10, 2006)*
Diabetes mellitus with acute keto-acidosis; neutropenia; deferox-amine rx	Rhizopus sp. (mucor), aspergillus	*Treat 5-10 days. Adult doses in footnote[46] & Comment; See Table 11, pages 97 & 106.* Ref.: *NEJM 337:254, 1997*		
Hospitalized + nasotracheal or nasogastric intubation	Gm-neg. bacilli 47% (pseu-domonas, acinetobacter, E. coli common), Gm+ (S. aureus) 35%, yeasts 18%. Polymicrobial in 80%	Remove nasotracheal tube and if fever persists, recom-mend sinus aspiration for C/S prior to empiric therapy **DORI** 500 mg IV q8h (1-hr infusion) or **IMP** 0.5 gm IV q6h or **MER** 1 gm IV q8h. Add vanco for MRSA if Gram stain suggestive.	**(Ceftaz** 2 gm IV q8h + **vanco)** or **(CFP** 2 gm IV q12h + **vanco).**	After 7 days of nasotracheal or gastric tubes, 95% have x-ray "sinusitis" (fluid in sinuses), but on transnasal puncture only 38% culture + *(AJRCCM 150:776, 1994).* For pts requiring mechanical ventilation with nasotracheal tube for ≥1 wk, bacterial sinusitis occurs in <10% *(CID 27:851, 1998).* May need fluconazole if yeast on Gram stain of sinus aspirate. Review: *CID 27:463, 1998*
Sinusitis, chronic Adults	Prevotella, anaerobic strep, & fusobacterium—common anaerobes. Strep sp., haemophilus, P. aeruginosa, S. aureus, & moraxella—aerobes. *(CID 35:428, 2002)*	Antibiotics usually not effective	Otolaryngology consultation. If acute exacerbation, treat as acute	Pathogenesis unclear and may be polyfactorial: damage to ostiomeatal complex during acute bacterial disease, allergy ± polyps, occult immunodeficiency, and/or odontogenic disease (periodontitis in maxillary teeth).
SKIN				
Acne vulgaris *(JAMA 292:726, 2004; NEJM 352:1463, 2005; Ln 364:2188, 2004; In the Clinic, AnIM, July 1, 2008).* Comedonal acne, "blackheads," "whiteheads," earliest form, no inflammation	Excessive sebum production & gland obstruction. No Propionibacterium acnes	Once-q24h: Topical **tretinoin** (cream 0.025 or 0.05%) or (gel 0.01 or 0.025%)	All once-q24h: Topical **adapalene** 0.1% gel OR **azelaic acid** 20% cream or **tazarotene** 0.1% cream	Goal is prevention. ↓ number of new comedones and create an environment unfavorable to P. acnes. Adapalene causes less irritation than tretinoin. Azelaic acid less potent but less irritating than retinoids. Expect 40–70% ↓ in comedones in 12 weeks.

[45] *Pediatric doses for sinusitis (all oral):* **Amoxicillin** high dose 90 mg per kg per day div. q12h, **AM-CL-ES** (extra strength) pediatric susp.: 90 mg **amox** component per kg per day div. q12h, **azithro** 10 mg per kg times 1, then 5 mg per kg per day times 3 days, **clarithro** 15 mg per kg per day div. q12h, **cefpodoxime** 10 mg per kg per day (max. 400 mg) div. q12–24h, **cefuroxime axetil** 30 mg per kg per day div. q12h, **cefdinir** 14 mg per kg per day once q24h or divided bid, **TMP-SMX** 8–12 mg TMP/40–60 SMX per kg per day. q12h.

[46] *Adult doses for sinusitis (all oral):* **AM-CL-ER** 2000/125 **mg** bid, **amox high-dose (HD)** 1 gm tid, **clarithro** 500 mg bid or **clarithro ext. release** 1 gm q24h, **doxy** 100 mg bid, **respiratory FQs (Gati** 400 mg q24h[NUS] due to hypo/hyperglycemia; **Gemi** 320 mg q24h (*not FDA indication but should work),* **Levo** 750 mg q24h x 5 days, **Moxi** 400 mg q24h); **O Ceph (cefdinir** 300 mg q12h or 600 mg q24h, **cefpodoxime** 200 mg bid, **cefprozil** 250–500 mg bid, **cefuroxime** 250–500 mg bid, **TMP-SMX** 1 double-strength (TMP 160 mg) bid (results after 3- and 10-day rx similar).

Abbreviations on page 3. NOTE: All dosage recommendations are for adults (unless otherwise indicated) and assume normal renal function.

TABLE 1A (44)

ANATOMIC SITE/DIAGNOSIS/ MODIFYING CIRCUMSTANCES	ETIOLOGIES (usual)	SUGGESTED REGIMENS*		ADJUNCT DIAGNOSTIC OR THERAPEUTIC MEASURES AND COMMENTS
		PRIMARY	ALTERNATIVE§	
SKIN/Acne vulgaris *(continued)*				
Mild inflammatory acne: small papules or pustules	Proliferation of P. acnes + abnormal desquamation of follicular cells	Topical **erythro** 3% + **benzoyl peroxide** 5%, bid	Can substitute **clinda** 1% gel for erythro	In random. controlled trial, topical benzoyl peroxide + erythro of equal efficacy to oral minocycline & tetracycline and not affected by antibiotic resistance of propionibacteria *(Ln 364:2188, 2004)*.
Inflammatory acne: comedones, papules & pustules. Less common: deep nodules (cysts)	Progression of above events	(Topical **erythro** 3% + **benzoyl peroxide** 5% bid) ± oral antibiotic. *See Comment for mild acne*	Oral drugs: (**doxy** 100 mg bid) or (**minocycline** 50 mg bid). Others: **tetracycline**, **erythro**, **TMP-SMX**, **clinda**. Expensive extended release **once-daily minocycline** (Solodyn) 1 mg/kg/d *(Med Lett 48:95, 2006)*.	Systemic **isotretinoin** reserved for pts with severe widespread nodular cystic lesions that fail oral antibiotic rx; 4–5 mo. course of 0.1–1 mg per kg per day. Aggressive/violent behavior reported. Tetracyclines stain developing teeth. Doxy can cause photosensitivity. Minocycline side-effects: urticaria, vertigo, pigment deposition in skin or oral mucosa. Rare induced autoimmunity in children: fever; polyarthralgia, positive ANCA *(J Peds 153:314, 2008)*.
Acne rosacea	Skin mite: Demodex folliculorum	**Azelaic acid gel** bid, topical or **Metro** topical cream bid	Any of variety of low dose oral tetracycline regimens *(Med Lett 49:5, 2007)*.	
Anthrax, cutaneous, inhalation **To report bioterrorism event: 770-488-7100; For info: www.bt.cdc.gov** Refs.: *JAMA 281:1735, 1999, & MMWR 50:909, 2001*	B. anthracis *See Lung, page 40, and Table 1B, page 61*	**Adults (including pregnancy) and children >50 kg: CIP** 500 mg po bid or **Levo** 500 mg IV/po q24h) x 60 days **Children <50 kg: CIP** 20–30 mg/kg day div q12h po (to max. 1 gm per day) or **levo** 8 mg/kg po q12h x 60 days	**Adults (including pregnancy): Doxy** 100 mg po bid x 60 days. **Children: Doxy** >8 y/o & >45 kg: 100 mg po bid; >8 y/o & ≤45 kg: 2.2 mg/kg po bid; ≤8 y/o: 2.2 mg/kg po bid All for 60 days	1. If penicillin susceptible, then: **Adults: Amox** 500 mg po q8h times 60 days. **Children: Amox** 80 mg per kg per day div. q8h (max. 500 mg q8h). 2. Usual treatment of cutaneous anthrax is 7–10 days; 60 days in setting of bioterrorism with presumed aerosol exposure 3. Other **FQs** (Levo, Moxi) should work based on in vitro susceptibility data
Bacillary angiomatosis: For other Bartonella infections, see *Cat-scratch disease lymphadenitis, page 43, and Bartonella systemic infections, page 53.* In immunocompromised (HIV-1, bone marrow transplant) patients *Also see SANFORD GUIDE TO HIV/AIDS THERAPY*	Bartonella henselae and quintana	**Clarithro** 500 mg po bid or ext. release 1 gm po q24h or **azithro** 250 mg po q24h or **CIP** 500–750 mg po bid (see Comment)	**Erythro** 500 mg po qid or **doxy** 100 mg po bid	In immunocompromised pts with severe disease: doxy 100 mg po/IV bid + RIF 300 mg po bid reported effective *(IDC No. Amer 12:37, 1998; Adv PID 11:1, 1996)*.
Bite: Remember tetanus prophylaxis—*see Table 20.* **See Table 20D for rabies prophylaxis**				
Bat, raccoon, skunk	Strep & staph from skin; rabies	**AM-CL** 875/125 mg po bid or 500/125 mg po tid	**Doxy** 100 mg po bid	In Americas, **antirabies rx indicated**: rabies immune globulin + vaccine. (See, Table 20D, page 191)
Cat: 80% get infected, culture & treat empirically.	**Pasteurella multocida**, Staph. aureus	**AM-CL** 875/125 mg po bid or 500/125 mg po tid	**Cefuroxime axetil** 0.5 gm po q12h or **doxy** 100 mg po bid. **Do not use cephalexin.** Sens. to FQs in vitro.	**P. multocida resistant to dicloxacillin, cephalexin, clinda; many strains resistant to erythro** (most sensitive to azithro but no clinical data). P. multocida infection develops within 24 hrs. Observe for osteomyelitis. If culture + for only P. multocida, can switch to pen G IV or pen VK po. See Dog Bite.
Cat-scratch disease: *page 43*				
Catfish sting	Toxins	See *Comments*		Presents as immediate pain, erythema and edema. Resembles strep cellulitis. May become secondarily infected; AM-CL is reasonable choice for prophylaxis.
Dog: Only 5% get infected; treat only if bite severe or bad co-morbidity (e.g. diabetes).	**P. multocida**, S. aureus, Bacteroides sp., Fusobacterium sp., EF-4, Capnocytophaga	**AM-CL** 875/125 mg po bid or 500/125 mg po tid	**Clinda** 300 mg po qid + **FQ** (adults) or **clinda** + **TMP-SMX** (children)	Consider antirabies prophylaxis: rabies immune globulin + vaccine (*TABLE 20B*). Capnocytophaga in splenectomized pts may cause local eschar, sepsis with DIC. **P. multocida resistant to diclox, cephalexin, clinda and erythro**; sensitive to ceftriaxone, cefuroxime, cefprodoxime and FQs.

Abbreviations on page 3.   *NOTE: All dosage recommendations are for adults (unless otherwise indicated) and assume normal renal function.*

TABLE 1A (45)

ANATOMIC SITE/DIAGNOSIS/ MODIFYING CIRCUMSTANCES	ETIOLOGIES (usual)	SUGGESTED REGIMENS*		ADJUNCT DIAGNOSTIC OR THERAPEUTIC MEASURES AND COMMENTS
		PRIMARY	ALTERNATIVE§	
SKIN/Bite (continued)				
Human For bacteriology, see CID 37:1481, 2003	Viridans strep 100%, Staph epidermidis 53%, coryne-bacterium 41%, **Staph. aureus 29%, eikenella 15%**, bacteroides 82%, peptostrep 26%	**Early** (not yet infected): **AM-CL** 875/125 mg po bid times 5 days. **Later:** Signs of infection (usually in 3–24 hrs): **(AM-SB** 1.5 gm IV q6h or **cefoxitin** 2 gm IV q8h) or **(TC-CL** 3.1 gm IV q6h) or **(PIP-TZ** 3.375 gm IV q6h or 4.5 gm q8h or 4-hr infusion of 3.375 gm q8h). Pen allergy: **Clinda** + (either **CIP** or **TMP-SMX**)		Cleaning, irrigation and debridement most important. For clenched fist injuries, x-rays should be obtained. Bites inflicted by hospitalized pts, consider aerobic Gm-neg. bacilli. **Eikenella resistant to clinda, nafcillin/oxacillin, metro, P Ceph 1, and erythro; susceptible to FQs and TMP-SMX.**
Pig (swine)	Polymicrobic: Gm+ cocci, Gm-neg, bacilli, anaerobes, Pasteurella sp.	**AM-CL** 875/125 mg po bid	**P Ceph 3** or **TC-CL** or **AM-SB** or **IMP**	Information limited but infection is common and serious (Ln 348:888, 1996).
Prairie dog	Monkeypox	See Table 14A, page 145. No rx recommended		
Primate, non-human	Microbiology. Herpesvirus simiae	**Acyclovir:** See Table 14B, page 148		CID 20:421, 1995
Rat	Spirillum minus & Strepto-bacillus moniliformis	**AM-CL** 875/125 mg po bid	**Doxy**	Antirabies rx not indicated.
Seal	Marine mycoplasma	Tetracycline times 4 wks		Can take weeks to appear after bite (Ln 364:448, 2004)
Snake: pit viper (Ref.: NEJM 347:347, 2002)	Pseudomonas sp., Enterobacteria-midis, Clostridium sp.	**Primary therapy is antivenom.** Ceftriaxone should be more effective. Tetanus prophylaxis indicated. Ref: CID 43:1309, 2006.		Penicillin generally used but would not be effective vs organisms isolated.
Spider bite: Most necrotic ulcers attributed to spiders are probably due to another cause, e.g., cutaneous anthrax (Ln 364:549, 2004) or **MRSA infection** (spider bite painful; anthrax not painful.)				
Widow (Latrodectus)	Not infectious	None		May be confused with "acute abdomen." Diazepam or calcium gluconate helpful to control pain, muscle spasm. Tetanus prophylaxis.
Brown recluse (Loxosceles) NEJM 352:700, 2005	Not infectious. Overdiagnosed! Spider distribution limited to S. Central & desert SW of US	Bite usually self-limited & self-healing. No therapy of proven efficacy.	**Dapsone** 50 mg po q24h often used despite marginal supportive data	Dapsone causes hemolysis (check for G6PD deficiency). Can cause hepatitis; baseline & weekly liver panels suggested.
Boils—Furunculosis—Subcutaneous abscesses in drug addicts ("skin poppers"). Carbuncles = multiple connecting furuncles; Emergency Dept Perspective (IDC No Amer 22:89, 2008).				
Active lesions See Table 6, page 75 Community-associated MRSA widespread & I&D mainstay of therapy: Ref: CID 46:1032, 2008	Staph. aureus, both MSSA & MRSA—concern for community-associated MRSA (See Comments)	**If afebrile & abscess <5 cm in diameter: I&D**, culture, hot packs. No drugs. **If ≥5 cm in diameter: TMP-SMX-DS** 1-2 tabs po bid times 5-10 days. Alternatives (Adult dosage): **clinda** 300-600 mg po q6-8h or **doxy** or **minocycline** 100 mg po q12h	**Febrile, large &/or multiple abscesses; outpatient care: I&D**, culture abscess & maybe blood, hot packs. **(TMP-SMX-DS** 1-2 tabs po bid) + **RIF** 300 mg bid) times 10 days	Why 1-2 **TMP/SMX-DS**? See discussion Table 6 (MRSA). **TMP/SMX** activity vs streptococci uncertain. Usually clear clinical separation of strep "cellulitis" (erysipelas) from S. aureus abscess. If unclear or strep, use **clinda** or **TMP/SMX** plus **beta-lactam**. **Rifampin** Consider with severe infection after **I&D**, and in combination with **TMP/SMX** (or other drugs). Few days of **TMP/SMP** alone first. Other options: (1) **Linezolid** 600 mg po bid x 10 days; (2) **Fusidic acid**[NUS] 250-500 mg po q8-12h ± **RIF** (CID 42:394, 2006); (3) **FQs** only if in vitro susceptibility known
		Incision and Drainage mainstay of therapy!		
To lessen number of furuncle recurrences	MSSA & MRSA	Guided by in vitro suscep-tibilities: (**Diclox** 500 mg po qid or **TMP-SMX-DS** 1-2 tabs po bid) + **RIF** 300 mg po q12h, all x 10 days	**Plus:** Nasal & under fingernail treatment with **mupirocin ointment** bid (See comment)	**Plus:** Shower with Hibiclens q24h times 3 days & then 3 times per week. Others have tried 5% povidone-iodine cream intranasal qid. times 5 days. Reports of S. aureus resistant to mupirocin. Triple antibiotic ointment is active vs S.epidermis and S.aureus (DMID 54:63, 2006). Mupirocin prophylaxis of non-surgical hosp. pts had no effect on S. aureus infection in placebo-controlled study (AnIM 140:419 & 484, 2004).

Abbreviations on page 3.   NOTE: All dosage recommendations are for adults (unless otherwise indicated) and assume normal renal function.

TABLE 1A (46)

ANATOMIC SITE/DIAGNOSIS/ MODIFYING CIRCUMSTANCES	ETIOLOGIES (usual)	SUGGESTED REGIMENS*		ADJUNCT DIAGNOSTIC OR THERAPEUTIC MEASURES AND COMMENTS
		PRIMARY	ALTERNATIVE§	
SKIN/Boils—Furunculosis—Subcutaneous abscesses in drug addicts (continued)				
Hidradenitis suppurativa	Lesions secondarily infected: S. aureus, Enterobacteriaceae, pseudomonas, anaerobes	Aspirate, base therapy on culture	Many pts ultimately require surgical excision.	Caused by keratinous plugging of apocrine glands of axillary and/or inguinal areas.
Burns. For overall management: NEJM 350:810, 2004—step-by-step case outlined & explained				
Initial burn wound care (CID 37:543, 2003& BMJ 332:649, 2006). Topical therapy options: NEJM 359:1037, 2008.	Not infected	Early excision & wound closure; shower hydrotherapy. Role of topical antimicrobics unclear.	**Silver sulfadiazine** cream, 1%, apply 1–2 times per day or 0.5% **silver nitrate** solution or **mafenide acetate** cream. Apply bid.	Marrow-induced neutropenia can occur during 1st wk of sulfadiazine but resolves even if use is continued. Silver nitrate leaches electrolytes from wounds & stains everything. Mafenide inhibits carbonic anhydrase and can cause metabolic acidosis.
Burn wound sepsis Variety of skin grafts and skin substitutes: see JAMA 283:717, 2000 & Adv Skin Wound Care 18:323, 2005.	Strep. pyogenes, Enterobacter sp., S. aureus, S. epidermidis, E. faecalis, E. coli, P. aeruginosa. Fungi rare. Herpesvirus rare.	(**Vanco** 1 gm IV q12h) + (**amikacin** 10 mg per kg loading dose then 7.5 mg per kg IV q12h) + [**PIP** 4 gm IV q4h (give ½ q24h dose of **piperacillin** into subeschar tissues with surgical eschar removal within 12 hours)]. Can use **PIP-TZ** if PIP not available.		**Monitor serum levels as T½ of most antibiotics ↓.** Staph. aureus tend to remain localized to burn wound; if toxic, consider toxic shock syndrome. Candida sp. colonize but seldom invade. Pneumonia is the major infectious complication, often staph. Complications include septic thrombophlebitis. Dapto (4 mg per kg IV q24h) alternative for vanco.
Cellulitis, erysipelas: Be wary of macrolide (erythro)-resistant) S. pyogenes. Review: NEJM 350:904, 2004. **NOTE:** Consider diseases that masquerade as cellulitis (AnIM 142:47, 2005)				
Extremities, non-diabetic For diabetes, see below	Group A strep, occ. Group B, C, G; Staph. aureus, including MRSA reported.	**Pen G** 1–2 million units IV q6h or (**Nafcillin** or **oxacillin** 2 gm IV q4h). If not severe, **dicloxacillin** 500 mg po q6h or **cefazolin** 1 gm IV q8h. See Comment	**Erythro** or **cefazolin** or **AM-CL** or **azithro** or **clarithro** or **tigecycline** or **dapto** 4 mg/kg/d IV or **ceftobiprole** (CFB) 500 mg IV q12h. (Dosage, see footnote page 31 or Table 10C.)	"Spontaneous" erysipelas of leg in non-diabetic is usually due to strep, Gps A,B,C or G. Hence OK to **start with IV pen G 1–2 million units q6h** & observe for localized S. aureus infection. Look for tinea pedis with fissures, a common portal of entry; can often culture strep from between toes. For rx of pts with lymphedema & recurrent erysipelas, see prophylaxis, Table 15. Reports of CA-MRSA presenting as erysipelas rather than furunculosis. If MRSA is a concern, use empiric **vanco, dapto** or **linezolid**.
Facial, adult (erysipelas)	Group A strep, Staph. aureus (to include MRSA), S. pneumo	**Vanco** 1 gm IV q12h; if over 100 kg, 1.5 gm IV q12h	**Dapto** 4 mg/kg IV q 24h **or Linezolid** 600 mg IV q 12h See Comment	**Choice of empiric therapy must have activity vs S. aureus.** S. aureus erysipelas of face can mimic S. pyogenes erysipelas of an extremity. Forced to treat empirically for MRSA until in vitro susceptibilities available.
Diabetes mellitus and erysipelas (See Foot, "Diabetic", page 15)	Group A strep, Staph. aureus, Enterobacteriaceae; clostridia (rare)	**Early mild: TMP-SMX-DS** 1–2 tabs po bid + **RIF** 300 mg bid po. **For severe disease: IMP** or **MER** or **ERTA** IV + (**linezolid** 600 mg IV/po bid or **vanco** IV or **dapto** 4 mg/kg IV q 24h). Dosage, see page 15, Diabetic foot		Prompt surgical debridement indicated to rule out necrotizing fasciitis and to obtain cultures. If septic, consider x-ray of extremity to demonstrate gas. **Prognosis dependent on blood supply: assess arteries. See diabetic foot, page 15.**
Erysipelas 2° to lymphedema (congenital = Milroy's disease); post-breast surgery with lymph node dissection	S. pyogenes, Groups A, C, G	**Benzathine pen G** 1.2 million units IM q4 wks [of minimal benefit in reducing recurrences in pts with underlying predisposing conditions (CID 25:685, 1997)]		Indicated only if pt is having frequent episodes of cellulitis. Pen V 250 mg po bid should be effective but not aware of clinical trials. In pen-allergic pts: erythro 500 mg po q24h, azithro 250 mg po q24h, or clarithro 500 mg po q24h.
Dandruff (seborrheic dermatitis)	Malassezia species	**Ketoconazole shampoo** 2% or **selenium sulfide** 2.5% (see page 10, chronic external otitis)		
Decubitus or venous stasis or arterial insufficiency ulcers: with sepsis	Polymicrobic: S. pyogenes (Gps A,C,G), enterococci, anaerobic strep, Enterobacteriaceae, Pseudomonas sp. Bacteroides sp., Staph. aureus	**IMP** or **MER** or **DORI** or **TC-CL** or **PIP-TZ** or **ERTA**	**CIP, Levo**, or **Moxi**) + (**clinda** or **metro**)	Without sepsis or extensive cellulitis local care may be adequate. Debride as needed. Topical mafenide or silver sulfadiazine adjunctive. R/O underlying osteomyelitis. May need wound coverage with skin graft or skin substitute (JAMA 283:716, 2000).
		Dosages, see footnotes pages 15, 23, 28, 57		
Erythema multiforme	H. simplex type 1, mycoplasma, Strep. pyogenes, drugs (sulfonamides, phenytoin, penicillins)			**Rx: Acyclovir** if due to H. simplex

Abbreviations on page 3.   NOTE: All dosage recommendations are for adults (unless otherwise indicated) and assume normal renal function.

TABLE 1A (47)

ANATOMIC SITE/DIAGNOSIS/ MODIFYING CIRCUMSTANCES	ETIOLOGIES (usual)	SUGGESTED REGIMENS*		ADJUNCT DIAGNOSTIC OR THERAPEUTIC MEASURES AND COMMENTS
		PRIMARY	ALTERNATIVE§	
SKIN (continued)				
Erythema nodosum	Sarcoidosis, inflammatory bowel disease, M. tbc, coccidioidomycosis, yersinia, sulfonamides			**Rx: NSAIDs; glucocorticoids** if refractory.
Erythrasma	Corynebacterium minutissimum	**Erythro** 250 mg po q6h times 14 days		Coral red fluorescence with Wood's lamp. Alt: 2% aqueous clinda topically.
Folliculitis	Many etiologies: S. aureus, candida, P. aeruginosa, malassezia, demadex	See *individual entities.* See *Whirlpool folliculitis, page 52.*		
Furunculosis	Staph. aureus	See *Boils, page 49*		
Hemorrhagic bullous lesions Hx of sea water-contaminated abrasion or eating raw seafood, shock	**Vibrio vulnificus, V. damsela** (CID 37:272, 2003)	**Ceftazidime** 2 gm IV q8h + **doxy** 100 mg IV/po bid	Either **cefotaxime** 2 gm IV q8h or (**CIP** 750 mg po bid or 400 mg IV bid)	¾ pts have chronic liver disease with mortality in 50% (NEJM 312:343, 1985). In Taiwan, where a number of cases are seen, the impression exists that ceftazidime is superior to tetracyclines (CID 15:271, 1992), hence both.
Herpes zoster (shingles): See Table 14				
Impetigo, ecthyma—usually children "Honey-crust" lesions (non-bullous)	**Group A strep impetigo**; crusted lesions can be Staph. aureus + streptococci	Mupirocin ointment 2% tid or fusidic acid cream^(NUS) 2% times 7–12 days or retapamulin ointment, 1% bid times 5 days *For dosages, see Table 10C for adults and Table 16, page 178 for children*	**Azithro** or **clarithro** or **erythro** or **O Ceph 2**	In meta-analysis that combined strep & staph impetigo, mupirocin had higher cure rates than placebo. Mupirocin superior to oral erythro. Penicillin inferior to erythro. Few placebo-controlled trials. Ref.: *Cochrane Database Systemic Reviews, 2004 (2): CD003261.*
Bullous (if ruptured, thin "varnish-like" crust)	**Staph. aureus impetigo** MSSA & MRSA	**For MSSA:** po therapy with **dicloxacillin, oxacillin, cephalexin, AM-CL, azithro, clarithro,** or **mupirocin** ointment or **retapamulin** ointment	**For MRSA: Mupirocin** ointment or po therapy with, **TMP-SMX-DS, minocycline, doxy, clinda**	46% of USA-300 CA-MRSA isolates carry gene encoding resistance to Mupirocin (Ln 367:731, 2006). **Note:** While resistance to Mupirocin continues to evolve, over-the-counter triple antibiotic ointment (Neomycin, polymyxin B, Bacitracin) remains effective (DMID 54:63, 2006).
Infected wound, extremity—Post-trauma *(for bites, see page 48; for post-operative, see below)*—**Gram stain negative**		*For dosages, see Table 10C*	**—Gram stain negative**	
Mild to moderate; uncomplicated	Polymicrobic: S. aureus (MSSA & MRSA), Group A & anaerobic strep, Enterobacteriaceae, Cl. Perfringens, Cl. tetani; if water exposure, Pseudomonas sp., Aeromonas sp. Acinetobacter in soldiers in Iraq (see CID 47:444, 2008).	**TMP-SMX-DS** 1-2 tabs po bid or **clinda** 300–450 mg po tid (see Comment)	**Minocycline** 100 mg po bid or **linezolid** 600 mg po bid (see Comment)	**Culture & sensitivity, check Gram stain. Tetanus toxoid if indicated. Mild infection:** Suggested drugs focus on S. aureus & Strep species. If suspect Gm-neg. bacilli, add **AM-CL-ER** 1000/62.5 two tabs po bid. If MRSA is erythro-resistant, may have inducible resistance to clinda.
Febrile with sepsis—hospitalized In random double-blind trial, ceftibiprole as effective as vanco + ceftaz (CID 46:647, 2008).		[**AM-SB** or **TC-CL** or **PIP-TZ** or **DORI**^(NFDA-1) or **IMP** or **MER** or **ERTA** (*Dosage, page 23*)] + **vanco** 1 gm IV q12h	**Vanco** 1 gm IV q12h or **dapto** 6 mg/kg IV q 24h or **ceftobiprole** 500 mg IV q8h (2-hr infusion) if mixed gm-neg & gm-pos; q12h over 1 hr. if only gm-pos) + (**CIP** or **Levo** IV—dose in Comment)	**Fever—sepsis:** Another alternative is **linezolid** 600 mg IV/po q12h. If Gm-neg. bacilli & severe pen allergy, **CIP** 400 mg IV q12h (q8h if P. aeruginosa) or **Levo** 750 mg IV q24h. Why 1-2 **TMP/SMX-DS**? See discussion Table 6 (MRSA). **TMP/SMX** not predictably active vs strep species. Another option: **telavancin**^(INV) 10 mg/kg IV q24h if S. aureus a concern.

Abbreviations on page 3.   NOTE: All dosage recommendations are for adults (unless otherwise indicated) and assume normal renal function.

TABLE 1A (48)

ANATOMIC SITE/DIAGNOSIS/ MODIFYING CIRCUMSTANCES	ETIOLOGIES (usual)	SUGGESTED REGIMENS*		ADJUNCT DIAGNOSTIC OR THERAPEUTIC MEASURES AND COMMENTS
		PRIMARY	ALTERNATIVE§	
SKIN (continued)				
Infected wound, post-operative—Gram stain negative: for Gram stain positive cocci – see below				
Surgery not involving GI or female genital tract				
Without sepsis (mild)	Staph. aureus, Group A, B, C or G strep	**TMP-SMX-DS** 1-2 tabs po bid	**Clinda** 300–450 mg po tid	Check Gram stain of exudate. If Gm-neg. bacilli, **add** β-lactam/β-lactamase inhibitor: AM-CL-ER po or (ERTA or PIP-TZ or TC-CL) IV. *Dosage on page 23.* Why 1-2 **TMP/SMX-DS**? See discussion Table 6 (MRSA) **TMP/SMX** not predictably active vs strep species.
With sepsis (severe)		**Vanco** 1 gm IV q12h; if >100 kg, 1.5 gm q12h.	**Dapto** 6 mg per kg IV q24h or **ceftobiprole** 500 mg IV q12h (1-hr infusion)	
Surgery involving GI tract (includes oropharynx, esophagus) or female genital tract—fever, neutrophilia	MSSA/MRSA, coliforms, bacteroides & other anaerobes	**[PIP-TZ** or (**P Ceph 3** + **metro** or **DORI** or **ERTA** or **IMP** or **MER]** + (**vanco** 1 gm IV q12h or **dapto** 6 mg/kg IV q 24h) **if severely ill.** **Mild infection: AM-CL-ER** 2 tabs po bid. Add **TMP-SMX-DS** 1-2 tabs po bid if Gm+ cocci on Gram stain. *Dosages Table 10C & footnote.*		For all treatment options, see *Peritonitis, page 44.* Most important: Drain wound & get cultures. Can sub **linezolid** for vanco. Can sub **CIP or Levo** for β-lactams. Why 2 **TMP/SMX-DS**? See *discussion Table 6 (MRSA)*
Meleney's synergistic gangrene *See Necrotizing fasciitis, page 52*				
Infected wound, febrile patient—Gram stain: Gram-positive cocci in clusters	S. aureus, possibly MRSA	**Do culture & sensitivity** **Oral: TMP-SMX-DS** 1-2 tabs po bid or **clinda** 300–450 mg po tid (see Comment)	**IV: Vanco** 1 gm IV q12h or **dapto** 4 mg/kg IV q24h or 6 mg/kg q24h	Need culture & sensitivity to verify MRSA. Other po options for CA-MRSA inc minocycline 100 mg po q12h (inexpensive) & linezolid 600 mg po q12h (expensive). If MRSA clinda-sensitive but erythro-resistant, watch out for inducible clinda resistance. Other IV alternatives: **tigecycline** 100 mg times 1 dose, then 50 mg IV q12h; **ceftobiprole** 500 mg IV q12h; **telavancin**[IV] 10 mg/kg IV q24h.
Necrotizing fasciitis ("flesh-eating bacteria") Post-surgery, trauma, streptococcal skin infections *See Gas gangrene, page 43, & Toxic shock, pages 58–59 Ref.: CID 44:705, 2007*	**4 types:** (1) Streptococci, Grp A, C, G; (2) Clostridia sp.; (3) polymicrobic: aerobic + anaerobic (if S. aureus + anaerobic strep = Meleney's synergistic gangrene); (4) Community- associated MRSA	*For treatment of clostridia, see Muscle, gas gangrene, page 43.* The terminology of **polymicrobic** wound infections is not precise: Meleney's synergistic gangrene, Fournier's gangrene, necrotizing fasciitis have common pathophysiology. **All require prompt surgical debridement** + antibiotics. Dx of necrotizing fasciitis req incision & probing. If no resistance to probing subcut (fascial plane), diagnosis = necrotizing fasciitis. **Need Gram stain/culture** to determine if etiology is strep. clostridia, polymicrobial, or S. aureus. **Treatment: Pen G** if strep or clostridia; **DORI**[NFDA⁻], **IMP** or **MER** if polymicrobial, add **vanco OR dapto** if MRSA suspected. **NOTE:** If strep necrotizing fasciitis, reasonable to treat with penicillin & clinda; if clostridia ± gas gangrene, add clinda to penicillin *(see page 43).* MRSA ref.: *NEJM 352:1445, 2005*		
Puncture wound—nail	Through tennis shoe: P. aeruginosa	Local debridement to remove foreign body & tetanus prophylaxis		Osteomyelitis evolves in only 1–2% of plantar puncture wounds.
Staphylococcal scalded skin syndrome Ref.: *PIDJ 19:819, 2000*	Toxin-producing S. aureus	**Nafcillin** or **oxacillin** 2 gm IV q4h (children: 150 mg/kg/day div. q6h) x 5–7 days for MSSA; **vanco** 1 gm IV q12h (children 40–60 mg/kg/day div. q6h) for MRSA		Toxin causes **intraepidermal split** and positive Nikolsky sign. Biopsy differentiates: drugs cause epiderm/dermal split, **called toxic epidermal necrolysis—**more serious *(Ln 351:1417, 1998).* Biopsy differentiates.
Ulcerated skin lesions	Consider: anthrax, tularemia, P. aeruginosa (ecthyma gangrenosum), plague, blastomycosis, venous stasis, and others.	Usually self-limited, treatment not indicated		Consider: anthrax, tularemia, P. aeruginosa (ecthyma gangrenosum), plague, blastomycosis, leishmania, mycobacteria, arterial insufficiency, venous stasis, and others.
Whirlpool (Hot Tub) folliculitis *See Folliculitis, page 51*	Pseudomonas aeruginosa	Usually self-limited, treatment not indicated		Decontaminate hot tub: drain and chlorinate. Also associated with exfoliative beauty aids (loofah sponges).

Abbreviations on page 3.   *NOTE: All dosage recommendations are for adults (unless otherwise indicated) and assume normal renal function.*

TABLE 1A (49)

ANATOMIC SITE/DIAGNOSIS/ MODIFYING CIRCUMSTANCES	ETIOLOGIES (usual)	SUGGESTED REGIMENS*		ADJUNCT DIAGNOSTIC OR THERAPEUTIC MEASURES AND COMMENTS
		PRIMARY	ALTERNATIVE§	
SPLEEN. For post-splenectomy prophylaxis, see *Table 15B, page 169*; for *Septic Shock Post-Splenectomy, see Table 1, pg 58.*				
Splenic abscess				
Endocarditis, bacteremia	Staph. aureus, streptococci	**Nafcillin** or **oxacillin** 2 gm IV q4h if MSSA	**Vanco** 1 gm IV q12h if MRSA	Burkholderia (Pseudomonas) pseudomallei is common cause of splenic abscess in SE Asia.
Contiguous from intra-abdominal site	Polymicrobic	*Treat as Peritonitis, secondary, page 44*		
Immunocompromised	Candida sp.	**Amphotericin B** *(Dosage, see Table 11, page 99)*	**Fluconazole, caspofungin**	
SYSTEMIC FEBRILE SYNDROMES				
Spread by infected **TICK, FLEA, or LICE**: Epidemiologic history crucial. **Babesiosis, Lyme disease, & Anaplasma (Ehrlichiosis)** have same reservoir & tick vector.				
Babesiosis: see *CID 43:1089, 2006*. Do not treat if asymptomatic, young, has spleen, and immunocompetent; can be fatal in lymphoma pts *(CID 46:370, 2008)*.	Etiol.: B. microti et al. Vector: Usually Ixodes ticks Host: White-footed mouse & others	[**(Atovaquone** 750 mg po q12h) + (**azithro** 500 mg po day 1, then 250 mg per day) times 7 days] OR [**clinda** 1.2 gm IV bid or 600 mg po tid times 7 days + **quinine** 650 mg po tid times 7 days. **Ped. dosage: Clinda** 20–40 mg per kg per day and **quinine** 25 mg per kg per day] plus **exchange transfusion**		Seven diseases with pathogen visible in peripheral blood smear: African/American trypanosomiasis; babesia; bartonellosis; filariasis; malaria; relapsing fever. Dx: Giemsa-stained blood smear; antibody test available. PCR under study. **Rx: Exchange transfusions successful adjunct, used early, in severe disease.**
Bartonella infections: *CID 35:684, 2002*; for *B. Quintana – EID 12:217, 2006*; Review *EID 12:389, 2006*				
Asymptomatic bacteremia	B. quintana	**Doxy** 100 mg po/IV times 15 days		Can lead to endocarditis &/or trench fever: found in homeless, esp. if lice/leg pain.
Cat-scratch disease	B. henselae	**Azithro** or symptomatic only—*see page 43*: usually lymphadenitis, can involve CNS, liver in immunocompetent pts		
Bacillary angiomatosis; Peliosis hepatis—pts with AIDS	B. henselae, B. quintana	(**Clarithro** 500 mg bid or **clarithro ER** 1 gm po q24h or **azithro** 250 mg po q24h or **CIP** 500–750 mg po bid) times 8 wks	(**Erythro** 500 mg po qid or **doxy** 100 mg po bid) times 8 wks or if severe, combination of **doxy** 100 mg po/IV bid + **RIF** 300 mg po bid	**Manifestations of Bartonella infections: Immunocompetent Patient:** Bacteremia/endocarditis/FUO encephalitis Cat scratch disease Vertebral osteo Trench fever Parinaud's oculoglandular syndrome **HIV/AIDS Patient:** Bacillary angiomatosis Bacillary peliosis Bacteremia/endocarditis/FUO
Bacteremia, immunocompetent pts	Blood PCR for B. henselae	Mild illness: No treatment	Moderate illness: **Azithro**	Person with arthropod & animal exposure: *EID 13:938, 2007*
Endocarditis *(see page 25) (Circ 111:3167, 2005)*	B. henselae, B. quintana	[**Ceftriaxone** 2 gm IV once daily x 6 wks +**Gentamicin** 1 mg/kg IV q8h x 14 days] with or without **doxy** 100 mg IV/po bid x 6 wks.	**Gentamicin** 1 mg/kg IV q8h x 14 days] with or without **doxy** 100 mg	Hard to detect with automated blood culture systems. Need lysis-centrifugation and/or blind subculture onto chocolate agar at 7 & 14 days. Diagnosis often by antibody titer ≥1:800. NOTE: Only aminoglycosides are bactericidal.
Oroya fever	B. bacilliformis	**CIP** IV or po—*Dosage see Table 10C*	**Chloro** 1 gm IV or po q6h. **RIF** for eruptive phase: *CID 33:772, 2001.*	Oroya fever transmitted by sandfly bite in Andes Mtns. Related Bartonella (B. rochalimae) caused bacteremia, fever and splenomegaly *(NEJM 356:2346 & 2381, 2007)*.
Trench fever (FUO)	B. quintana	**Doxy** 100 mg po bid (doxy alone if **no** endocarditis)		
Ehrlichiosis[47]. CDC def. is one of: (1) 4x ↑ IFA antibody. (2) detection of Ehrlichia DNA in blood or CSF by PCR, (3) visible morulae in WBC and IFA ≥1:64				
Human monocytic ehrlichiosis (HEM) *(MMWR 55(RR-4), 2006; CID 43:1089, 2006)*	Ehrlichia chaffeensis (Lone Star tick is vector)	**Doxy** 100 mg po/IV bid times 7–14 days	**Tetracycline** 500 mg po qid x 7–14d. No current rec. for children or pregnancy	30 states: mostly SE of line from NJ to Ill. to Missouri to Oklahoma to Texas. History of outdoor activity and tick exposure. April-Sept. Fever, rash (36%), leukopenia and thrombocytopenia. Blood smears no help. PCR for early dx.

[47] In endemic area (New York), high % of both adult ticks and nymphs were jointly infected with both Anaplasma (HGE) and B. burgdorferi *(NEJM 337:49, 1997)*.

Abbreviations on page 3.   *NOTE: All dosage recommendations are for adults (unless otherwise indicated) and assume normal renal function.*

TABLE 1A (50)

ANATOMIC SITE/DIAGNOSIS/ MODIFYING CIRCUMSTANCES	ETIOLOGIES (usual)	SUGGESTED REGIMENS* PRIMARY	ALTERNATIVE§	ADJUNCT DIAGNOSTIC OR THERAPEUTIC MEASURES AND COMMENTS
SYSTEMIC FEBRILE SYNDROMES/Spread by infected TICK, FLEA, or LICE/Ehrlichiosis			*(continued)*	
Human Anaplasmosis (formerly known as Human granulocytic ehrlichiosis)	Anaplasma (Ehrlichia) phagocytophilum (Ixodes sp. ticks are vector). Dog variant is Ehrlichia ewingii (NEJM 341:148 & 195, 1999)	**Doxy** 100 mg bid po or IV times 7–14 days	**Tetracycline** 500 mg po qid times 7–14 days. Not in children or pregnancy See Comment	Upper Midwest, NE, West Coast & Europe. H/O tick exposure. April-Sept. Febrile flu-like illness after outdoor activity. No rash. Leukopenia/ thrombocytopenia common. **Dx:** Up to 80% have + blood smear. Antibody test for confirmation. **Rx:** RIF successful in pregnancy (CID 27:213, 1998) but worry about resistance developing. Based on in vitro studies, no clear alternative rx— Levo activity marginal (AAC 47:413, 2003).
Lyme Disease NOTE: Think about concomitant tick-borne disease—e.g., babesiosis, ehrlichiosis or Lyme. **Guideline CID 43:1089, 2006.**				
Bite by ixodes-infected tick in an endemic area	Borrelia burgdorferi **ISDA guideline CID 43:1089, 2006**	**If endemic area,** if nymphal partially engorged deer tick: **doxy** 200 mg po times 1 dose with food	**If not endemic area,** not engorged, not deer tick: No treatment	Prophylaxis study in endemic area: erythema migrans developed in 3% of the control group and 0.4% doxy group (NEJM 345:79 & 133, 2001).
Early (erythema migrans) See Comment	Western blot diagnostic criteria: **IgM**—Need 2 of 3 positive of kiladaltons (KD): 23, 39, 41	**Doxy** 100 mg po bid, or **amoxicillin** 500 mg po tid or **cefuroxime axetil** 500 mg po bid times 14–21 days	**Doxy** 100 mg po tid or **cefuroxime axetil** 500 mg po bid or **erythro** 250 mg po qid. All regimens for 14–21 days. (10 days as good as 20: AnIM 138:697, 2003) See Comment for peds doses	High rate of clinical failure with azithro & erythro (Drugs 57:157, 1999) **Peds** (all po for 14–21 days): **Amox** 50 mg per kg per day in 3 div. doses or **cefuroxime axetil** 30 mg per kg per day in 2 div. doses or **erythro** 30 mg per. kg per day in 3 div. doses. Lesions usually homogenous—not target-like (AnIM 136:423, 2002).
Carditis See Comment	**IgG**—Need 5 of 10 positive of KD: 18, 21, 28, 30, 39, 41, 45, 58, 66, 93	**(Ceftriaxone** 2 gm IV q24h) or **(cefotaxime** 2 gm IV q4h) or **(pen G** 24 million units IV q24h) times 14–21 days	**Doxy** (see Comments) 100 mg po bid times14–21 days or **amoxicillin** 500 mg po tid times14–21 days.	First degree AV block: Oral regimen. High degree AV block (PR >0.3 sec.): IV therapy—permanent pacemaker not necessary.
Facial nerve paralysis (isolated finding, early)	For chronic lyme disease discussion see: CID 45:143, 2007	**(Doxy** 100 mg po bid) or **(amoxicillin** 500 mg po) tid times 14–21 days	**Ceftriaxone** 2 gm IV q24h times 14–21 days	LP suggested to exclude neurologic disease. If LP neg., oral regimen OK. If abnormal or not done, suggest parenteral regimen.
Meningitis, encephalitis For encephalopathy, see Comment		**Ceftriaxone** 2 gm IV q24h times 14–28 days	**(Pen G** 20 million units IV q24h in div. dose) or **(cefotaxime** 2 gm IV q8h) times 14–28 days	Encephalopathy: memory difficulty, depression, somnolence, or headache, CSF abnormalities. 89% had objective CSF abnormalities. 18/18 pts improved with ceftriaxone 2 gm per day times 30 days (JID 180:377, 1999). No compelling evidence that prolonged treatment has any benefit in post-Lyme syndrome (Neurology 69:1, 2007).
Arthritis		**(Doxy** 100 mg po bid) or **amoxicillin** 500 mg po qid), both times 30–60 days. Choice should **not** include doxy; **amoxicillin** 500 mg po tid times 21 days.	**(Ceftriaxone** 2 gm IV q24h) or **pen G** 20–24 million units per day IV) times 14–28 days	
Pregnant women			**If pen. allergic: (azithro** 500 mg po q24h times 7–10 days) or **(erythro** 500 mg po qid times 14–21 days)	
Asymptomatic seropositivity and symptoms post-rx		None indicated		No benefit from treatment (NEJM 345:85, 2001).
Relapsing fever (EID 12:369, 2006)	Borrelia recurrentis, B. hermsii, & other borrelia sp.	**Doxy** 100 mg po bid	**Erythro** 500 mg po qid	Jarisch-Herxheimer (fever, ↑ pulse, ↑ resp., ↓ blood pressure) in most patients (occurs in ~2 hrs). Not prevented by prior steroids. **Dx: Examine peripheral blood smear during fever for spirochetes.** Can relapse up to 10 times. Post-exposure **doxy** pre-emptive therapy highly effective (NEJM 355:148, 2006)

Abbreviations on page 3.   *NOTE: All dosage recommendations are for adults (unless otherwise indicated) and assume normal renal function.*

TABLE 1A (51)

ANATOMIC SITE/DIAGNOSIS/ MODIFYING CIRCUMSTANCES	ETIOLOGIES (usual)	SUGGESTED REGIMENS*		ADJUNCT DIAGNOSTIC OR THERAPEUTIC MEASURES AND COMMENTS
		PRIMARY	ALTERNATIVE§	
SYSTEMIC FEBRILE SYNDROMES. Spread by infected **TICK, FLEA or LICE/Relapsing fever** *(continued)*				
Rickettsial diseases. Review—Disease in travelers *(CID 39:1493, 2004)*				
Spotted fevers (NOTE: Rickettsial pox not included)				
Rocky Mountain spotted fever (RMSF) *(LnID 7:724, 2007 and MMWR 55 (RR-4), 2007)*	R. rickettsii (Dermacentor ticks)	**Doxy** 100 mg po/IV bid times 7 days or for 2 days after temp. normal	**Chloro** use found as risk factor for fatal RMSF *(JID 184:1437, 2001)*	Fever, rash (95%), petechiae 40–50%. **Rash spreads from distal extremities to trunk.** Dx: Immunohistology on skin biopsy; confirmation with antibody titers. Highest incidence in Mid-Atlantic states; also seen in Oklahoma, S. Dakota, Montana. **NOTE: Only 3–18% of pts present with fever, rash, and hx of tick exposure; esp. in children many early deaths & empiric doxy reasonable** *(MMWR 49: 888, 2000).*
NOTE: Can mimic ehrlichiosis. Pattern of rash important—*see Comment*				
Other spotted fevers, e.g., Boutonneuse fever: *LnID 3:557, 2003*	6 species: R. conorii et al. (multiple ticks). In sub-Saharan Africa, R. africae	**Doxy** 100 mg po bid times 7 days	**Chloro** 500 mg po/IV qid times 7 days Children <8 y.o.: **azithro** or **clarithro** *(see Comment)*	Clarithro 7.5 mg per kg q12h & azithro 10 mg per kg per day times 1 for 3 days equally efficacious in children with Mediterranean spotted fever *(CID 34:154, 2002)*. R. africae review: *CID 36:1411, 2003.* R. parkeri in U.S: *CID 47:1188, 2008.*
Typhus group—Consider in returning travelers with fever				
Louse-borne: epidemic typhus Ref: *LnID 8:417, 2008.*	R. prowazekii (body louse)	**Doxy** 100 mg IV/po bid times 7 days	**Chloro** 500 mg IV/po qid times 7 days	**Brill-Zinsser disease** *(Ln 357:1198, 2001)* is a relapse of remote past infection, e.g., WW II. Truncal rash spreads centrifugally—opposite of RMSF. A winter disease.
Murine typhus (cat flea typhus similar): *EID 14:1019, 2008*	R. typhi (rat reservoir and flea vector) *CID 46:913, 2008*	**Doxy** 100 mg IV/po bid times 7 days	**Chloro** 500 mg IV/po qid times 7 days	Most U.S. cases south Texas and southern Calif. Flu-like illness. Pox rash in <50%. Dx based on suspicion; confirmed serologically.
Scrub typhus	O. tsutsugamushi [rodent reservoir; vector is larval stage of mites (chiggers)]	**Doxy** 100 mg IV/po bid times 7 days. NOTE: Reports of doxy and chloro resistance from northern Thailand *(Ln 348:86, 1996).* In prospective random trial, single 500 mg dose of **azithro** as effective as **doxy** *(AAC 51:3259, 2007).*		Limited to Far East (Asia, India). Cases imported into U.S. Evidence of chigger bite; flu-like illness. Rash like louse-borne typhus. **RIF** alone 450 mg po times 7 days reported effective *(Ln 356:1057, 2000).* Worry about RIF resistance.
Tularemia, typhoidal type Ref. **bioterrorism**: *see Table 1B, page 62, & JAMA 285:2763, 2001*	Francisella tularensis. (Vector depends on geography; ticks, biting flies, mosquitoes identified)	**Gentamicin or tobra** 5 mg per kg per day div. q8h IV times 7–14 days	Add **chloro** if evidence of meningitis. **CIP** reported effective in 12 children *(PIDJ 19:449, 2000).*	Typhoidal form in 5–30% pts. No lymphadenopathy. Diarrhea, pneumonia common. Dx: blood cultures. Antibody confirmation. Rx: Jarisch-Herxheimer reaction may occur. Clinical failures with rx with P Ceph 3 *(CID 17:976, 1993).*
Other Zoonotic Systemic Bacterial Febrile Illnesses: Obtain careful epidemiologic history				
Brucellosis Review: *NEJM 352:2325, 2005; Ref on vertebral osteo due to Brucella: CID 46:426, 2008.*				
Adult or child >8 years	Brucella sp. B. abortus—cattle B. suis—pigs B. melitensis—goats B. canis—dogs	[**Doxy** 100 mg po bid times 6 wks + **gentamicin** times 7 days *(see Table 10D, page 96)]* or [**doxy** times 6 wks + **streptomycin** 1 gm IM q24h times 2–3 wks)] *See Comment*	[**Doxy** + **RIF** 600–900 mg po q24h, both times 6 wks] or [**TMP-SMX** 1 DS tab (160 mg TMP) po qid times 6 wks + **gentamicin** times 2 wks]	**Clinical disease:** Protean. Fever in 91%. **Malodorous perspiration almost pathognomic.** Osteoarticular disease in approx. 20%%; epididymitis/orchitis 6%. **Lab:** Mild hepatitis. Leukopenia & relative lymphocytosis. **Diagnosis:** Serology, bone marrow culture, real-time PCR if available. **Treatment:** Drugs must penetrate macrophages & act in acidic milieu. **Pregnancy:** TMP-SMX-DS + RIF reasonable. Prospective random. Study documents **doxy** + 7 days of **gent** as effective as **doxy + streptomycin** x 14 days *(CID 42:1075, 2006).* Review of **FQs** (in combination) as alternative therapy *(AAC 50:22, 2006).*
CDC: All positive rapid serologies require confirmation with Brucella-specific agglutination *(MMWR 57:603, 2008).*				
Child <8 years		**TMP-SMX** 5 mg per kg TMP po q12h times 6 wks + **genta-micin** 2 mg per kg IV/IM q8h times 2 wks		
Leptospirosis *(CID 36:1507 & 1514, 2003; LnID 3:757, 2003)*	Leptospira—in urine of domestic livestock, dogs, small rodents	**Doxy** 100 mg IV/po q12h or **AMP** 0.5–1 gm IV q6h	**Pen G** 1.5 million units IV q6h or **ceftriaxone** 1 gm q24h. Duration: 7 days	**Severity varies.** Two-stage mild anicteric illness to severe icteric disease (Weil's disease) with renal failure and myocarditis. **Rx:** Penicillin, doxy, & cefotaxime of equal efficacy in severe lepto *(CID 39:1417, 2004).*

Abbreviations on page 3.   NOTE: All dosage recommendations are for adults (unless otherwise indicated) and assume normal renal function.

TABLE 1A (52)

ANATOMIC SITE/DIAGNOSIS/ MODIFYING CIRCUMSTANCES	ETIOLOGIES (usual)	SUGGESTED REGIMENS*		ADJUNCT DIAGNOSTIC OR THERAPEUTIC MEASURES AND COMMENTS
		PRIMARY	ALTERNATIVE§	
SYSTEMIC FEBRILE SYNDROMES/Other Zoonotic Systemic Bacterial Febrile Illnesses (continued)				
Salmonella bacteremia (enteric fever most often caused by S. typhi)	Salmonella enteritidis— a variety of serotypes	**CIP** 400 mg IV q12h times 14 days (switch to po 750 mg bid when clinically possible)	**Ceftriaxone** 2 gm IV q24h times 14 days (switch to po **CIP** when possible)	Usual exposure is contaminated poultry and eggs. Many others. Myriad of complications to consider, e.g., mycotic aneurysm (10% of adults over age 50. *AJM 110:60, 2001)*, septic arthritis, osteomyelitis, septic shock. Sporadic reports of resistance to CIP. Ref.: *LnID 5:341, 2005*
Miscellaneous Systemic Febrile Syndromes				
Kawasaki syndrome 6 weeks to 12 yrs of age, peak at 1 yr of age; 85% below age 5. (*Ln 364:533, 2004*)	Acute self-limited vasculitis with ↑ temp., rash, conjunctivitis, stomatitis, cervical adenitis, red hands/feet & coronary artery aneurysms (25% if untreated)	**IVIG** 2 gm per kg over 12 hrs + **ASA** 20-25 mg per kg qid THEN **ASA** 3-5 mg per kg per day po q24h times 6-8 wks	If still febrile after 1st dose of IVIG, some give 2nd dose (*PIDJ 17:1144, 1998*)	IV gamma globulin (2 gm per kg over 10 hrs) in pts rx before 10th day of illness ↓ coronary artery lesions (*Ln 347:1128, 1996*). See *Table 14B, page 138* for IVIG adverse effects. Pulsed steroids of NO value: *NEJM 356:659 & 663, 2007*.
Rheumatic Fever, acute Ref.: *Ln 366:155, 2005* **Prophylaxis** Primary prophylaxis	Post-Group A strep pharyngitis (not Group B, C, or G) (see *Pharyngitis, p. 45*)			(1) Symptom relief: **ASA** 80-100 mg per kg per day in children; 4-8 gm per day in adults. (2) Eradicate Group A strep: **Pen** times 10 days (see *Pharyngitis, page 45*). (3) Start prophylaxis: see below
	Benzathine pen G 1.2 million units IM			**Penicillin** for 10 days, prevents rheumatic fever even when started 7-9 days after onset of illness (*see page 45*). **Alternative: Penicillin V** 250 mg po bid or **sulfadiazine (sulfisoxazole)** 1 gm po q24h or **erythro** 250 mg po bid.
Secondary prophylaxis (previous documented rheumatic fever)	**Benzathine pen G** 1.2 million units IM q3-4 wks			**Duration?** No cardits: 5 yr or age 21, whichever is longer; carditis without residual heart disease: 10 yr; carditis with residual valvular disease: 10 yr since last episode & at least age 40 (*PEDS 96:758, 1995*).
Typhoidal syndrome (typhoid fever, enteric fever) (*Ln 366:749, 2005; LnID 5:623, 2005*) NOTE: In vitro resistance to nalidixic acid often predicts clinical failure of CIP (FQs) (*Ln 366:749, 2005*). Decreased CIP susceptibility in S. paratyphi isolates from S.E. Asia (*CID 46:1656, 2008*).	Salmonella typhi, S. paratyphi	(**CIP** 500 mg po bid times 10 days) or (**ceftriaxone** 2 gm IV q24h times 14 days). If associated shock, give **dexamethasone** a few minutes before antibiotic (See Comment)	**Azithro** 1 gm po day 1, then 500 mg po times 6 days (*AAC 43: 1441, 1999*) or 1 gm po q24h times 5 days (*AAC 44: 1855, 2000*) (See Comment)	**Dexamethasone dose:** 3 mg per kg then 1 mg per kg q6h times 8 doses ↓ mortality (*NEJM 310:82, 1984*). **Complications:** perforation of terminal ileum &/or cecum, osteo, septic arthritis, **mycotic aneurysm** (approx. 10% over age 50, *AJM 110:62, 2001)*, meningitis. **Other rx options:** Controlled trial of CIP vs chloro. Efficacy equivalent. After 5 days, blood culture positive: CIP 18%, chloro 36% (*AAC 47:1727, 2003*). **Children & adolescents: Ceftriaxone** (75 mg per kg per day) and **azithro** (20 mg per kg per day to 1 gm max.) equal efficacy. More relapses with ceftriaxone (*CID 38:951, 2004*).
Sepsis: Following suggested **empiric** therapy assumes pt is bacteremic; mimicked by viral, fungal, rickettsial infections and pancreatitis (*Intensive Care Medicine 34:17, 2008; IDC No Amer 22:1, 2008*).			In children, CIP superior to ceftriaxone (*LnID 3:537, 2003*)	
Neonatal—early onset <1 week old	Group B strep, E. coli, klebsiella, enterobacter, Staph. aureus (uncommon), listeria (rare in U.S.)	**AMP** 25 mg per kg IV q8h + **cefotaxime** 50 mg per kg q12h	(**AMP** + **gent** 2.5 mg per kg IV/IM q12h) or (**AMP** + **ceftriaxone** 50 mg per kg IV/IM q24h)	Blood cultures are key but only 5-10% +. Discontinue antibiotics after 72 hrs if cultures and course do not support diagnosis. In Spain, listeria predominates; in S. America, salmonella.
Neonatal—late onset 1-4 weeks old	As above + H. influenzae & S. epidermidis	(**AMP** 25 mg per kg IV q6h + **cefotaxime** 50 mg per kg q8h) or (**AMP** + **ceftriaxone** 75 mg per kg IV q24h)	**AMP** + **gent** 2.5 mg per kg q8h IV or IM	If MSSA/MRSA a concern, add vanco.
Child; not neutropenic	Strep. pneumoniae, meningococci, Staph. aureus (MSSA & MRSA), H. influenzae now rare	**Cefotaxime** 50 mg per kg IV q8h or **ceftriaxone** 100 mg per kg IV q24h) + **vanco** 15 mg per kg IV q6h	**Aztreonam** 7.5 mg per kg IV q6h + **linezolid** (see *Table 16, page 178 for dose*)	Major concerns are S. pneumoniae & community-associated MRSA. Coverage for Gm-neg. bacilli included but H. influenzae infection now rare. Meningococcemia mortality remains high (*Ln 356:961, 2000*).

Abbreviations on page 3.   NOTE: All dosage recommendations are for adults (unless otherwise indicated) and assume normal renal function.

TABLE 1A (53)

ANATOMIC SITE/DIAGNOSIS/ MODIFYING CIRCUMSTANCES	ETIOLOGIES (usual)	SUGGESTED REGIMENS* PRIMARY	ALTERNATIVE§	ADJUNCT DIAGNOSTIC OR THERAPEUTIC MEASURES AND COMMENTS
SYSTEMIC FEBRILE SYNDROMES/Sepsis (continued)				
Adult; not neutropenic; NO HYPOTENSION but LIFE-THREATENING!—For Septic shock, see page 58 Source unclear—consider intra-abdominal or skin source. **Life-threatening.**	Aerobic Gm-neg. bacilli; S. aureus; streptococci; others	**(DORI** or **ERTA** or **IMP** or **MER) + vanco** Could substitute linezolid for vanco or dapto; however, linezolid bacteriostatic vs S. aureus.	**(Dapto** 6 mg per kg IV q24h) **+ (P Ceph 3/4** or **PIP-TZ** or **TC-CL)** _Dosages in footnote[48]_	Systemic inflammatory response syndrome **(SIRS):** 2 or more of the following: 1. Temperature >38°C or <36°C 2. Heart rate >90 beats per min. 3. Respiratory rate >20 breaths per min. 4. WBC >12,000 per mcL or >10% bands **Sepsis:** SIRS + a documented infection (+ culture) **Severe sepsis:** Sepsis + organ dysfunction: hypotension or hypoperfusion abnormalities (lactic acidosis, oliguria, ↓ mental status) **Septic shock:** Sepsis-induced hypotension (systolic BP <90 mmHg) not responsive to 500 mL IV fluid challenge + peripheral hypoperfusion.
If suspect biliary source (_see p.11_)	Enterococci + aerobic Gm-neg. bacilli	**AM-SB, PIP-TZ,** or **TC-CL**	**P Ceph 3 + metro; (CIP** or **Levo) + metro.** Dosages-footnote[48]	
If community-acquired pneumonia	**S. pneumoniae; MRSA, Legionella, Gm-neg. bacillus**	**(Levo** or **moxi) + (PIP-TZ) + Vanco**	**Aztreonam + (Levo** or **moxi) + linezolid**	Many categories of CAP, _page 36_. Suggestions based on most severe CAP, e.g., MRSA after influenza or Klebsiella pneumonia in an alcoholic.
If illicit use IV drugs	S. aureus	**Vanco** if high prevalence of MRSA.	**Do NOT use empiric vanco + oxacillin pending organism ID.** In vitro nafcillin increased production of toxins by CA-MRSA (_JID 195:202, 2007_). **Dosages—footnote[48]**	
If suspect intra-abdominal source	Mixture aerobic & anaerobic Gm-neg. bacilli	See _secondary peritonitis, page 44_		
If suspect Nocardia	Nocardia sp.	See _haematogenous brain abscess, page 7_		
If petechial rash	Meningococcemia	**Ceftriaxone** 2 gm IV q12h (until sure no meningitis); consider Rocky Mountain spotted fever—_see page 55_		
If suspect urinary source	Aerobic Gm-neg. bacilli & enterococci	See _pyelonephritis, page 31_		
Neutropenia: Child or Adult (absolute PMN count <500 per mm3) in cancer and transplant patients. Guideline: _CID 34:730, 2002_ **Prophylaxis—afebrile**				
Post-chemotherapy—impending neutropenia	Aerobic Gm-neg. bacilli, pneumocystis (PCP)	Meta-analysis demonstrates substantive reduction in mortality with **CIP** 500 mg po bid (_AnIM 142:979, 2005_). Similar results in observational study using **Levo** 500 mg po q24h (_CID 40:1087 & 1094, 2005_). Also _NEJM 353:977, 988 & 1052, 2005._		
Post-chemotherapy in AIDS patient	↑ risk pneumocystis	**TMP-SMX-DS** po once daily—adults; 10 mg per kg per day div bid po—children		Need TMP-SMX to prevent PCP. Hard to predict which leukemia/lymphoma/solid tumor pt at ↑ risk of PCP
Allogeneic hematopoietic stem-cell transplant	↑ risk pneumocystis, herpes viruses, candida	**TMP-SMX** as above + [either **acyclovir** or **ganciclovir**] + **fluconazole]**		Combined regimen justified by combined effect of neutropenia and immuno-suppression.
Empiric therapy—febrile neutropenia (≥38.3°C x 1 or ≥38°C for ≥1 hr) **Low-risk adults** Peds data pending (_Def. low risk in Comment_)	As above	**CIP** 750 mg po bid + **AM-CL** 875 mg po bid	**Treat as outpatients with 24/7 access to inpatient care if: no focal findings, no hypotension, no COPD, no fungal infection, no dehydration, age <60 & >16.**	

[48] **P Ceph 3 (cefotaxime** 2 gm IV q8h, use q4h if life-threatening; **cefotaxime** 2 gm IV q12h), **AP Pen (piperacillin** 3 gm IV q4h, **ceftriaxone** 2 gm IV q4h; **ceftizoxime** 2 gm IV q6h, **Aminoglycosides** (see _Table 10D, page 96_), **AMP** 30 mg per kg IV q4h, **ticarcillin** 3 gm IV q4h), **TC-CL** 3.1 gm IV q4h, **PIP-TZ** 3.375 gm IV q4h or 4-hr infusion of 3.375 gm q8h, **AM-SB** 3 gm IV q6h, **clinda** 900 mg IV q8h, **IMP** 0.5 gm IV q6h, **MER** 1 gm IV q8h, **ERTA** 1 gm q24h, **DORI** 500 mg IV q8h (1-hr infusion), **Nacfillin** or **oxacillin** 2 gm IV q8h), **P Ceph 3 AP (ceftazidime** 2 gm IV q8h), **P Ceph 4 [CFP (cefepime** 2 gm IV q12h, **aztreonam** 2 gm IV q8h, **metro** 1 gm loading dose then 0.5 gm q6h or 1 gm IV q12h, **vanco** 1 gm IV q12h, **cefpirome**[NUS] 2 gm IV q12h], **CIP** 400 mg IV q12h, **levo** 750 mg IV q24h, **linezolid** 600 mg IV q12h.

Abbreviations on page 3. NOTE: _All dosage recommendations are for adults (unless otherwise indicated) and assume normal renal function._

TABLE 1A (54)

ANATOMIC SITE/DIAGNOSIS/ MODIFYING CIRCUMSTANCES	ETIOLOGIES (usual)	SUGGESTED REGIMENS*		ADJUNCT DIAGNOSTIC OR THERAPEUTIC MEASURES AND COMMENTS
		PRIMARY	ALTERNATIVE§	
SYSTEMIC FEBRILE SYNDROMES/Sepsis/Neutropenia: Child or Adult: Empiric therapy—febrile neutropenia (≥38.3°C x 1 or ≥38°C for ≥1 hr) *(continued)*				
High-risk adults and children Oral "mucositis" can falsely elevate oral temperature readings (CID 46:1859, 2008).	Aerobic Gm-neg. bacilli; cephalosporin-resistant viridans strep, MRSA	**Monotherapy:** ceftaz or IMP or MER or CFP or PIP-TZ *Dosages: Footnote[48] page 57 and Table 10* **Include empiric vanco** if: suspect IV access infected; colonized with drug-resistant S. pneumo or MRSA; blood culture pos. for Gm-pos. cocci; pt hypotensive	**Combination therapy:** **(Gent or tobra) + (TC-CL or PIP-TZ)**	Increasing resistance of viridans streptococci to penicillins, cephalosporins & FQs (CID 34:1469 & 1524, 2002). **What if severe IgE-mediated β-lactam allergy?** No formal trials, but [aminoglycoside (or CIP) + aztreonam] ± vanco should work. In meta-analysis of monotherapies, **cefepime** (CFP) associated with higher 30 days all cause mortality; individual pt assessments pending (JAC 57:176, 2006). In another study, PIP-TZ & CFP of equal efficacy (CID 43:447, 2006)
Persistent fever and neutropenia after 5 days of empiric antibacterial therapy—see CID 34:730, 2002—General guidelines	Candida species, aspergillus	Add either **caspofungin** 70 mg IV day 1, then 50 mg IV q24h **OR voriconazole** 6 mg per kg IV q12h times 2 doses, then 3 mg per kg IV q12h		Conventional **ampho B** causes more fever & nephrotoxicity & lower efficacy than lipid-based ampho B; both **caspofungin** & **voriconazole** better tolerated & perhaps more efficacious than lipid-based ampho B (NEJM 346:225, 2002 & 351:1391 & 1445, 2005).
Shock syndromes **Septic shock: Fever & hypo-tension** **Bacteremic shock, endotoxin shock** Antimicrobial therapy: CCM 32 (Suppl):S495, 2004 & Surviving Sepsis Campaign: CCM 36:296, 2008 & Intensive Care Med 34:17, 2008.	Bacteremia with aerobic Gm-neg. bacteria or Gm+ cocci	**Proven therapy: (1) Replete intravascular volume, (2) correct, if possible, disease that allowed bloodstream invasion, (3) appropriate empiric antimicrobial rx:** see *suggestions under life-threatening sepsis, page 56*. **(4)** Decreased indication for recombinant **activated Protein C** (drotrecogin alfa), see Comment. **(5) Low-dose steroids:** No benefit from hydrocortisone, 50 mg IV q6h, regardless of results of ACTH stimulation test (NEJM 358:111, 2008). **(6) Blood glucose control:** Target is unclear: 150-180 mg/dL reasonable. **(7) Vasopressors:** Target MAP of ≥ 65 mm Hg.		**Activ. Protein C: Drotrecogin (Xigris):** In a double-blind placebo-controlled trial (DBPCT) (NEJM 344:699, 2001), 28-days. mortality ↓ from 31 to 25% in sickest pts. In less ill pts (APACHE II score <25) showed no benefit. Xigris not indicated in pts with single organ dysfunction & surgery within last 30 days: evidence of increased mortality (NEJM 353:1332 & 1398, 2005). **Hemorrhage** is major adverse event. **Dose:** 24 mcg per kg per hr over 96 hrs by continuous IV infusion. Stop 2 hrs before & restart 12 hrs after surgery. **Low-dose steroids:** Surviving sepsis campaign endorses only if no response to fluids and vasopressors. **Low-dose vasopressin:** No benefit in trial vs. nor-epinephrine (NEJM 358:877, 2008). **Targeted glucose levels:** Tight plasma glucose control, 80-110 mg/dL, resulted in unacceptable frequency of hypoglycemia (NEJM 358:125, 2008; JAMA 300:933 & 963, 2008). **IVIG:** No clear evidence of benefit (CCM 35:2677, 2686, 2693 & 2852, 2007).
Septic shock: post-splenectomy (asplenia)	S. pneumoniae, N. meningi-tidis, H. influenzae, Capno-cytophaga (DF-2)	**Ceftriaxone** 2 gm IV q24h (↑ to 2 gm q12h if meningitis) *Other management as per Septic shock, above*	**(Levo** 750 mg or **Moxi** 400 mg) all once IV q24h	Howell-Jolly bodies in peripheral blood smear confirm absence of functional spleen. Often results in **symmetrical peripheral gangrene of digits** due to severe DIC. For prophylaxis, see Table 15A, page 168
Toxic shock syndrome, Clostridium sordellii Post-partum, post-abortion, post-mifepristone, IUD CID 43:1436 & 1447, 2006	Clostridium sordellii Mortality 69%!	Fluids, aq. **penicillin G** 18-20 million units per day div. q4-6h + **clindamycin** 900 mg IV q8h		Several deaths reported after use to abortifacient regimen of mifepristone (RU486) & misoprostol. Clinically: often afebrile, rapid progression, hypotension, hemoconcentration (high Hct), neutrophilia. Leukemoid reaction (WBC>50,000) induced by neuraminidase (JID 195:1838, 2007).
Toxic shock syndrome, staphylococcal. Superantigen review: LnID 2:156, 2002 Colonization by toxin-producing Staph. aureus of: vagina (tampon-assoc.), surgical/traumatic wounds, endometrium, burns	Staph. aureus (toxic shock toxin-mediated)	**(Nafcillin** or **oxacillin** 2 gm IV q4h) or (if MRSA, **vanco** 1 gm IV q12h) + **IVIG**	**(Cefazolin** 1–2 gm IV q8h) or (if MRSA, **vanco** 1 gm IV q12h OR **dapto** 6 mg/kg IV q24h) + **IVIG**	**IVIG reasonable** (see Streptococcal TSS)— dose 1 gm IV per kg day 1, then 0.5 gm per kg days 2 & 3—antitoxin antibodies present. If suspect, "turn off" toxin production with clinda; report of success with **linezolid** (JID 195:202, 2007). Exposure of MRSA to nafcillin increased toxin production in vitro: JID 195:202, 2007.

Abbreviations on page 3.   NOTE: All dosage recommendations are for adults (unless otherwise indicated) and assume normal renal function.

TABLE 1A (55)

ANATOMIC SITE/DIAGNOSIS/ MODIFYING CIRCUMSTANCES	ETIOLOGIES (usual)	SUGGESTED REGIMENS*		ADJUNCT DIAGNOSTIC OR THERAPEUTIC MEASURES AND COMMENTS
		PRIMARY	ALTERNATIVE§	
SYSTEMIC FEBRILE SYNDROMES/Shock syndromes (continued)				
Toxic shock syndrome, streptococcal. NOTE: For Necrotizing fasciitis without toxic shock, see page 52				
Associated with invasive disease, i.e., erysipelas, necrotizing fasciitis; secondary strep infection of varicella. Secondary cases TSS reported (NEJM 335:547 & 590, 1996; CID 27:150, 1998).	Group A, B, C, & G Strep. pyogenes	(**Pen G** 24 million units per day IV in div. doses) + (**clinda** 900 mg IV q8h) **IVIG** associated with ↓ in sepsis-related organ failure (CID 37:333 & 341, 2003). IVIG dose: 1 gm per kg day 1, then 0.5 gm per kg days 2 & 3. IVIG preps vary in neutral. Antibody content (CID 43:743, 2006)	**Ceftriaxone** 2 gm IV q24h + **clinda** 900 mg IV q8h	**Definition:** Isolation of Group A strep, hypotension and ≥2 of: renal impairment, coagulopathy, liver involvement, ARDS, generalized rash, soft tissue necrosis (JAMA 269:390, 1993). Associated with invasive disease. **Surgery usually required.** Mortality with fasciitis 30–50%, myositis 80% even with early rx (CID 14:2, 1992). Clinda ↓ toxin production. Use of NSAID may predispose to TSS. For reasons pen G may fail in fulminant S. pyogenes infections (see JID 167:1401, 1993).
Other Toxin-Mediated Syndromes—no fever unless complicated				
Botulism (CID 41:1167, 2005. As **biologic weapon:** JAMA 285:1059, 2001; Table 1B, page 61; www.bt.cdc.gov)				
	C. botulinum	For all types: Follow vital capacity; other supportive care	Trivalent (types A, B, E) equine serum antitoxin—State Health Dept. or CDC (see Comment)	**Equine antitoxin:** Obtain from State Health Depts. or CDC (404-639-2206 M-F OR 404-639-2888 evenings/weekends). Skin test first & desensitize if necessary. One vial IV and one vial IM.
Food-borne Dyspnea at presentation bad sign (CID 43:1247, 2006)		If no ileus, purge GI tract		**Antimicrobials:** May make infant botulism worse. Untested in wound botulism. When used, pen G 10–20 million units per day usual dose. If complications
Infant		Human botulinum immunoglobulin (BIG) IV, single dose. Call 510-540-2646.	No antibiotics; may lyse C. botulinum in gut and ↑ load of toxin	(pneumonia, UTI) occur, avoid antimicrobials with assoc. neuromuscular blockade, i.e., aminoglycosides, tetracycline, polymyxins. **Differential dx:** Guillain-Barré, myasthenia gravis, tick paralysis, organophosphate toxicity, West Nile virus
Wound		Débridement & anaerobic cultures. No proven value of local antitoxin. Role of antibiotics untested.	Trivalent equine antitoxin (see Comment)	Can result from spore contamination of tar heroin. Ref: CID 31:1018, 2000.
Tetanus	C. tetani	(**Pen G** 24 million units per day in div. dose or **doxy** 100 mg IV q12h) times 7–10 days	**Metro** 500 mg po q6h or 1 gm IV q12h times 7–10 days (See Comment)	Multifaceted treatment: Wound debridement, tetanus immunoglobulin (250–500 units IM), antimicrobics & tetanus toxoid (tetanus does not confer immunity). Options for control of muscle spasms: continuous infusion of midazolam, IV propofol, and/or intrathecal baclofen (CID 38:321, 2004).
VASCULAR				
Cavernous sinus thrombosis	Staph. aureus, Group A strep, H. influenzae, aspergillus/mucor/rhizopus	**Vanco** 1 gm IV q12h + **ceftriaxone** 2 gm IV q24h	(**Dapto** 6 mg per kg IV q24hNFDA4 or **linezolid** 600 mg IV q12h) + **ceftriaxone** 2 gm IV q24h	CT or MRI scan for diagnosis. **Heparin indicated.** If patient diabetic with ketoacidosis or post-deferoxamine iron chelation or neutropenic, consider fungal etiology: aspergillus, mucor, rhizopus, see Table 11A, pages 97 & 106.

Abbreviations on page 3.   NOTE: All dosage recommendations are for adults (unless otherwise indicated) and assume normal renal function.

TABLE 1A (56)

ANATOMIC SITE/DIAGNOSIS/ MODIFYING CIRCUMSTANCES	ETIOLOGIES (usual)	SUGGESTED REGIMENS*		ADJUNCT DIAGNOSTIC OR THERAPEUTIC MEASURES AND COMMENTS
		PRIMARY	ALTERNATIVE$	
VASCULAR (continued)				
IV line infection (see LnID 7:645, 2007): **Treatment:** (For Prevention, see below). **Diagnosis of infected line** without removal of IV catheter? See CID 44:820 & 827, 2007.				
Heparin lock, midline catheter, non-tunneled central venous catheter (subclavian, internal jugular), peripherally inserted central catheter (PICC) Avoid femoral vein if possible: ↑ risk of infection and/or thrombosis (JAMA 286:700, 2001)– especially if BMI >28.4 (JAMA 299:2413, 2008)	Staph. epidermidis, Staph. aureus (MSSA/MRSA)	**Vanco** 1 gm IV q12h. **Linezolid alternative—see Comment.** Other rx and duration: **(1) If S. aureus**, remove catheter. Can use TEE result to determine if 2 or 4 wks of therapy (JAC 57:1172, 2006). **(2) If S. epidermidis**, can try to "save" catheter. 80% cure after 7–10 days of therapy. If need to "salvage" the IV line can try "lock" solution of 3 mg/mL of minocycline + 30 mg/mL of EDTA in 25% ethanol. Use 2 mL per catheter lumen; dwell time minimum of 2 hrs (AAC 51:78, 2007). If IV minocycline not available, tigecycline should work but expensive.		If no response to, or intolerant of, **vanco**: switch to **daptomycin** 6 mg per kg IV q24h. **Quinupristin-dalfopristin** an option: 7.5 mg per kg IV q8h via central line. Culture removed catheter. With "roll" method, >15 colonies (NEJM 312:1142, 1985) suggests infection. Lines do not require "routine" changing when not infected. When infected, do not insert new catheter over a wire. Antimicrobial-impregnated catheters may ↓ infection risk; the debate is lively (CID 37:65, 2003 & 38:1287, 2004 & 39:1829, 2004).
Tunnel type indwelling venous catheters and ports (Broviac, Hickman, Groshong, Quinton), dual lumen hemodialysis catheters (Perma-cath). For prevention, see below.	Staph. epidermidis, Staph. aureus. (Candida sp.). Rarely: leuconostoc or lactobacillus—both resistant to vanco (see Table 2, page 63)			If subcutaneous tunnel infected, very low cure rates; need to remove catheter.
Impaired host (burn, neutropenic)	As above + Pseudomonas sp., Enterobacteriaceae, Corynebacterium jeikeium, aspergillus, rhizopus	**(Vanco + P Ceph 3 AP)** or **(vanco + AP Pen)** or **IMP** or **(P Ceph 3 + aminoglycoside)** (Dosage, see page 57)		Usually have associated septic thrombophlebitis: biopsy of vein to rule out fungi. If fungal, surgical excision + amphotericin B. Surgical drainage, ligation or removal often indicated.
Hyperalimentation	As with tunnel, Candida sp. common (see Table 11, resistant Candida species)	If candida, **voriconazole** or an **echinocandin (anidulafungin, micafungin, caspofungin)** if clinically stable. Dosage: see Table 11B, page 108.		Remove venous catheter and discontinue antimicrobial agents if possible. Ophthalmologic consultation recommended. **Rx all patients with + blood cultures.** See Table 11A, Candidiasis, page 99
Intravenous lipid emulsion	Staph. epidermidis Malassezia furfur	**Vanco** 1 gm IV q12h **Fluconazole** 400 mg IV q24h		Discontinue intralipid AJM 90:129, 1991
Prevention of Infection of Long-Term IV Lines NEJM 355:2725 & 2781, 2006; LnID 7:645, 2007	To minimize risk of infection: **Hand washing and** 1. Maximal sterile barrier precautions during catheter insertion 2. Use 2% chlorhexidine for skin antisepsis 3. If infection rate high despite #1 & 2, use either chlorhexidine/silver sulfadiazine or minocycline/rifampin-impregnated catheters or "lock" solutions (see Comment). 4. If possible, use subclavian vein, avoid femoral vessels			**IV line "lock" solutions.** In vitro 25% ethanol + EDTA (30 mg/mL) + minocycline (3 mg/mL) most active. IV minocycline not available. Meta-analysis of 7 prospective randomized trials favored a variety of lock solutions (Am J Kid Dis 51:233, 2008). 70% ethanol/water superior to heparin in prospective randomized double-blind study (JAC 62:809, 2008). In meta-analysis, both topical & intraluminal antibiotics decreased incidence of bacteremia & catheter removal in hemodialysis patients (AnIM 148:596, 2008; CID 47:83, 2008).
Septic pelvic vein thrombophlebitis (with or without septic pulmonary emboli) Postpartum or postabortion or postpelvic surgery	Streptococci; bacteroides, Enterobacteriaceae	**Metro + P Ceph 3; cefoxitin; TC-CL; PIP-TZ;** or **AM-SB** Dosages: Table 10C, page 88	**IMP** or **MER** or **ERTA** or **[clinda + (aztreonam or gent)]**	Use heparin during antibiotic regimen. Continued oral anticoagulation not recommended. Cefotetan less active than cefoxitin vs non-fragilis bacteroides. Cefotetan has methyltetrazole side-chain which is associated with hypoprothrombinemia (prevent with vitamin K).

Abbreviations on page 3.   NOTE: All dosage recommendations are for adults (unless otherwise indicated) and assume normal renal function.

TABLE 1B – PROPHYLAXIS AND TREATMENT OF ORGANISMS OF POTENTIAL USE AS BIOLOGICAL WEAPONS
(See page 3 for abbreviations)

DISEASE	ETIOLOGY	SUGGESTED EMPIRIC TREATMENT REGIMENS		SPECIFIC THERAPY AND COMMENTS
		PRIMARY	**ALTERNATIVE**	
Anthrax **Cutaneous, inhalational, gastrointestinal** Refs.: *NEJM 345:1607 & 1621, 2001; CID 35:851, 2002; AnIM 144:270, 2006* or *www.bt.cdc.gov* *See updated guidelines from a conference summary in on-line version of Emerg Infect Dis; April 2008* *(http://www.cdc.gov/eid/content/14/4/e1.htm)* *See also Table 1A, pages 40 & 48* To report bioterrorism event: 770-488-7100	Bacillus anthracis Post-exposure **prophylaxis**	**Adults (including pregnancy) and children >50 kg: (CIP** 500 mg po bid or **Levo** 500 mg po q24h) times 60 days **Children <50 kg: CIP** 20–30 mg per kg per day div q12h x 60 days or **levo** 8 mg/kg po q12h x 60 days	**Adults (including pregnancy): Doxy** 100 mg po bid times 60 days. **Children** (*see Comment*): **Doxy** >8 y/o & >45 kg: 100 mg po bid; >8 y/o & ≤45 kg: 2.2 mg per kg po bid; ≤8 y/o: 2.2 mg per kg po bid. All for 60 days.	1. Once organism shows susceptibility to penicillin, switch children to **amoxicillin** 80 mg per kg per day div. q8h (max. 500 mg q8h); switch pregnant pt to **amoxicillin** 500 mg po tid. 2. Do **not** use cephalosporins or TMP-SMX. 3. Other **FQs** (Gati, Moxi) & clarithro should work but no clinical experience. 4. CDC also recommends a 3-dose series of anthrax vaccine adsorbed (AVA), BioThrax (BioPort Corporation, Lansing, MI, USA) administered at 2-week intervals. AVA is not FDA-approved for PEP and therefore would be available under an Investigational New Drug (IND) protocol in the event of an act of bioterrorism. 5. A 60 day duration is recommended to prevent late relapse which may occur with inhalational exposure.
	Treatment— **Cutaneous** anthrax Skin lesions not painful	**Adults (including pregnancy):** (**CIP** 500 mg po bid or **Levo** 500 mg po q24h) times 60 days **Children: CIP** 20–30 mg per kg per day div q12h po (to max. 1 gm per day) times 60 days	**Adults (including pregnancy): Doxy** 100 mg po bid times 60 days **Children: Doxy** >8 y/o & >45 kg: 100 mg po bid; >8 y/o & ≤45 kg: 2.2 mg per kg po bid ≤8 y/o: 2.2 mg per kg po bid All for 60 days.	1. If penicillin susceptible, then: **Adults: Amox** 500 mg po q8h times 60 days **Children: Amox** 80 mg per kg per day div. q8h (max. 500 mg q8h) 2. Usual treatment of cutaneous anthrax is 7–10 days; 60 days in setting of bioterrorism with presumed aerosol exposure 3. Other **FQs** (Gati, Levo, Moxi) should work based on in vitro susceptibility data 4. AVA is also recommended in cutaneous disease occurring as a consequence of and act of bioterrorism. 5. Shorter courses of therapy are effective for naturally acquired cutaneous anthrax, but inhalational exposure is presumed to accompany cutaneous anthrax acquired from bioterrorism.

	Treatment—**Inhalational**, gastrointestinal, or oropharyngeal
	
	Characteristic signs & symptoms—**Present**: Dyspnea, N/V; **Absent**: Rhinorrhea, sore throat
		Adults (including pregnancy): (**CIP** 400 mg IV q12h) or **Levo** 500 mg IV q24h) or (**doxy** 100 mg IV q12h) **+ RIF** 300 mg IV q8h **+ clinda** 900 mg IV q8h. Switch to po when able & ↓ **CIP** to 500 mg po bid; **clinda** to 450 mg po q8h; & **RIF** 300 mg po bid.
		Treat times 60 days. See *Table 2, page 63 for other alternatives.*
			Children: (**CIP** 10 mg per kg IV q12h or 15 mg per kg po q12h) or **levo** 8 mg/kg po q12h or (**Doxy** >8 y/o & >45 kg: 100 mg IV q12h; >8 y/o & ≤45 kg: 2.2 mg per kg IV q12h; ≤8 y/o: 2.2 mg per kg IV q12h) **plus clindamycin** 7.5 mg per kg IV q6h **plus RIF** 20 mg per kg (max. 600 mg) IV qd. Treat times 60 days. See *Table 16, page 178 for oral dosage.*	1. Clinda may block toxin production.
				2. Rifampin penetrates CSF & intracellular sites.
				3. If isolate shown penicillin-susceptible:
				  a. **Adult: Pen G** 4 million units IV q4h
				  b. **Child: Pen G** <12 y/o: 50,000 units per kg IV q6h; >12 y/o: 4 million units IV q4h
				  c. Constitutive & inducible β-lactamases—do not use pen or AMP alone.
				4. Do not use cephalosporins or TMP-SMX.
				5. Meropenem also has good CNS penetration.
				6. Drainage of pleural effusions recommended.
				7. Erythro, azithro activity borderline; clarithro active.
				8. No person-to-person spread.

Botulism: *CID 41:1167, 2005; JAMA 285:1059, 2001* **Food-borne** *See Table 1A, page 59*	Clostridium botulinum	Purge GI tract if no ileus. **Trivalent antitoxin** (types A, B, & E): single 10 mL vial per pt. diluted in saline IV (slowly)	Antibiotics have no effect on toxin. Call state health dept for antitoxin.	Supportive care for all types. Follow vital capacity. Submit suspect food for toxin testing. Ref.: *www.bt.cdc.gov*

TABLE 1B (2)

DISEASE	ETIOLOGY	SUGGESTED EMPIRIC TREATMENT REGIMENS		SPECIFIC THERAPY AND COMMENTS
		PRIMARY	ALTERNATIVE	
Hemorrhagic fever viruses Ref.: *JAMA 287:2391, 2002* *See Table 14, page 137*	Ebola, Lassa, Hanta, yellow fever, & others	Fluid/electrolyte balance. Optimize circulatory volume.	For Lassa & Hanta: **Ribavirin** dose same as Adults. Pregnancy. Children: LD 30 mg per kg (max. 2 gm) IV times 1, then 16 mg per kg IV (max. 1 gm per dose) q6h times 4 days, then 8 mg per kg IV (max. 500 mg) q8h times 6 days	Ribavirin active in vitro; not FDA-approved for this indication. NOTE: Ribavirin contraindicated in pregnancy. However, in this setting, the benefits outweigh the risks.
Plague Ref.: *JAMA 283:2281, 2000* **Inhalation pneumonic plague** Both **gentamicin** and **doxy** alone efficacious *(CID 42:614, 2006)* **Treatment**	Yersinia pestis	**Gentamicin** 5 mg per kg IV q24h or **streptomycin** 15 mg per kg IV bid. Tobramycin should work.	**(Doxy** 200 mg IV times 1, & then 100 mg po or IV bid) or **CIP** 500 mg po bid or 400 mg IV q12h) or **gentamicin** plus **doxy.** 3rd generation cephalosporins reported to work. Ref.: *CID 38:663, 2004*	1. **Chloro** also active: 25 mg per kg IV qid. 2. In mass casualty situation, may have to treat po 3. Pediatric doses: *see Table 16, page 178* 4. Pregnancy: *as for non-pregnant adults* 5. Isolate during first 48 hrs of treatment
Post-exposure prophylaxis		**Doxy** 100 mg po bid times 7 days	**CIP** 500 mg po bid times 7 days	For community with pneumonic plague epidemic. Pediatric doses: *see Table 16, page 178.* Pregnancy: *As for non-pregnant adults*
Smallpox Ref.: *NEJM 346:1300, 2002* *See Table 14, page 147*	Variola virus	Smallpox vaccine up to 4 days after exposure; isolation; gloves, gown; & NAS respirator	**Cidofovir** protected mice against aerosol cowpox *(JID 181:10, 2000)*. Maybe **adefovir.**	*Immediately notify* **State Health Dept.** & State notifies CDC (770-488-7100). Vaccinia immune globulin of no benefit. For vaccination complications, see *JAMA 288:1901, 2002.*
Tularemia **Inhalational tularemia** Ref.: *JAMA 285:2763, 2001&* www.bt.cdc.gov *See Table 1A, page 55* **Treatment**	Francisella tularemia	**(Streptomycin** 15 mg per kg IV bid) or **(gentamicin** 5 mg per kg IV qd) times 10 days	**Doxy** 100 mg IV or po bid times 14–21 days or **CIP** 400 mg IV (or 750 mg po) bid times 14–21 days	For pediatric doses, see *Table 16, page 178.* Pregnancy: *as for non-pregnant adults.* **Tobramycin** should work.
Post-exposure prophylaxis		**Doxy** 100 mg po bid times 14 days	**CIP** 500 mg po bid times 14 days	For pediatric doses, see *Table 16, page 178.* Pregnancy: *As for non-pregnant adults*

TABLE 2 – RECOMMENDED ANTIMICROBIAL AGENTS AGAINST SELECTED BACTERIA

BACTERIAL SPECIES	ANTIMICROBIAL AGENT (See page 3 for abbreviations)		
	RECOMMENDED	ALTERNATIVE	ALSO EFFECTIVE[1] (COMMENTS)
Alcaligenes xylosoxidans (Achromobacter xylosoxidans)	IMP, MER, AP Pen	TMP-SMX. Some strains susc. to ceftaz (AAC 32: 276, 1988)	Resistant to APAG; P Ceph 1, 2, 3, 4; aztreonam; FQ (AAC 40:772, 1996)
Acinetobacter calcoaceticus—baumannii complex	IMP or MER or Dori or [FQ + (amikacin or ceftaz)]	AM-SB (CID 24:932, 1997; CID 34:1425, 2002). Sulbactam[NUS] also effective (JAC 42:793, 1998); colistin (CID 36:1111, 2003)	Up to 10% isolates resistant to IMP, MER; resistance to FQs, amikacin increasing. Doxy + amikacin effective in animal model (JAC 45: 493, 2000). Minocycline, tigecycline also effective against many strains (IDCP 16:16, 2008; JAC 62:45, 2008) (See Table 5, pg 74)
Actinomyces israelii	AMP or Pen G	Doxy, ceftriaxone	Clindamycin, erythro
Aeromonas hydrophila	FQ	TMP-SMX or (P Ceph 3, 4)	APAG; ERTA; IMP; MER; tetracycline (some resistant to carbapenems)
Arcanobacterium (C.) haemolyticum	Erythro	Benzathine Pen G	Sensitive to most drugs, resistant to TMP-SMX (AAC 38:142, 1994)
Bacillus anthracis (anthrax): inhalation	See Table 1B, page 61		
Bacillus cereus, B. subtilis	Vancomycin, clinda	FQ, IMP	
Bacteroides fragilis (ssp. fragilis)	Metronidazole	Cefoxitin, Dori, ERTA, IMP, MER, TC-CL, PIP-TZ, AM-SB, cefotetan, AM-CL	Resist to clindamycin, cefotetan limit utility against B.frag. (JAC 53(Suppl2):ii29, 2004; CID 35:S126, 2002).
"DOT" group of bacteroides			(not cefotetan)
Bartonella (Rochalimaea) henselae, quintana See Table 1A, pg 43, 48, 53	Azithro, clarithro, CIP (bacillary angiomatosis), azithro (cat-scratch) (PIDJ 17:447, 1998; AAC 48:1921, 2004)	Erythro or doxy	Other drugs: TMP-SMX (IDC N.Amer 12: 137, 1998). Consider doxy + RIF for severe bacillary angiomatosis (IDC N.Amer 12: 137, 1998); doxy + gentamicin optimal for endocarditis (AAC 47:2204, 2003)
Bordetella pertussis	Erythro	TMP-SMX	An erythro-resistant strain reported in Arizona (MMWR 43:807, 1994)
Borrelia burgdorferi, B. afzelii, B. garinii	Ceftriaxone, cefurox-ime axetil, doxy, amox (See Comments)	Penicillin G (HD), cefotaxime	Clarithro. Choice depends on stage of disease, Table 1A, pg 54
Borrelia sp.	Doxy	Erythro	Penicillin G
Brucella sp.	Doxy + either gent or SM (IDCP 7, 2004; CID 42:1075, 2006)	(Doxy + RIF) or (TMP-SMX + gentamicin)	FQ + RIF (AAC 41:80,1997; EID 3: 213, 1997; CID 21:283,1995). Mino + RIF (J Chemother 15:248, 2003).
Burkholderia (Pseudomonas) cepacia	TMP-SMX or MER or CIP	Minocycline or chloramphenicol	(Usually resist to APAG, AG, polymyxins) (AAC 37: 123, 1993 & 43:213, 1999; Inf Med 18:49, 2001) (Some resist to carbapenems). May need combo rx (AJRCCM 161:1206, 2000).
Burkholderia (Pseudomonas) pseudomallei See Table 1A, pg 38, & Ln 361:1715, 2003	Initially, IV ceftaz or IMP (CID 29:381, 1999; CID 41:1105, 2005)	Then po TMP-SMX + doxy x 3 mo ± chloro (AAC 49:4020, 2005)	(Thai, 12–80% strains resist to TMP-SMX). FQ active in vitro. Combo chloro, TMP-SMX, doxy ↑ effective than doxy alone for maintenance (CID 29:375, 1999). MER also effective (AAC 48: 1763, 2004)
Campylobacter jejuni	Erythro	FQ (↑ resistance, NEJM 340:1525,1999)	Clindamycin, doxy, azithro, clarithro (see Table 5, pg 74)
Campylobacter fetus	Gentamicin	P Ceph 3	AMP, chloramphenicol
Capnocytophaga ochracea (DF-1) and	Clinda or AM-CL	CIP, Pen G	P Ceph 3, IMP, cefoxitin, FQ, (resist to APAG, TMP-SMX). C. haemolytica & C. granulosa oft resist to β-lactams & amino-glycosides [CID 35 (Suppl.1): S17, 2002].
canimorsus (DF-2)	AM-CL		
Chlamydophila pneumoniae	Doxy	Erythro, FQ	Azithro, clarithro
Chlamydia trachomatis	Doxy or azithro	Erythro	
Chryseobacterium meningo-septicum (now Elizabethkingae meningoseptica)	Vancomycin ± RIF (CID 26:1169, 1998)	CIP, levofloxacin	In vitro susceptibilities may not correlate with clinical efficacy (AAC 41:1301, 1997; CID 26:1169, 1998)
Citrobacter diversus (koseri), C. freundii	AP Pen	FQ	APAG
Clostridium difficile	Metronidazole (po)	Vancomycin (po)	Bacitracin (po); nitazoxanide (CID 43:421, 2006; JAC 59:705, 2007). Rifaximin (CID 44:846, 2007). See also Table 1A re severity of disease.
Clostridium perfringens	Pen G ± clindamycin	Doxy	Erythro, chloramphenicol, cefazolin, cefoxitin, AP Pen, CARB
Clostridium tetani	Metronidazole or Pen G	Doxy	AP Pen
Corynebacterium jeikeium	Vancomycin	Pen G + APAG	
C. diphtheriae	Erythro	Clindamycin	RIF. Penicillin reported effective (CID 27:845, 1998)
Coxiella burnetii (Q fever) acute disease	Doxy (see Table 1A, page 28)	Erythro	In meningitis consider FQ (CID 20: 489, 1995). Endocarditis: doxy + hydroxy-chloroquine (JID 188:1322, 2003; LnID 3:709, 2003).
chronic disease	(CIP or doxy) + RIF	FQ + doxy x 3 yrs (CID 20:489, 1995)	CQ + doxy (AAC 37:1773, 1993). ? gamma interferon (Ln 20:546, 2001)

TABLE 2 (2)

BACTERIAL SPECIES	ANTIMICROBIAL AGENT *(See page 3 for abbreviations)*		
	RECOMMENDED	**ALTERNATIVE**	**ALSO EFFECTIVE[1] (COMMENTS)**
Ehrlichia chaffeensis, Ehrlichia ewubguum Anaplasma (Ehrlichia) phagocytophilium	Doxy	Tetracycline, RIF *(CID 27:213, 1998)*	CIP, oflox, chloramphenicol also active in vitro. Resist to clinda, TMP-SMX, IMP, AMP, erythro, & azithro *(AAC 41:76, 1997)*.
Eikenella corrodens	Penicillin G or AMP or AM-CL	TMP-SMX, FQ	Doxy, cefoxitin, cefotaxime, IMP (Resistant to clinda, cephalexin, erythro, & metro)
Enterobacter species	Recommended agents vary with clinical setting. *See Table 1A & Table 5*		
Enterococcus faecalis	*See Table 5, pg 73*		
Enterococcus faecium, β-lactamase +, high-level aminoglycoside resist., vancomycin resist.: *See Table 5, pg 73*			
Erysipelothrix rhusiopathiae	Penicillin G or AMP	P Ceph 3, FQ	IMP, AP Pen (vancomycin, APAG, TMP-SMX resistant)
Escherichia coli	Recommended agents vary with clinical setting. *See Table 1A & Table 4*		
Francisella tularensis (tularemia) *See Table 1B, pg 62*	Gentamicin, tobramy-cin, or streptomycin	Doxy or CIP	Chloramphenicol, RIF. Doxy/chloro bacteriostatic → relapses
Gardnerella vaginalis (bacterial vaginosis)	Metronidazole	Clindamycin	*See Table 1A, pg 24 for dosage*
Hafnia alvei	*Same as Enterobacter spp.*		
Helicobacter pylori	*See Table 1A, pg 19*		Drugs effective in vitro often fail in vivo.
Haemophilus aphrophilus	[(Penicillin or AMP) ± gentamicin] or [AM-SB ± gentamicin]	P Ceph 2, 3 ± gentami-cin	(Resistant to vancomycin, clindamycin, methicillin)
Haemophilus ducreyi (chancroid)	Azithro or ceftriaxone	Erythro, CIP	Most strains resistant to tetracycline, amox, TMP-SMX
Haemophilus influenzae Meningitis, epiglottitis & other life-threatening illness	Cefotaxime, ceftriax-one	TMP-SMX, AP Pen, FQs (AMP if β-lactamase neg) (US 25–30% AMP resist, Japan 35%)	Chloramphenicol (downgrade from 1st choice due to hematotoxicity). 9% US strains resist to TMP-SMX *(AAC 41:292, 1997)*
non-life threatening illness	AM-CL, O Ceph 2/3, TMP-SMX, AM-SB		Azithro, clarithro, telithro
Klebsiella ozaenae/ rhinoscleromatis	FQ	RIF + TMP-SMX	*(Ln 342:122, 1993)*
Klebsiella species	Recommended agents vary with clinical setting. *See Table 1A & Table 5*		
Lactobacillus species	(Pen G or AMP) ± gentamicin	Clindamycin, erythro	**May be resistant to vancomycin**
Legionella sp. *(42 species & 60 serotypes recognized) (Sem Resp Inf 13:90, 1998)*	FQ, or azithro, or (erythro ± RIF)	Clarithro	TMP-SMX, doxy. Most active FQs in vitro: Gemi, Levo, Moxi. *See AnIM 129:328, 1998.* Telithro active in vitro.
Leptospira interrogans	Penicillin G	Doxy	Ceftriaxone *(CID 36:1507, 2003)*, cefotaxime *(CID 39:1417, 2004)*.
Leuconostoc	Pen G or AMP	Clinda, erythro, minocycline	APAG **NOTE: Resistant to vancomycin**
Listeria monocytogenes	AMP	TMP-SMX	Erythro, penicillin G (high dose), APAG may be synergistic with β-lactams. **Cephalosporin-resistant!**
Moraxella (Branhamella) catarrhalis	AM-CL or O Ceph 2/3, TMP-SMX	Azithro, clarithro, dirithromycin, telithro	Erythro, doxy, FQs
Morganella species	Recommended agents vary with clinical setting. *See Table 1A & Table 4*		
Mycoplasma pneumoniae	Erythro, azithro, clari-thro, FQ	Doxy	(Clindamycin & ß lactams NOT effective)
Neisseria gonorrhoeae (gonococcus)	Ceftriaxone, cefixime, cefpodoxime	Ofloxacin & other FQs *(Table 1A, pg 20–21)*, spectinomycin, azith	High prevalence of FQ resistance in Asia. FQ resistance now so high in U.S. that FQs are no longer recommended *(MMWR 56:332, 2007; AIM 148:606, 2008)*.
Neisseria meningitidis (meningococcus)	Penicillin G	Ceftriaxone, cefuroxime, cefotaxime	Sulfonamide (some strains), chloramphen-icol. Chloro-resist strains in SE Asia *(NEJM 339:868, 1998)* (Prophylaxis: pg 9)
Nocardia asteroides	TMP-SMX, sulfona-mides (high dose),	Minocycline	Amikacin + (IMP or ceftriaxone or cefuroxime) for brain abscess
Nocardia brasiliensis	TMP-SMX, sulfona-mides (high dose)	AM-CL	Amikacin + ceftriaxone
Pasteurella multocida	Pen G, AMP, amox	Doxy, AM-CL	Ceftriaxone, cefpodoxime, FQ (active in vitro), azithro (active in vitro) *(DMID 30:99, 1998; AAC 43:1475, 1999)*; resistant to cephalexin, oxacillin, clindamycin.
Plesiomonas shigelloides	CIP	TMP-SMX	AM-CL, P Ceph 1,2,3,4, IMP, MER, tetracycline, aztreonam
Proteus mirabilis (indole–)	AMP	TMP-SMX	Most agents except nafcillin/oxacillin. β-lactamase (including ESBL) production now being described in P. mirabilis *(J Clin Micro 40:1549, 2002)*
vulgaris (indole +)	P Ceph 3 or FQ	APAG	Aztreonam, BL/BLI, AP-Pen
Providencia sp.	Amikacin, P Ceph 3, FQ	TMP-SMX	AP-Pen + amikacin, IMP

TABLE 2 (3)

BACTERIAL SPECIES	ANTIMICROBIAL AGENT *(See page 3 for abbreviations)*		
	RECOMMENDED	**ALTERNATIVE**	**ALSO EFFECTIVE[1] (COMMENTS)**
Pseudomonas aeruginosa	AP Pen, AP Ceph 3, Dori, IMP, MER, tobramycin, CIP, aztreonam. For serious inf., use AP β-lactam + tobramycin or CIP *(LnID 4:519, 2004)*	For UTI, single drugs usually effective: AP Pen, AP Ceph 3, cefepime, IMP, MER, APAG, CIP, aztreonam	Resistance to ß-lactams (IMP, ceftaz) may emerge during rx. β-lactam inhibitor adds nothing to activity of TC or PIP against P. aeruginosa. Clavulanic acid antag TC in vitro *(AAC 43:882, 1999)*. *(See also Table 5).* Recommend combination therapy for serious infections, but value of combos controversial *(LnID 5:192, 2005).*
Rhodococcus (C. equi)	IMP, APAG, erythro, vanco, or RIF (Consider 2 agents)	CIP (variable)[resistant strains in SE Asia *(CID 27:370, 1998)*], TMP-SMX, tetra, or clinda	Vancomycin active in vitro but intracellular location of R. equi may impair efficacy *(Sem Resp Inf 12:57, 1997; CID 34:1379, 2002)*
Rickettsiae species	Doxy	Chloramphenicol	FQ; clari, azithro effective for Mediterranean spotted fever in children *(CID 34:154, 2002).*
Salmonella typhi	FQ, ceftriaxone	Chloramphenicol, amox, TMP-SMX, azithro (for uncomplicated disease: *AAC 43:1441, 1999)*	Multi drug resistant strains (chloramphenicol, AMP, TMP-SMX) common in many developing countries, seen in immigrants. FQ resistance now being reported *(AJTMH 61:163, 1999).*
Serratia marcescens	P Ceph 3, ERTA, IMP, MER, FQ	Aztreonam, gentamicin	TC-CL, PIP-TZ
Shigella sp.	FQ or azithro	TMP-SMX and AMP (resistance common in Middle East, Latin America). Azithro ref.: *AnIM 126:697, 1997*	
Staph. aureus, methicillin-susceptible	Oxacillin/nafcillin	P Ceph 1, vanco, teicoplanin[NUS], clinda	ERTA, IMP, MER, BL/BLI, FQ, erythro, clarithro, azithro, telithro, quinu-dalfo, linezolid, dapto. Investigational drugs with good activity include oritavancin, telavancin, ceftobiprole.
Staph. aureus, methicillin-resistant (health-care associated)	Vancomycin	Teicoplanin[NUS], TMP-SMX (some strains resistant), quinu-dalfo, linezolid, daptomycin	Fusidic acid[NUS]. >60% CIP-resistant in U.S. (Fosfomycin + RIF), novobiocin. Partially vancomycin-resistant strains (GISA, VISA) & highly resistant strains now described— *see Table 6, pg 75*. Investigational drugs with good activity include oritavancin, telavancin, ceftobiprole.
Staph. aureus, methicillin-resistant [community- associated (CA-MRSA)]			CA-MRSA usually not multiply-resistant *(Ln 359: 1819, 2002; JAMA 286: 1201, 2001)*. Oft resist. to erythro & variably to FQ. Vanco, teico[NUS] or daptomycin can be used in pts requiring hospitalization *(see Table 6, pg 75).*[2]
Mild-moderate infection	(TMP-SMX or doxy or mino) ± RIF *(CID 40: 1429, 2005)*	Clinda (if D-test neg— *see Table 5 & 6)*	
Severe infection	Vanco or teico[NUS]	Linezolid or daptomycin	
Staph. epidermidis	Vancomycin ± RIF	RIF + (TMP-SMX or FQ), daptomycin *(AAC 51:3420, 2007)*	Cephalothin or nafcillin/oxacillin if sensitive to nafcillin/oxacillin but 75% are resistant. FQs. *(See Table 5).*[2]
Staph. haemolyticus	TMP-SMX, FQ, nitrofurantoin	Oral cephalosporin	Recommendations apply to UTI only.
Staph. lugdunensis	Oxacillin/nafcillin or penicillin G (if β-lactamase neg.) *(Inf Dis Alert 22:193, 2003)*	P Ceph 1 or vancomycin or teico[NUS]	Approx. 75% are penicillin-susceptible. Usually susceptible to gentamicin, RIF *(AAC 32:2434, 1990).*
Staph. saprophyticus (UTI)	Oral cephalosporin or AM-CL	FQ	Suscept to most agents used for UTI; occ. failure of sulfonamides, nitrofurantoin reported *(JID 155:170, 1987).* Resist to fosfomycin.
Stenotrophomonas (Xanthomonas, Pseudomonas) maltophilia	TMP-SMX	TC-CL or (aztreonam + TC-CL) *(AAC 41:2612, 1997)*	Minocycline, doxy, ceftaz. [In vitro synergy (TC-CL + TMP-SMX) & (TC-CL + CIP), *AAC 39:2220, 1995; CMR 11:57, 1998]*
Streptobacillus moniliformis	Penicillin G or doxy	Erythro, clindamycin	
Streptococcus, anaerobic (Peptostreptococcus)	Penicillin G	Clindamycin	Erythro, doxy, vancomycin
Streptococcus pneumoniae penicillin-susceptible	Penicillin G	Multiple agents effective, e.g., amox	*See footnote 8 pg 11*
penicillin-resistant (MIC ≥2.0)	(Vancomycin ± RIF) or (Gemi, Gati, Levo, or Moxi). *See footnote 3 pg 8 and Table 5, pg 74*		For non-meningeal infec: P Ceph 3/4, AP Pen, quinu-dalfo, linezolid, telithro
Streptococcus pyogenes, Groups A, B, C, G, F, **Strep. milleri** (constellatus, intermedius, anginosus)	Penicillin G or V (some add genta for serious Group B infec & some add clinda for serious invasive Group A) *(SMJ 96:968, 2003)*	All ß lactams, erythro, azithro, clarithro, telithro	Macrolide resistance increasing.
Vibrio cholerae	Doxy, FQ	TMP-SMX	Strain 0139 is resistant to TMP-SMX
Vibrio parahemolyticus	Antibiotic rx does not ↓ course		Sensitive in vitro to FQ, doxy
Vibrio vulnificus, alginolyticus, damsela	Doxy + ceftaz	Cefotaxime, FQ (eg, levo, *AAC 46:3580, 2002)*	APAG often used in combo with ceftaz
Yersinia enterocolitica	TMP-SMX or FQ	P Ceph 3 or APAG	*CID 19:655, 1994*
Yersinia pestis (plague)	*See Table 1B, pg 61*		

[1] Agents are more variable in effectiveness than "Recommended" or "Alternative." Selection of "Alternative" or "Also Effective" based on in vitro susceptibility testing, pharmacokinetics, host factors such as auditory, renal, hepatic function, & cost.

[2] Investigational drugs with good activity include oritavancin, telavancin, ceftobiprole.

TABLE 3 – SUGGESTED DURATION OF ANTIBIOTIC THERAPY IN IMMUNOCOMPETENT PATIENTS[1,2]

SITE	CLINICAL SITUATION / CLINICAL DIAGNOSIS	DURATION OF THERAPY (Days)
Bacteremia	Bacteremia with removable focus (no endocarditis)	10–14 *(CID 14:75, 1992) (See Table 1A)*
Bone	Osteomyelitis, adult; acute	42
	adult; chronic	Until ESR normal (often > 3 months)
	child; acute; staph. and enterobacteriaceae[3]	21
	child; acute; strep, meningococci, haemophilus[3]	14
Ear	Otitis media with effusion	<2 yr: 10 (or 1 dose ceftriaxone).; ≥2 yr: 5–7
	Recent meta-analysis suggests 3 days of azithro *(JAC 52:469, 2003)* or 5 days of "short-acting" antibiotics effective for uncomplicated otitis media *(JAMA 279:1736, 1998)*, but may be inadequate for severe disease *(NEJM 347:1169, 2002)*.	
Endocardium	Infective endocarditis, native valve	
	Viridans strep	14 or 28 *(See Table 1A, page 25)*
	Enterococci	28 or 42 *(See Table 1A, page 26)*
	Staph. aureus	14 (R-sided only) or 28 *(See Table 1A, page 27)*
Gastrointestinal *Also see Table 1A*	Bacillary dysentery (shigellosis)/traveler's diarrhea	3
	Typhoid fever (S. typhi): Azithro	5 (children/adolescents)
	Ceftriaxone	14*
	FQ	5–7
	Chloramphenicol	14
		*[Short course ↓ effective *(AAC 44:450, 2000)*]
	Helicobacter pylori	10–14
	Pseudomembranous enterocolitis (C. difficile)	10
Genital	Non-gonococcal urethritis or mucopurulent cervicitis	7 days doxy or single dose azithro
	Pelvic inflammatory disease	14
Heart	Pericarditis (purulent)	28
Joint	Septic arthritis (non-gonococcal) Adult	14–28 *(Ln 351:197, 1998)*
	Infant/child	Rx as osteomyelitis above
	Gonococcal arthritis/disseminated GC infection	7 *(See Table 1A, page 21)*
Kidney	Cystitis (bladder bacteriuria)	3 (Single dose extended-release cipro also effective) *(AAC 49:4137, 2005)*
	Pyelonephritis	14 (7 days if CIP used; 5 days if levo 750 mg)
	Recurrent (failure after 14 days rx)	42
Lung	Pneumonia, pneumococcal	Until afebrile 3–5 days (minimum 5 days)
	Community-acquired pneumonia	Minimum 5 days and afebrile for 2-3 days *(CID 44:S55, 2007; AJM 120:783, 2007)*
	Pneumonia, enterobacteriaceae or pseudomonal	21, often up to 42
	Pneumonia, staphylococcal	21–28
	Pneumocystis carinii, in AIDS;	21
	other immunocompromised	14
	Legionella, mycoplasma, chlamydia	7–14
	Lung abscess	Usually 28–42[4]
Meninges[5] *(CID 39:1267, 2004)*	N. meningitidis	7
	H. influenzae	7
	S. pneumoniae	10–14
	Listeria meningoencephalitis, gp B strep, coliforms	21 (longer in immunocompromised)
Multiple systems	Brucellosis *(See Table 1A, page 55)*	42 (add SM or gent for 1st 7–14 days)
	Tularemia *(See Table 1A, pages 42, 55)*	7–14
Muscle	Gas gangrene (clostridial)	10
Pharynx *Also see Pharyngitis, Table 1A, page 45*	Group A strep pharyngitis	10
		O Ceph 2/3, azithromycin effective at 5 days *(JAC 45, Topic TI 23, 2000; JIC 14:213, 2008)*. 3 days less effective *(Inf Med 18:515, 2001)*
	Diphtheria (membranous)	7–14
	Carrier	7
Prostate	Chronic prostatitis (TMP/SMX)	30–90
	(FQ)	28–42
Sinuses	Acute sinusitis	5–14[6]
Skin	Cellulitis	Until 3 days after acute inflamm disappears
Systemic	Lyme disease	*See Table 1A, page 54*
	Rocky Mountain spotted fever *(See Table 1A, page 55)*	Until afebrile 2 days

[1] It has been shown that early change from parenteral to oral regimens (about 72 hours) is cost-effective with many infections, i.e., intra-abdominal *(AJM 91:462, 1991)*.
[2] The recommended duration is a minimum or average time and should not be construed as absolute.
[3] These times are with proviso: sx & signs resolve within 7 days and ESR is normalized *(J.D. Nelson, APID 6:59, 1991)*.
[4] After patient afebrile 4-5 days, change to oral therapy.
[5] In children relapses seldom occur until 3 days or more after termination of rx. Practice of observing in hospital for 1 or 2 days after rx is expensive and non-productive. For meningitis in children, *see Table 1A, page 8.*
[6] Duration of therapy dependent upon agent used and severity of infection. Longer duration (10-14 days) optimal for beta-lactams and patients with severe disease. For sinusitis of mild-moderate severity shorter courses of therapy (5-7 days) effective with "respiratory FQ's" (including gemifloxacin, levofloxacin 750 mg), azithromycin. Courses as short as 3 days reported effective for TMP-SMX and azithro and one study reports effectiveness of single dose extended-release azithro. Authors feel such "super-short" courses should be restricted to patients with mild-mod disease *(JAMA 273:1015, 1995; AAC 47:2770, 2003; Otolaryngol-Head Neck Surg 133:194, 2005; Otolaryngol-Head Neck Surg 127:1, 2002; Otolaryngol-Head Neck Surg 134:10, 2006).*

TABLE 4 – COMPARISON OF ANTIMICROBIAL SPECTRA
(These are generalizations; major differences exist between countries/areas/hospitals depending on antibiotic usage—verify for individual location. See Table 5 for resistant bacteria)

Organisms	Penicillins		Antistaphylococcal Penicillins			Amino-Penicillins			Anti-Pseudomonal Penicillins				Carbapenems				Aztreonam	Fluoroquinolones						
	Penicillin G	Penicillin V	Methicillin	Nafcillin/Oxacillin	Cloxacillin[NUS]/Diclox.	AMP/Amox	Amox/Clav	AMP-Sulb	Ticarcillin	Ticar-Clav	Pip-Tazo	Piperacillin	Doripenem	Ertapenem	Imipenem	Meropenem	Aztreonam	Ciprofloxacin	Ofloxacin	Pefloxacin[NUS]	Levofloxacin	Moxifloxacin	Gemifloxacin	Gatifloxacin
GRAM-POSITIVE:																								
Strep, Group A,B,C,G	+	+	+	+	+	+	+	+	+	+	+	+	+	+	+	+	0	±	±	0	+	+	+	+
Strep. pneumoniae	+	+	+	+	+	+	+	+	+	+	+	+	+	+	+	+	0	±	±	0	+	+	+	+
Viridans strep	±	±	±	±	±	±	±	±	±	±	±	±	+	+	+	+	0	0	0	0	+	+	+	+
Strep. milleri	+	+	+	+	+	+	+	+	+	+	+	+	+	+	+	+	0	0	0	0	+	+	+	+
Enterococcus faecalis	+	+	0	0	0	+	+	+	±	±	+	+	±	0	+	±	0	**	**	0	+	±	±	±
Enterococcus faecium	0	0	0	0	0	+	+	+	±	±	±	±	0	0	±	0	0	0	0	0	0	±	±	±
Staph. aureus (MSSA)	0	0	+	+	+	0	+	+	0	+	+	+	+	+	+	+	0	+	+	+	+	+	+	+
Staph. aureus (MRSA)	0	0	0	0	0	0	0	0	0	0	0	0	0	0	0	0	0	0	0	0	0	±	±	±
Staph. aureus (CA-MRSA)	0	0	0	0	0	0	0	0	0	0	0	0	0	0	0	0	0	±	+	+	±	±	±	±
Staph. epidermidis	0	0	±	±	±	0	+	+	±	±	+	0	+	+	+	+	0	0	0	0	±	+	+	+
C. jeikeium	0	0	0	0	0	0	0	0	0	0	0	0			0	0	0	+	0	+	+	+	+	+
L. monocytogenes	+	0	0	0	0	+	0	+	+	0	+	+	+	±	+	+	0	+	0	0	+	+	+	+
GRAM-NEGATIVE:																								
N. gonorrhoeae	0	0	0	0	0	0	+	+	+	+	+	+	+	+	+	+	+	+[1]	+[1]	+[1]	+[1]	+[1]		+[1]
N. meningitidis	+	0	0	0	0	+	+	+	+	+	+	+	+	+	+	+	+	+	+	+	+	+		+
M. catarrhalis	0	0	0	0	0	0	+	+	±	+	+	±	+	+	+	+	+	+	+	+	+	+	+	+
H. influenzae	0	0	0	0	0	±	+	+	±	+	+	±	+	+	+	+	+	+	+	+	+	+	+	+
E. coli	0	0	0	0	0	±	+	+	±	+	+	+	+	+	+	+	+	+	+	+	+	+	+	+
Klebsiella sp.	0	0	0	0	0	0	+	+	0	+	+	0	+	+	+	+	+	+	+	+	+	+	+	+
E. coli/Klebs sp ESBL+	0	0	0	0	0	0	0	0	0	±	±	+	+	+	+	+	0	0	0		0	+		+
Enterobacter sp.	0	0	0	0	0	0	0	0	+	+	+	+	+	+	+	+	+	+	+	+	+	+		+
Serratia sp.	0	0	0	0	0	0	0	0	±	±	+	0	+	+	+	+	+	+	+	+	+	+		+
Salmonella sp.	0	0	0	0	0	±	0	0	+	+	+	+	+	+	+	+	+	+	+	+	+	+		+
Shigella sp.	0	0	0	0	0	±	+	0	+	+	+	0	+	+	+	+	+	+	+	+	+	+	+	+
Proteus mirabilis	0	0	0	0	0	+	+	+	+	+	+	+	+	+	+	+	+	+	+	+	+	+	+	+

+ = **usually effective clinically or >60% susceptible**; ± = clinical trials lacking or 30–60% susceptible; 0 = not effective clinically or <30% susceptible; blank = data not available

** Most strains ±, can be used in UTI, not in systemic infection

[1] Prevalence of quinolone-resistant GC varies worldwide from <1% to 30.9% in Europe and >90% in Taiwan. In US in 2006 it was 6.7% overall and as a result, CDC no longer recommends FQs for first line therapy of GC (*MMWR 56:332, 2007; JAC 58:587, 2006; CID 40:188, 2005; AnIM 147:81, 2007*).

TABLE 4 (2)

Organisms	Penicillins		Antistaphylococcal Penicillins			Amino-Penicillins			Anti-Pseudomonal Penicillins				Carbapenems					Fluoroquinolones						
	Penicillin G	Penicillin V	Methicillin	Nafcillin/Oxacillin	Cloxacillin[NUS]/Diclox.	AMP/Amox	Amox/Clav	AMP-Sulb	Ticarcillin	Ticar-Clav	Pip-Tazo	Piperacillin	Doripenem	Ertapenem	Imipenem	Meropenem	Aztreonam	Ciprofloxacin	Ofloxacin	Pefloxacin[NUS]	Levofloxacin	Moxifloxacin	Gemifloxacin	Gatifloxacin
Proteus vulgaris	0	0	0	0	0	0	+	+	+	+	+	+	+	+	+	+	+	+	+	+	+	+	+	+
Providencia sp.	0	0	0	0	0	0	±	+	+	+	+	+	+	+	+	+	+	+	+	+	+	+		+
Morganella sp.	0	±	0	0	0	0	0	0	+	+	+	+	+	+	+	+	+	+	+	+	+	+		+
Citrobacter sp.	0	±	0	0	0	0	0	+	+	+	+	+	+	+	+	+	+	+	+	+	+	+		+
Aeromonas sp.	0	0	0	0	0	0	0	0	+	+	+	+	+	+	+	+	+	+	+	+	+	+		+
Acinetobacter sp.	0	0	0	0	0	0	0	0	0	±	±	0	±	0	±	±	0	±	±	0	±	±	±	±
Ps. aeruginosa	0	0	0	0	0	0	0	0	+	+	+	+	+	0	+	+	+	+	±	+	±	±		±
B. (Ps.) cepacia	0	0	0	0	0	0	0	0	0	±	±	±	±	0	0	0	0	0	0	0	±	0		0
S. (X.) maltophilia	0	0	0	0	0	0	0	0	0	±	±	0	0	0	0	0	0	0	0		±	0		
Y. enterocolitica	0	0	0	0	0	0	0	±	0	+	±	±	0	+	+	+	+	+	+	+	+	+		+
Legionella sp.	0	0	0	0	0	0	0	0	+	+	+	+			0	0	0	+	+	+	+	+	+	+
P. multocida	+	+	0	0	0	+	+	+	0	+	0	0	+	+	+	+	+	+	+	+	+	+		+
H. ducreyi	+	+	+	+	+	0	+	+	+	+	+	+	+	+	+	+	+	+	+	+	+	+		+
MISC.: Chlamydophila sp	0	0	0	0	0	0	0	0	0	0	0	0	0	0	0	0	0	+	+	+	+	+	+	+
M. pneumoniae	0	0	0	0	0	0	0	0	0	0	0	0	0	0	0	0	0	+	+	+	+	+	+	+
ANAEROBES: Actinomyces	+	+	0	0	0	+	+	+	0	+	+	+	+	+	+	+	0	0	±	0	0	+		+
Bacteroides fragilis	0	0	0	0	0	0	+	+	0	+	+	0	+	+	+	+	0	0	0	0	0	+	±	±
P. melaninogenica	+[1]		0	0	0	+	+	+[1]	+	+	+	+[1]	+	+	+	+	0	0	±		+	+		+
Clostridium difficile	+	+	+	+	+	+	+	+	+	+	+	+	+	+	+	+	0	0	0	0	0	0	0	0
Clostridium (not difficile)	+	+	+	+	+	+	+	+	+	+	+	+	+	+	+	+	0	±	±		+	+		+
Peptostreptococcus sp.	+	+	+	+	+	+	+	+	+	+	+	+	+	+	+	+	0	±	±		+	+		+

+ = usually effective clinically or >60% susceptible; ± = clinical trials lacking or 30–60% susceptible; 0 = not effective clinically or <30% susceptible; blank = data not available

[1] No clinical evidence that penicillins or fluoroquinolones are effective for C. difficile enterocolitis (but they may cover this organism in mixed intra-abdominal and pelvic infections).

TABLE 4 (3)

CEPHALOSPORINS

Organisms	1st Gen: Cefazolin	2nd Gen: Cefotetan	2nd Gen: Cefoxitin	2nd Gen: Cefuroxime	3rd/4th Gen: Cefotaxime	Ceftizoxime	Ceftriaxone	Ceftobiprole	Ceftazidime	Cefepime	Oral 1st: Cefadroxil	Cephalexin	Oral 2nd: Cefaclor/Loracarbef*	Cefprozil	Cefuroxime axetil	Oral 3rd: Cefixime	Ceftibuten	Cefpodox/Cefdinir/Cefditoren
GRAM-POSITIVE:																		
Strep, Group A,B,C,G	+	+	+	+	+	+	+	+	+	+	+	±	+	+	+	+	+	+
Strep. pneumoniae[1]	+	+	+	+	+	+	+	+	±[1]	+	+	±	+	+	+	+	±	+
Viridans strep	+	+	+	+	+	+	+	+	±	+	+	+	+	+	+	+	+	+
Enterococcus faecalis	0	0	0	0	0	0	0	+	0	0	0	0	0	0	0	0	0	0
Staph. aureus (MSSA)	+	+	+	+	+	+	+	+	±	+	+	+	+	+	+	0	0	+
Staph. aureus (MRSA)	0	0	0	0	0	0	0	+	0	0	0	0	0	0	0	0	0	0
Staph. aureus (CA-MRSA)	0	0	0	0	0	0	0	+	0	0	0	0	0	0	0	0	0	0
Staph. epidermidis	±	±	±	±	±	±	±	+	±	±	±	±	±	±	±	0	0	±
C. jeikeium	0	0	0	0	0	0	0		0	0	0	0	0	0	0	0	0	0
L. monocytogenes	0	0	0	0	0	0	0		0	0	0	0	0	0	0	0	0	0
GRAM-NEGATIVE																		
N. gonorrhoeae	+	±	±	+	±	±	+	+	±	+	0	0	±	±	±	+	+	+
N. meningitidis	0	±	±	+	+	+	+	+	±	+	0	0	±	±	±	±	±	±
M. catarrhalis	±	+	+	+	+	+	+	+	+	+		0	±	+	+	+	+	+
H. influenzae	+	+	+	+	+	+	+	+	+	+	+	+	+	+	+	+	+	+
E. coli	+	+	+	+	+	+	+	+	+	+	0	+	+	+	+	+	+	+
Klebsiella sp.	0	+	0	+	+	+	+	+	+	+	0	0	0	0	0	+	0	0
E. coli/Klebs sp ESBL+	0	±	0	0	0	0	0	0	0	0	0	0	0	0	0	0	±	0
Enterobacter sp.		+	0	±	+	+	+	+	+	+	0	0	0	0	0	0	±	0
Serratia sp.		+	0	0	+	+	+	+	+	+	0	0	0	0	0	±	±	+
Salmonella sp.		+			+	+	+	+	+	+	0	0	0	0	0	+	+	+
Shigella sp.		+			+	+	+	+	+	+	0	+	0	0	0	+	+	+
Proteus mirabilis	+	+	+	+	+	+	+	+	+	+	+	+	+	+	+	+	+	+
Proteus vulgaris	0	+	+	0	+	+	+	+	+	+	0	0	0	0	0	+	+	+
Providencia sp.	0	+	+	0	+	+	+	+	+	+	0	0	0	0	0	+	+	±
Morganella sp.	0	+	+	±	+	+	+	+	+	+	0	0	0	0	±	0	0	0

+ = **usually effective clinically or >60% susceptible; ± = clinical trials lacking or 30–60% susceptible; 0 = not effective clinically or <30% susceptible; blank = data not available**

* A 1-carbacephem best classified as a cephalosporin

[1] Ceftaz 8–16 times less active than cefotax/ceftriax, effective only vs Pen-sens. strains (AAC 39:2193, 1995). Oral cefuroxime, cefprozil, cefpodoxime most active in vitro vs resistant S. pneumo (PIDJ 14:1037, 1995).

TABLE 4 (4)

CEPHALOSPORINS

Organisms	1st Gen. Cefazolin	2nd Generation Cefotetan	2nd Gen. Cefoxitin	2nd Gen. Cefuroxime	3rd/4th Gen. Cefotaxime	3rd/4th Gen. Ceftizoxime	3rd/4th Gen. Ceftriaxone	3rd/4th Gen. Ceftobiprole	3rd/4th Gen. Ceftazidime	3rd/4th Gen. Cefepime	Oral 1st Gen. Cefadroxil	Oral 1st Gen. Cephalexin	Oral 2nd Gen. Cefaclor/Loracarbef*	Oral 2nd Gen. Cefprozil	Oral 2nd Gen. Cefuroxime axetil	Oral 3rd Gen. Cefixime	Oral 3rd Gen. Ceftibuten	Oral 3rd Gen. Cefpodox/Cefdinir/Cefditoren
C. freundii	0	0	0	0	+	0	+		0	+	0	0	0	0	0	0	0	0
C. diversus	0	±	±	±	+	+	+	+	+	+	0	0	0	0	±	+	+	+
Citrobacter sp.	0	±	±	+	+	+	+	+	+	+			±	0	±	+	+	
Aeromonas sp.	0	+	±	+	+	+	+	+	+	+						+	+	
Acinetobacter sp.	0	0	0	0	0	0	0	±	±	±	0	0	0	0	0	0	0	0
Ps. aeruginosa	0	0	0	0	±	±	±	+	+	+	0	0	0	0	0	0	0	0
B. (Ps.) cepacia	0	0	0	0	±	±	±	0	+	±	0	0	0	0	0	0	0	0
S. (X.) maltophilia	0	0	0	0	0	0	0	0	+	±	0	0	0	0	0	0		
Y. enterocolitica	0	±	±	±	+	+	+	0	±	0	0	0	0	0	0	0	0	
Legionella sp.	0	0	0	0	0	0	0	0	0	0	0	0	0	0	0	0	0	0
P. multocida		+	0	+	+	+	+		+	+						+		+
H. ducreyi		+	+	+	+	+	+		+	+		+	+	+	+	+		+
ANAEROBES:																		
Actinomyces	0			0	0		+		0	0	0	0	0	0	0	0	0	
Bacteroides fragilis	0	±¹	+	0	0	±	0	0	0	0		0				0		
P. melaninogenica		+	+	+	+	+	±		+			+		+	+	+		+
Clostridium difficile		0	0	0	0	0	0	0	+	0				+	+	0		0
Clostridium (not difficile)		+	+	+	+	+	+		+			+	+	+	+	0		+
Peptostreptococcus sp.		+	+	+	+	+	+		+	+		+	+		+	+		+

+ = **usually effective clinically or >60% susceptible**; ± = clinical trials lacking or 30–60% susceptible; 0 = not effective clinically or <30% susceptible; blank = data not available

* A 1-carbacephem best classified as a cephalosporin

1 Cefotetan is less active against B. ovatus, B. distasonis, B. thetaiotamicron

TABLE 4 (5)

Legend: **+** = usually effective clinically or >60% susceptible; **±** = clinical trials lacking or 30–60% susceptible; **0** = not effective clinically or <30% susceptible; **S** = synergistic with penicillins (ampicillin); blank = data not available. Antimicrobials such as azithromycin have high tissue penetration and some such as clarithromycin are metabolized to more active compounds, hence in vivo activity may exceed in vitro activity.

Organism column key (Gram-positive then Gram-negative):

- **GRAM-POSITIVE:** G1 = Strep Group A,B,C,G · G2 = Strep. pneumoniae · G3 = Enterococcus faecalis · G4 = Enterococcus faecium · G5 = Staph.aureus (MSSA) · G6 = Staph.aureus (MRSA) · G7 = Staph.aureus (CA-MRSA) · G8 = Staph. epidermidis · G9 = C. jeikeium · G10 = L. monocytogenes
- **GRAM-NEGATIVE:** N1 = N. gonorrhoeae · N2 = N. meningitidis · N3 = M. catarrhalis · N4 = H. influenzae · N5 = Aeromonas · N6 = E. coli · N7 = Klebsiella sp. · N8 = E. coli/Klebs sp ESBL+ · N9 = Enterobacter sp. · N10 = Salmonella sp. · N11 = Shigella sp. · N12 = Serratia marcescens

Class	Drug	G1	G2	G3	G4	G5	G6	G7	G8	G9	G10	N1	N2	N3	N4	N5	N6	N7	N8	N9	N10	N11	N12
MISCELLANEOUS	Colistimethate (Colistin)	0	0	0	0	0	0	0	0	0	0	0	0				+	+	+	+			0
	Daptomycin	+	+[2]	+	+	+	+	+	+	+	±	0	0	0	0	0	0	0	0	0	0	0	0
	Linezolid	+	+	+	+	+	+	+	+	+	+	0	±	±	0	0	0	0	0	0	0	0	0
	Quinupristin-dalfopristin	+	+	0	+	+	+	+	+	+	+	+	0	±	+	0	0	0	0	0	0	0	0
	Metronidazole	0	0	0	0	0	0	0	0	0	0	0	0	0	0	0	0	0	0	0	0	0	0
	Rifampin	+	+	±	0	+	+	+	+	+	+	+	+	+	0	0	0	0	0	0	0	0	0
AGENTS URINARY TRACT	Fosfomycin		+	±								+					+	±		±			±
	Nitrofurantoin	+	+	+	+	+	+	+		0		+					+	±		±	+	+	0
	TMP-SMX	+[1]	+	+[1]	0	+	+	+	±	0	+	±	+	±	+	±	±	±		±	±	±	±
	Trimethoprim	+	±		0	±	±	+		0	+	0	±		±		+	±	±	±	±	±	
	Fusidic Acid NUS	±	±	+			+	+	+	+	+		+	+		0	0	0	0	0	0	0	0
GLYCOPEPTIDES	Telavancin	+	+	+	+	+	+	+	+	+	+	0	0		0		0	0	0	0	0	0	0
	Teicoplanin NUS	+	+	+	±	+	+	+	±	+	+	0	0		0		0	0	0	0	0	0	0
	Vancomycin	+	+	+	±	+	+	+	+	+	+	0	0		0		0	0	0	0	0	0	0
GLYCYL-CYCLINE	Tigecycline	+	+	+	+	+	+	+	+	+	+	+		+	+	+	+	+	+	+	+	+	+
TETRA-CYCLINES	Minocycline	+	+	0	0	+	±	+	0	0	+	±	+	+	+	+	+	±	±	±	0	±	0
	Doxycycline	±	+	0	0	±	±	+	0	0	+	±	+	+	+	+	+	±	±	±	0	±	0
KETOLIDE	Telithromycin	+	+	±	0	+	0	±	0	0	+	+	+	+	+	0	0	0	0	0	0	0	0
MACROLIDES	Clarithromycin	±	+	0	0	+	0	±	0	0	+	±		+	+	0	0	0	0	0	0	0	0
	Azithromycin	±	+	0	0	+	0	±	0	0	+	±	+	+	+	0	0	0	0	0	±	±	0
	Erythro	±	+	0	0	+	0	±	±	0	+	±	+	+	±	0	0	0	0	0	0	0	0
	Clindamycin	+	+	0	0	+	0	±	0	0		0	0	0	0		0	0	0	0	0	0	0
	Chloramphenicol	+	+	±	±	±	0		0	0	+	+	+	+	+	+	±	±	±	+	0	+	0
AMINO-GLYCOSIDES	Amikacin	0	0	S	0	+	0		±	0	S	0	0	+	+	+	+	+			+		+
	Tobramycin	0	0	S	0	+	0		±	0	S	0	0	+	+	+	+	+			+		+
	Gentamicin	0	0	S	S	+	0		±	0	S	0	0	+	0	+	+	+			+		+

[1] Although active in vitro, TMP-SMX is not clinically effective for Group A strep pharyngitis or for infections due to E. faecalis.

[2] Although active in vitro, daptomycin is not clinically effective for pneumonia caused by strep pneumonia.

TABLE 4 (6)

Class	Drug	Proteus vulgaris	Acinetobacter sp.	Ps. aeruginosa	B. (Ps.) cepacia	S. (X.) maltophilia	Y. enterocolitica	F. tularensis	Brucella sp.	Legionella sp.	H. ducreyi	V. vulnificus	Chlamydophila sp.	M. pneumoniae	Rickettsia sp.	Mycobacterium avium	Actinomyces	Bacteroides fragilis	P. melaninogenica	Clostridium difficile	Clostridium (not difficile)**	Peptostreptococcus sp.
MISCELLANEOUS	Colistimethate (Colistin)	0	+	+	0	±																
	Daptomycin	0	0	0	0	0	0	0	0	0	0	0										
	Linezolid	0	0	0	0	0	0	0	0							0	+	0		±	+	+
	Quinupristin-dalfopristin			0													+	+	0		+	±
	Metronidazole	0	0	0	0	0	0	0	0	0	0	0	0	0	0	0	0	+	+	+	+	+
	Rifampin	0	0	0	0				+	+						+						
AGENTS URINARY TRACT	Fosfomycin	±																				
	Nitrofurantoin	0	0	0	0												0					
	TMP-SMX	0	±	0	+	+	+	+	+	+	±						0					
	Trimethoprim	0	0	0	+	0			+	+			0				+					
	Fusidic Acid NUS	0	0	0	0	0	0			±		0	0	0	0		+		+		+	+
GLYCOPEPTIDES	Telavancin	0	0	0	0	0			0							0	+	0		+	+	+
	Teicoplanin NUS	0	0	0	0	0			0							0				+	+	+
	Vancomycin	0	0	0	0	0			0	0						0	+	0		+	+	+
GLYCYL-CYCLINE	Tigecycline	±	±	0	±	+		+	+	0			+	+		0		+	+		+	+
TETRA-CYCLINES	Minocycline	0	0	0	±	0	0		+	+		+	+	+	+	0	+	±	+		+	+
	Doxycycline	0	0	0	0	0	0	+	+	+		+	+	+	+	0	+	±	+		+	+
KETOLIDE	Telithromycin	0	0	0	0	0	0		0	+			+	+	+							+
MACROLIDES	Clarithromycin	0	0	0	0	0	0		0	+			+	+	+	+	+	0	+		+	±
	Azithromycin	0	0	0	0	0	0		0	+	+		+	+	+	+	+	0	+		+	+
	Erythro	0	0	0	0	0	0		0	+	+		+	+	±	+	+	0			±	±
	Clindamycin	0	0	0	0	0	0		0			+	±	0			+	±	+			+
	Chloramphenicol	±	0	0	+	+	+	+	+		+	+	+	+		+	+	+	±	+	+	
AMINO-GLYCOSIDES	Amikacin	+	±	+	0	0	+				±		0	0	0	+	0	0	0	0		
	Tobramycin	+	0	+	0	0	+				±		0	0	0		0	0	0	0		
	Gentamicin	+	0	+	0	0	+	+	+		±		0	0	0		0	0	0	0		0

MISC.: Chlamydophila sp., M. pneumoniae, Rickettsia sp., Mycobacterium avium

ANAEROBES: Actinomyces, Bacteroides fragilis, P. melaninogenica, Clostridium difficile, Clostridium (not difficile)**, Peptostreptococcus sp.

+ = usually effective clinically or >60% susceptible; 0 = not effective clinically or <30% susceptible; blank = data not available.
± = clinical trials lacking or 30–60% susceptible; 0 = not effective clinically or <30% susceptible.

Antimicrobials such as azithromycin have high tissue penetration & some such as clarithromycin are metabolized to more active compounds, hence in vivo activity may exceed in vitro activity.

** Vancomycin, metronidazole given po active vs C. difficile; IV vancomycin not effective.

TABLE 5 – TREATMENT OPTIONS FOR SELECTED HIGHLY RESISTANT BACTERIA

(See page 3 for abbreviations)

ORGANISM/RESISTANCE	THERAPEUTIC OPTIONS	COMMENT[1]
E. faecalis. Resistant to:		
Vaco + strep/gentamicin (MIC >500 mcg per mL); β-lactamase neg. (JAC 40:161, 1997).	**Penicillin G or AMP** (systemic infections); **Nitrofurantoin**, **fosfomycin** (UTI only). Usually resistant to **quinu-dalfo**.	AMP + ceftriaxone effective for endocarditis due to E. faecalis with high level AG resistance (no comparator treated with AMP alone) but no data for therapy of VRE (AnIM 146:574, 2007). Non BL+ strains of E. faecalis resistant to penicillin and AMP described in Spain, but unknown (except BL+ strains) in U.S. and elsewhere (AAC 40:2420, 1996). Linezolid effective in 60–70% of cases (AnIM 138:135, 2003). Daptomycin, tigecycline, ceftobiprole active in vitro (JAC 52:123, 2003).
Penicillin (β-lactamase producers)	**Vanco, AM-SB**	Appear susceptible to AMP and penicillin by standard in vitro methods. Must use direct test for β-lactamase with chromogenic cephalosporin (nitrocefin) to identify. Rare since early 1990s. Ceftobiprole active in vitro (AAC 51:2043, 2007).
E. faecium. Resistant to:		
Vanco and high levels (MIC >500 mcg per mL) of streptomycin and gentamicin	**Penicillin G or AMP** (systemic infections); **fosfomycin, nitrofurantoin** (UTI only)	For strains with pen/AMP MICs of >8 ≤64 mcg per mL, anecdotal evidence that high-dose (300 mg per kg per day) AMP rx may be effective. Daptomycin, tigecycline active in vitro (JAC 52:123, 2003).
Penicillin, AMP, vanco. & high-level resist. to streptomycin and gentamicin (NEJM 342:710, 2000)	**Linezolid** 600 mg po or IV q12h and **quinu-dalfo** 7.5 mg per kg IV q8h are bacteriostatic against most strains of E. faecium. Can try combinations of cell wall-active antibiotics with other agents (including FQ, chloramphenicol, RIF, or **doxy**). Chloramphenicol alone effective in some cases of bacteremia (Clin Micro Inf 7:17, 2001). **Nitro-furantoin** or **fosfomycin** may work for UTI.	For strains with Van B phenotype (vanco R, teico S), teicoplanin[NUS], preferably in combination with strep-tomycin or gentamicin (if not highly AG resistant), may be effective. Synercid roughly 70% effective in clinical trials (CID 30:790, 2000 & 33:1816, 2001). Linezolid shows similar efficacy. Comparable but somewhat lower (58% linezolid, 43% QD) response rates in cancer pts (JAC 53:646, 2004). Emergence of resistance with therapeutic failure has occurred during monotherapy with either quinu-dalfo or linezolid (CID 30:790, 2000; Ln 357:1179, 2001). Nosocomial spread of linezolid-resistant E. faecium possible (NEJM 346:867, 2002). Daptomycin active in vitro against most strains (JAC 52:123, 2003) but therapeutic failure with or without development of resistance reported (CID 45:1343, 2007). Tigecycline also active in vitro (Circulation 111:e394, 2005). **Infectious disease consultation imperative!**
S. aureus. Resistant to:		
Methicillin (health-care associated) (CID 32:108, 2001) **For community-associated MRSA infections, see Table 6**	**Vanco** [For persistent bacteremia (≥7 days) on vanco or teicoplanin[NUS], see Table 6]	Alternatives: teicoplanin[NUS], daptomycin (AAC 49:770, 2005; NEJM 355:653, 2006), linezolid (Chest 124:1789, 2003), dalbavancin (EMID 48:137, 2004), TMP-SMX (test susceptibility first), minocycline & doxy (some strains)(NEJM 357:380, 2007), tigecycline [CID 41(Suppl 5):S303, 2005], or quinu-dalfo (CID 34:1481, 2002). Fusidic acid[NUS], fosfomycin, RIF may be active; use only in combination to prevent in vivo emergence of resistance. Staphylococci (incl. CA-MRSA) with inducible MLS_B resistance may appear susceptible to clin-damycin in vitro. Clinda therapy may result in therapeutic failure (CID 37:1257, 2003). Test for inducible resistance [double-disc ("D test")] before treating with clinda (J Clin Micro 42:2777, 2004). Investigational drugs with activity against MRSA include oritavancin (LY333328), telavancin, ceftobiprole, ceftaroline, iclaprim.
Vanco, methicillin (VISA & VRSA) (CID 32:108, 2001; MMWR 51:902, 2002; NEJM 348:1342, 2003; CID 46:668, 2008)	Unknown, but even high-dose vanco may fail. **Linezolid, quinu-dalfo, daptomycin** active in vitro.	VISA/GISA: Vanco-intermediate resistance of MRSA with MICs of ≤16 mcg/mL. Anecdotal data on treatment regimens. Most susceptible to TMP-SMX, minocycline, doxycycline, RIF and AGs (CID 32:108, 2001). RIF should always be combined with a 2nd therapeutic agent to prevent emergence of RIF resistance during therapy. VRSA: only 6 clinical isolates of truly vancomycin-resistant (MIC >64) MRSA described. Organisms still susceptible to TMP-SMX, chloro, linezolid, minocycline, quinu-dalfo, ceftobiprole (MMWR 51:902, 2002; NEJM 348:1342, 2003).
S. epidermidis. Resistant to:		
Methicillin	**Vanco** (+ **RIF** and **gentamicin** for prosthetic valve endocarditis)	
Methicillin, glycopeptides (AAC 49: 770, 2005)	**Quinu-dalfo** (see comments on E. faecium) generally active in vitro as are **linezolid** & **daptomycin**.	Vanco more active than teicoplanin[NUS] (Clin Micro Rev 8:585, 1995). New FQs (levofloxacin, gatifloxacin, moxifloxacin) active in vitro, but development of resistance is a potential problem.

[1] Guideline on prevention of resistance: CID 25:584, 1997

TABLE 5 (2)

ORGANISM/RESISTANCE	THERAPEUTIC OPTIONS	COMMENT[1]
S. pneumoniae. Resistant to: Penicillin G (MIC >0.1 ≤2.0)	**Ceftriaxone** or **cefotaxime**. High-dose penicillin (≥10 million units per day) or **AMP (amox)** likely effective for nonmeningeal sites of infection (e.g., pneumonia), **telithro**	IMP, ERTA, cefepime, cefpodoxime, cefuroxime also active (*IDCP 3:75, 1994*). MER less active than IMP (*AAC 38:898, 1994; DMID 31:45, 1998; Exp Opin Invest Drugs 8:123, 1999*). Gemi, moxi, levo also have good activity (*AAC 38:898, 1994*). High-dose cefotaxime (300 mg per kg per day, max. 24 gm per day) effective in meningitis due to strains with cefotaxime MICs as high as 2 mcg per mL (*AAC 40:218, 1996*). Review: *IDCP 6 (Suppl 2):S21, 1997*
Penicillin G (MIC ≥4.0)	**[Vanco ± RIF]**. Alternatives if non-meningeal infection: **ceftriax/cefotax, high-dose AMP, ERTA, IMP, MER**, or an active FQ: **(Gemi, moxi, levo)**, **telithro**	Note new CLSI breakpoints for penicillin susceptibilities. Meningeal isolates ≤0.06 = S; 0.12-1.0 = I; ≥2.0 = R. For non-meningeal isolates ≤2.0 = S; 4.0 = I; ≥8.0 = R.
Penicillin, erythro, tetracycline, chloramphenicol, TMP-SMX	**Vanco ± RIF**, **(Gemi, moxi, or levo)**; **telithro** (non-meningeal infections)	60–80% of strains susceptible to clindamycin (*DMID 25:201, 1996*).
Acinetobacter baumannii. Resistant to: IMP, P Ceph 3 AP, AP Pen, APAG, FQ (*see page 3 for abbreviations*)	**AM-SB** (*CID 34:1425, 2002*). Subactam alone is active against some A. baumannii *JAC 42:793, 1998*). **Colistin** effective most multi-resistant strains (*CID 36:1111, 2003; JAC 54:1085, 2004; CID 43:S89, 2006*). AM-SB appears more effective than colistin (*JAC 61:1369, 2008*).	6/8 patients with A. baumannii meningitis (7 organisms resistant to IMP) cured with AM/SB (*CID 24: 932, 1997*). Various combinations of FQs and AGs, IMP and AGs or RIF, or AP Pens or P Ceph 3 APs with AGs or RIF + colistin may show activity against **some** multiresistant strains (*CID 36:1268, 2003; JAC 61:417, 2008*). MER + subactam active in vitro & in vivo (*JAC 53:393, 2004*). Active in vitro: triple drug combinations of polymyxin B, IMP, & RIF (*AAC 48:753, 2004*), other colistin-containing combination regimens (*CID 43:S95, 2006; AAC 51:1621, 2007*) & tigecycline (*CID 41:S315, 2005*), but several studies document borderline activity of tigecycline against acinetobacter and emergence of resistance during therapy (*JAC 59:772, 2007; AAC 51: 376, 2007; CID 46:567, 2008*). Definitive data concerning its effectiveness not yet available (*JAC 62:45, 2008*). Minocycline effective in traumatic wound infections (*IDCP 16:16, 2008*).
Campylobacter jejuni. Resistant to: FQs	Erythro, azithro, clarithro, doxy, clindamycin	Resistance to **both** FQs & macrolides reported (*CID 22:868, 1996; EID 7:24, 2002; AAC 47:2358, 2003*).
Klebsiella pneumoniae (producing ESBL). Resistant to: Ceftazidime & other 3rd generation cephalosporins (*see Table 10C*), aztreonam	**IMP, MER.** (*CID 39:31, 2004*) (*See Comment*)	P Ceph 4, TC-CL, PIP-TZ show in vitro activity, but not proven entirely effective in animal models (*IJAA 8:37, 1997*); some strains which hyperproduce ESBLs are primarily resistant to TC-CL and PIP-TZ (*J Clin Micro 34:358, 1996*). Note: there are strains of ESBL-producing klebsiella sensitive in vitro to P Ceph 2, 3 but resistant to ceftazidime; infections with such strains do not respond to P Ceph 2 or 3 (*J Clin Micro 39:2206, 2001*). FQ may be effective if susceptible but many strains resistant. Note Klebsiella sp. with carbapenem resistance due to class A carbapenemase. Some of these organisms resistant to all antimicrobials except colistin (*CID 39:55, 2004*). Tigecycline active in vitro (*AAC 50:3166, 2006*). Ertapenem active against ESBL-producing E. coli in pharmacodynamic model (*JAC 61:643, 2008*).
Resistant to: Carbapenems, 2nd & 3rd generation cephalosporins due to KPC enzymes	**Colistin** (*AAC 48:4793, 2004*)	
Pseudomonas aeruginosa. Resistant to: IMP, MER	**CIP** (check susceptibility), **APAG** (check susceptibility). **Colistin** effective for multiresistant strains (*CID 28:1008, 1999; CMI 13:560, 2007*).	Many strains remain susceptible to aztreonam & ceftazidime or AP Pens (*JAC 36:1037, 1995*). Combinations of (AP Pen & APAG) or (AP Ceph 3 + APAG) may show in vitro activity (*AAC 39:2411, 1995*).

TABLE 6 – SUGGESTED MANAGEMENT OF SUSPECTED OR CULTURE-POSITIVE COMMUNITY-ASSOCIATED METHICILLIN-RESISTANT S. AUREUS (CA-MRSA) INFECTIONS (See footnote[1] for doses)

In the absence of definitive comparative efficacy studies, the Editors have generated the following guidelines. With the magnitude of the clinical problem and a number of new drugs, it is likely new data will require frequent revisions of the regimens suggested. (See page 3 for abbreviations).

CLINICAL ILLNESS	ABSCESS, AFEBRILE; & IMMUNOCOMPETENT: OUTPATIENT CARE	ABSCESS(ES) WITH FEVER; OUTPATIENT CARE	PNEUMONIA	BACTEREMIA OR POSSIBLE ENDOCARDITIS OR BACTEREMIC SHOCK	TREATMENT FAILURE (See footnote[2])
Management (for drug doses, see footnote)	**TMP-SMX-DS** or **doxycycline** or **minocycline** or **clindamycin** (CID 40:1429, 2005 & AAC 51:2628, 2007) **NOTE: I&D** alone may be sufficient (PIDJ 23:123, 2004; AAC 51:4044, 2007; NEJM 357:380, 2007).	**TMP-SMX-DS** ± **RIF** or **clindamycin** or **doxycycline** (do not use RIF alone as resistance develops rapidly) Culture abscess & maybe blood. **I&D** Hot packs. Close follow-up.	**Vanco** IV or **linezolid** IV	**Vanco** or **dapto** IV. **Dapto** not inferior to **vanco** in bacteremia trial (NEJM 355:653, 2006). No apparent benefit of adding RIF, maybe harm (AAC 52:2463, 2008). **Vanco** MICs ↑ing; disproportionate ↑ in MBCs (CID 42:513, 2006 & 44:1208, 2007). Ideal **vanco** trough level unclear. More nephrotoxicity with higher troughs (Curr Ther 29:107, 2007). If **vanco** MIC≥2 ug/mL, consider alternative therapy; ID consultation suggested.	Confirm adequate vanco troughs of 15-20 µg/ml and vancomycin susceptibility; search for deep focus of infection. Switch to alternative regimen if **vanco** MIC ≥ 2 µg/ml. **Dapto** resistance reported after **vanco** exposure & prior to **dapto** therapy (CID 45:601, 2007). **Dapto appears safe at doses of up to** 12 mg/kg/d (AAC 50:3245, 2006). For endocarditis or complicated bacteremia **dapto** 10 mg/kg IV once daily plus **gentamicin** 1 mg/kg IV every 8 hours or **RIF** 300-450 mg twice daily; 2nd choice **quinupristin-dalfopristin** (Q-D) ± with **vanco**. 3rd choice **linezolid** ± a second agent (JAC 58:273, 2006 & JAC 56:923, 2005).
Comments	Effective dose of **TMP-SMX-DS** is unclear. IV dose is 8-10 mg/kg/d; roughly equivalent to 2 tabs po bid. Anecdotally, most pts respond to I&D and 1 tab bid although failures may occur (see footnote 1).	Patients not responding after 2-3 days should be evaluated for complicated infection and switched to **vancomycin**.	**Linezolid** superior to **vanco** in retrospective subset analysis; prospective study in progress.	Efficacy of IV **TMP-SMX** vs CA-MRSA uncertain. IV **TMP-SMX** was inferior to **vanco** vs bacteremic MSSA (AnIM 117:390, 1992). **Dapto** failures associated with development of **dapto** resistance (NEJM 355:653, 2006).	If MRSA resistant to **erythro**, likely that Q-D will have bacteristatic & not bactericidal activity. Interest in Q-D + **vanco**, but no data. Do not add **linezolid** to **vanco**: no benefit & may be antagonistic (AAC 47:3002, 2003). Linezolid successful in compassionate use (JAC 50:1017, 2002) & in pts with reduced vanco in vitro suscept. (CID 38:521, 2004). New drugs likely available in 2009: ceftobiprole, ceftaroline and telavancin.

[1] **Clindamycin:** 300 mg po tid. **Daptomycin:** 6 mg/kg IV q24h is the standard dose; higher doses (10 mg/kg) and use of combination therapy recommended for vancomycin treatment failures. **Doxycycline or minocycline:** 100 mg po bid. **Linezolid:** 600 mg po/IV bid. **Quinupristin-dalfopristin (Q-D):** 7.5 mg per /kg IV q8h via central line. **Rifampin:** Long serum half-life justifies dosing 600 mg po q24h; however, frequency of nausea less with 300 mg po bid. **TMP-SMX-DS:** Standard dose 8–10 mg per kg per day. For 70 kg person = 700 mg TMP component per day. **TMP-SMX** contains 160 mg TMP and 800 mg SMX. The dose for treatment of CA-MRSA skin and soft tissue infecions (SSTI) is not established. In one small study 1 DS tablet twice daily was effective, although 3/14 subjects failed therapy (AAC 51:2628, 2007); therefore 2 DS tablets twice daily is recommended for treatment of patients with fever or complicated SSTI. **Vancomycin:** 1 gm IV q12h; up to 45–60 mg/kg/day in divided doses may be required to achieve target trough concentrations of 15-20 mcg/mL recommended for serious infections.

[2] The median duration of bacteremia in endocarditis is 7-9 days in patients treated with vancomycin (AnIM 115:674, 1991). Longer duration of bacteremia, greater likelihood of endocarditis (JID 190:1140, 2004). Definition of failure unclear. Clinical response should be factored in. **Unsatisfactory clinical response especially if blood cultures remain positive beyond 5-7 days is an indication for change in therapy.**

TABLE 7 – METHODS FOR PENICILLIN DESENSITIZATION
(CID 35:26, 2002; AJM 121:572, 2008)

(See Table 10C, page 95, for TMP/SMX desensitization)

Perform in ICU setting. Discontinue all β-adrenergic antagonists. Have IV line, ECG and spirometer (CCTID 13:131, 1993). Once desensitized, rx must not lapse or risk of allergic reactions ↑. A history of Stevens-Johnson syndrome, exfoliative dermatitis, erythroderma are nearly absolute contraindications to desensitization (use only as an approach to IgE sensitivity).

Oral Route: If oral prep available and pt has functional GI tract, oral route is preferred. 1/3 pts will develop transient reaction during desensitization or treatment, usually mild.

Step *	1	2	3	4	5	6	7	8	9	10	11	12	13	14
Drug (mg per mL)	0.5	0.5	0.5	0.5	0.5	0.5	0.5	5.0	5.0	5.0	50	50	50	50
Amount (mL)	0.1	0.2	0.4	0.8	1.6	3.2	6.4	1.2	2.4	4.8	1.0	2.0	4.0	8.0

* Interval between doses: 15 min. After Step 14, observe for 30 minutes, then 1.0 gm IV.

Parenteral Route:

Step **	1	2	3	4	5	6	7	8	9	10	11	12	13	14	15	16	17
Drug (mg per mL)	0.1	0.1	0.1	0.1	1.0	1.0	1.0	10	10	10	100	100	100	100	1000	1000	1000
Amount (mL)	0.1	0.2	0.4	0.8	0.16	0.32	0.64	0.12	0.24	0.48	0.1	0.2	0.4	0.8	0.16	0.32	0.64

** Interval between doses: 15 min. After Step 17, observe for 30 minutes, then 1.0 gm IV. *[Adapted from Sullivan, TJ, in Allergy: Principles and Practice, C.V. Mosby, 1993, p. 1726, with permission.]*

TABLE 8 – RISK CATEGORIES OF ANTIMICROBICS IN PREGNANCY

DRUG	FDA CATEGORIES*
Antibacterial Agents	
Aminoglycosides:	
Amikacin, gentamicin, isepamicin^NUS, netilmicin^NUS, streptomycin & tobramycin	D
Beta Lactams	
Penicillins; pens + BLI; cephalosporins; aztreonam	B
Imipenem/cilastatin	C
Meropenem, ertapenem, doripenem	B
Chloramphenicol	C
Ciprofloxacin, oflox, levoflox, gatiflox, gemiflox, moxiflox	C
Clindamycin	B
Colistin	C
Daptomycin	B
Fosfomycin	B
Fusidic acid[1]	See Footnote[1]
Linezolid	C
Macrolides:	
Erythromycins/azithromycin	B
Clarithromycin	C
Metronidazole	B
Nitrofurantoin	B
Rifaximin	C
Sulfonamides/trimethoprim	C
Telithromycin	C
Antibacterial Agents: *(continued)*	
Tetracyclines, tigecycline	D
Tinidazole	C
Vancomycin	C
Antifungal Agents: *(CID 27:1151, 1998)*	
Amphotericin B preparations	B
Anidulafungin	C
Caspofungin	C
Fluconazole, itraconazole, ketoconazole, flucytosine	C
Micafungin	C
Posaconazole	C
Terbinafine	B
Voriconazole	C
Antiparasitic Agents:	
Albendazole/mebendazole	C
Atovaquone/proguanil; atovaquone alone	C
Chloroquine	C
Eflornithine	C
Ivermectin	B
Mefloquine	C
Miltefosine	B
Nitazoxanide	B
Pentamidine	C
Praziquantel	B
Pyrimethamine/pyrisulfadoxine	C
Quinidine	C
Antimycobacterial Agents:	
Quinine	X
Capreomycin	C
Clofazimine/cycloserine	"avoid"
Dapsone	C
Ethambutol	"safe"
Ethionamide	"do not use"
INH, pyrazinamide	C
Rifabutin	B
Rifampin	C
Thalidomide	X
Antiviral Agents:	
Abacavir	C
Acyclovir	B
Adefovir	C
Amantadine	C
Atazanavir	B
Cidofovir	C
Darunavir	C
Delavirdine	C
Didanosine (ddI)	B
Efavirenz	D
Emtricitabine	B
Enfuvirtide	B
Entecavir	C
Etravirine	C
Famciclovir	C
Antiviral Agents: *(continued)*	
Fosamprenavir	C
Ganciclovir	C
Indinavir	C
Interferons	C
Lamivudine	C
Lopinavir/ritonavir	C
Maraviroc	B
Nelfinavir	B
Nevirapine	C
Oseltamivir	C
Raltegravir	C
Ribavirin	X
Rimantadine	C
Ritonavir	B
Saquinavir	B
Stavudine	C
Telbivudine	B
Tenofovir	B
Tipranavir	C
Valacyclovir	B
Valganciclovir	C
Zalcitabine	C
Zanamivir	C
Zidovudine	C

* **FDA Pregnancy Categories: A**—studies in pregnant women, no risk; **B**—animal studies no risk, but human not adequate or animal toxicity but human studies no risk; **C**—animal studies show toxicity, human studies inadequate but benefit of use may exceed risk; **D**—evidence of human risk, but benefits may outweigh; **X**—fetal abnormalities in humans, risk > benefit

[1] **Fusidic acid**: no problems reported

TABLE 9A – SELECTED PHARMACOLOGIC FEATURES OF ANTIMICROBIAL AGENTS (Footnotes at end of table)

DRUG	DOSE, ROUTE OF ADMINISTRATION	FOR PO DOSING—Take Drug[7] WITH FOOD	WITHOUT FOOD[8]	WITH OR WITHOUT FOOD	% AB[1]	PEAK SERUM LEVEL mcg per mL[6]	PROTEIN BINDING, %	AVERAGE SERUM T½, HOURS[2]	BILIARY EXCRETION, %[3]	CSF[4]/BLOOD, %	CSF LEVEL POTENTIALLY THERAPEUTIC[5]
PENICILLINS: Natural											
Benzathine Pen G	1.2 million units IM					0.15					
Penicillin G	2 million units IV					20	65		500	5–10	Yes for Pen-sens. S. pneumo
Penicillin V	500 mg po		X		60–73	5–6	65	0.5			
PEN'ASE-RESISTANT PENICILLINS											
Clox/Diclox	500 mg po		X		50	10–15	95–98	0.5			
Natcillin/Oxacillin	500 mg po		X		Erratic	10–15	90–94	0.5	>100/25	9–20	Yes-high-dose IV therapy
AMINOPENICILLINS											
Amoxicillin	500 mg po			X	80	6–10	17	1.2	100–3000	13–14	Yes
AM-CL	875/125 mg po	X		X		11.6/2.2	20/30	1.4/1.1	100–3000		
AM-CL-ER						17/2.1	18/25	1.3/1.0			
Ampicillin	2 gm IV					47	18–22	1.2	100–3000	13–14	Yes
AM-SB	3 gm IV					109–150	28/38	1.2			
ANTIPSEUDOMONAL PENICILLINS											
Indanyl carb.	382 mg po			X	35	6.5	50	1.0			
Piperacillin	4 gm IV					400	16–48	1.0	3000–6000	30	Not for P. aeruginosa; marginal for coliforms
PIP-TZ	3.375 gm IV					209	16–48	1.0	>100		
Ticarcillin	3 gm IV					260	45	1.2		40	Not for P. aeruginosa; marginal for coliforms
TC-CL	3.1 gm IV					330	45/25	1.2/1.0			
CEPHALOSPORINS—1st Generation											
Cefadroxil	500 mg po			X	90	16	20	1.5	22		
Cefazolin	1 gm IV					188	73–87	1.9	29–300	1–4	No
Cephalexin	500 mg po			X	90	18–38	5–15	1.0	216		
CEPHALOSPORINS—2nd Generation											
Cefaclor	500 mg po		X		93	9.3	22–25	0.8	≥60		
Cefaclor-CD	500 mg po		X			8.4	22–25	0.8	≥60		
Cefotetan	1 gm IV					124	78–91	4.2	2–21		
Cefoxitin	1 gm IV					110	65–79	0.8			
Cefprozil	500 mg po			X	95	10.5	36	1.5	280	3	No
Cefuroxime	1.5 gm IV					100	33–50	1.5	35–80		
Cefuroxime axetil	250 mg po			X	52	4.1	50	1.5		17–88	Marginal
Loracarbef			X		90	8	25	1.2			
CEPHALOSPORINS—3rd Generation											
Cefdinir	300 mg po			X	25	1.6	60–70	1.7			
Cefditoren pivoxil	400 mg po	X			16	4	88	1.6			
Cefixime	400 mg po			X	50	3–5	65	3.1	800		
Cefotaxime	1 gm IV					100	30–51	1.5	15–75	10	Yes
Cefpodoxime proxetil	200 mg po	X			46	2.9	40	2.3	115		
Ceftazidime	1 gm IV					60	<10	1.9	13–54	20–40	Yes
Ceftibuten	400 mg po		X		80	15	65	2.4			

TABLE 9A (2) (Footnotes at the end of table)

DRUG	DOSE, ROUTE OF ADMINISTRATION	FOR PO DOSING—Take Drug[7] WITH FOOD	WITHOUT FOOD[8]	WITH OR WITHOUT FOOD	% AB[1]	PEAK SERUM LEVEL mcg per mL[6]	PROTEIN BINDING, %	SERUM T½, HOURS[2]	BILIARY EXCRETION, %[3]	CSF[4]/BLOOD, %	CSF LEVEL POTENTIALLY THERAPEUTIC[5]
CEPHALOSPORINS—3rd Generation (continued)											
Ceftizoxime	1 gm IV					132	30	1.7	34-82		
Ceftriaxone	1 gm IV					150	85-95	8	200-500	8-16	Yes
CEPHALOSPORIN—4th Generation and anti-MRSA (ceftobiprole)											
Cefepime	2 gm IV					193	20	2.0	∝ 5	10	Yes
Ceftobiprole	500 mg IV					33-34.2	16	2.9-3.3			
CARBAPENEMS											
Doripenem	500 mg IV					23	8.1	1	117 (0-611)		
Ertapenem	1 gm IV					154	95	4	10		
Imipenem	500 mg IV					40	15-25	1	minimal	8.5	+[9]
Meropenem	1 gm IV					49	2	1	3-300	Approx. 2	+
MONOBACTAM											
Aztreonam	1 gm IV					125	56	2	115-405	3-52	±
AMINOGLYCOSIDES											
Amikacin, gentamicin, kanamycin, tobramycin—see Table 10D, page 96, for dose & serum levels											
Neomycin	po				<3	0	0-10	2.5	10-60	0-30	No; intrathecal dose: 5-10 mg
FLUOROQUINOLONES[10]											
Ciprofloxacin	750 mg po			X	70	1.8-2.8	20-40	4	2800-4500	26	1 mcg per mL: Inadequate for Strep. species (CID 31:1131, 2000).
	400 mg IV			X		4.6	20-40	4	2800-4500		
	500 mg ER po			X		1.6	20-40	6.6			
	1000 mg ER po			X		3.1	20-40	6.3			
Gatifloxacin	400 mg po/IV			X	96	4.2-4.6	20	7-8		36	
Gemifloxacin	320 mg po			X	71	0.7-2.6	55-73	7			
Levofloxacin	500 mg po/IV			X	99	5.7	24-38	7			
	750 mg po/IV			X	99	8.6	24-38	7		30-50	
Moxifloxacin	400 mg po/IV			X	89	4.5	30-50	10-14			
Ofloxacin	400 mg po/IV			X	98	4.6/6.2	32	7			
MACROLIDES, AZALIDES, LINCOSAMIDES, KETOLIDES											
Azithromycin	500 mg po			X	37	0.4	7-51	68	High		
	500 mg IV					3.6	7-51	12/68	High		
Azithromycin-ER	2 gm po		X		∝ 30	0.8	7-50	59	High		
Clarithromycin	500 mg po			X	50	3-4	65-70	5-7	7000		
	ER—500 mg po	X			∝ 50	2-3	65-70				
Erythromycin Oral (various)	500 mg po		X		18-45	0.1-2	70-74	2-4		2-13	No
Lacto/glucep	500 mg IV					3-4	70-74	2-4			
Telithromycin	800 mg po			X	57	2.3	60-70	10	7		
Clindamycin	150 mg po			X	90	2.5	85-94	2.4	250-300		No
	600 mg IV			X		10	85-94	2.4	250-300		No

See page 82 for all footnotes; see page 3 for abbreviations

TABLE 9A (3) (Footnotes at the end of table)

DRUG	DOSE, ROUTE OF ADMINISTRATION	FOR PO DOSING—Take Drug[7]			% AB[1]	PEAK SERUM LEVEL mcg per mL[6]	PROTEIN BINDING, %	SERUM T½, HOURS[2]	BILIARY EXCRETION, %[3]	CSF[4]/BLOOD, %	CSF LEVEL POTENTIALLY THERAPEUTIC[5]
		WITH FOOD	WITHOUT FOOD[8]	WITH OR WITHOUT FOOD							
MISCELLANEOUS ANTIBACTERIALS											
Chloramphenicol	1 gm po			X	High	11–18	25–50	4.1		45–89	Yes
Colistin	150 mg IV					5–7.5		2–3	0		No
Daptomycin	4–6 mg per kg IV					58–99	92	8–9			
Doxycycline	100 mg po			X		1.5–2.1	93	18	200–3200		No (26%)
Fosfomycin	3 gm po		X			26	<10	5.7			
Fusidic acid	500 mg po				91	30	95–99	5–15			
Linezolid	600 mg po/IV			X	100	15–20	31	5		60–70	
Metronidazole	500 mg po/IV			X		20–25	20	6–14	100	45–89	
Minocycline	200 mg po			X		2.0–3.5	76	16	200–3200		No
Polymyxin B	20,000 units per kg IV					1–8		4.3–6			
Quinu-Dalfo	7.5 mg per kg IV					5		1.5			
Rifampin	600 mg po		X			4–32	80	2–5	10,000		
Rifaximin	200 mg po			X	<0.4	0.004–0.01		7–12			
Sulfamethoxazole (SMX)	2 gm po				70–90	50–120					
Tetracycline	250 mg po		X			1.5–2.2		6–12	200–3200		No (7%)
Telavancin	10 mg/kg/q24h					87.5	90	7–8	Low		
Tigecycline	50 mg IV q12h					0.63	71–89	42	138		No
Trimethoprim (TMP)	100 mg po				80	1		8–15			
TMP-SMX-DS	160/800 mg po / 160/800 mg IV			X	85	1–2/40–60 / 9/105		6–12	100–200 / 40–70	50/40	Most meningococci resistant. Static vs coliforms
Vancomycin	1 gm IV					20–50	<10–55	4–6	50	7–14	Need high doses. See Meningitis, Table 1A, page 7
ANTIFUNGALS											
Amphotericin B											
Standard: 0.4–0.7 mg per kg IV						0.5–3.5		24		0	
Ampho B lipid complex (ABLC): 5 mg per kg IV						1–2.5		173			
Ampho B cholesteryl complex: 4 mg per kg IV						2.9		39			
Liposomal ampho B: 5 mg per kg IV						83		6.8 ± 2.1			
Azoles											
Fluconazole	400 mg po/IV		X		90	6.7	10	20–50		50–94	Yes
	800 mg po/IV		X		90	Approx. 14		20–50			
Itraconazole	Oral soln 200 mg po		X		Low	0.3–0.7	99.8	35		0	
Posaconazole	200 mg po	X				0.2–1.0	98–99	20–66			Yes (JAC 56:745, 2005)
Voriconazole	200 mg po		X		96	3	58	6		22–100	Yes (CID 37:728, 2003)
Anidulafungin	200 mg IV x 1, then 100 mg IV q24h					7.2	>99	26.5	100–200		No
Caspofungin	70 mg IV x 1, then 50 mg IV qd					9.9	97	9–11	40–70		No
Flucytosine	2.5 gm po			X	78–90	30–40		3–6		60–100	Yes
Micafungin	150 mg IV					16.4	>99	15–17			No

See page 82 for all footnotes; see page 3 for abbreviations

TABLE 9A (4) (Footnotes at the end of table)

DRUG	DOSE, ROUTE OF ADMINISTRATION	FOR PO DOSING—Take Drug[7] WITH FOOD	WITHOUT FOOD[8]	WITH OR WITHOUT FOOD	% AB[1]	PEAK SERUM LEVEL mcg per mL[6]	PROTEIN BINDING, %	SERUM T½, HOURS[2]	BILIARY EXCRETION, %[3]	CSF[4]/BLOOD, %	CSF LEVEL POTENTIALLY THERAPEUTIC[5]
ANTIMYCOBACTERIALS											
Ethambutol	25 mg per kg po	X			80	2–6	10–30	4		25–50	No
Isoniazid	300 mg po		X		100	3–5		0.7–4		90	Yes
Pyrazinamide	20–25 mg per kg po			X	95	30–50	5–10	10–16		100	Yes
Rifampin	600 mg po		X		70–90	4–32	80	1.5–5	10,000	7–56	Yes
Streptomycin	1 gm IV (see Table 10D, page 96)					25–50	0–10	2.5	10–60	0–30	No. Intrathecal: 5–10 mg
ANTIPARASITICS											
Albendazole	400 mg po	X				0.5–1.6	70				
Atovaquone suspension	750 mg po	X			47	15	99.9	67		<1	No
Dapsone	100 mg po		X		100	1.1		10–50			
Ivermectin	12 mg po		X			0.05–0.08					
Mefloquine	1.25 gm po	X				0.5–1.2	98	13–24 **days**			Ref: AAC52:2855, 2008
Miltefosine	50 mg po tid	X				31	95	7–31			
Nitazoxanide	500 mg po	X				3	99				
Proguanil[11]		X					75				
Pyrimethamine	25 mg po			X	"High"	0.1–0.3	87	96			
Praziquantel	20 mg per kg po	X			80	0.2–2.0		0.8–1.5			
Tinidazole	2 gm po	X			48		12	13			Chemically similar to metronidazole
ANTIVIRAL DRUGS—NOT HIV											
Acyclovir	400 mg po			X	10–20	1.21	9–33	2.5–3.5			
Adefovir	10 mg po			X	59	0.02	≤4	7.5			
Entecavir	0.5 mg po		X		100	4.2 ng/mL	13	128–149			
Famciclovir	500 mg po			X	77	3–4	<20	2–3			
Ganciclovir	5 mg per kg IV			X	75	8.3	1–2	3.5			
Oseltamivir	75 mg po			X	75	0.65/3.5[12]	3	1–3			
Ribavirin	600 mg po			X	64	0.8		44			
Rimantadine	100 mg po			X				25			
Telbivudine	600 mg po			X		0.1–0.4	3.3	40–49			
Valacyclovir	1000 mg po			X	55	5.6	13–18	3			
Valganciclovir	900 mg po	X			59	5.6	1–2	4			

DRUG	DOSE, ROUTE OF ADMINISTRATION	FOR PO DOSING—Take Drug[7] WITH FOOD	WITHOUT FOOD[8]	WITH OR WITHOUT FOOD	% AB[1]	PEAK SERUM LEVEL mcg per mL[6]	PROTEIN BINDING, %	INTRACELLULAR T½, HOURS[2]	SERUM T½, HOURS[2]	CYTOCHROME P450
ANTI-HIV VIRAL DRUGS										
Abacavir	600 mg po			X	83	3.0	50	12–26	1.5	
Atazanavir	400 mg po	X			"Good"	2.3	86		7	
Darunavir	600 mg with 100 mg ritonavir	X			82	3.5	95		15	
Delavirdine	400 mg po			X	85	19 ± 11	98		5.8	Inhibitor
Didanosine	400 mg EC[13] po		X		30–40	?	<5	25–40	1.4	
Efavirenz	600 mg po		X		42	13 mcM[14]	99		52–76	Inducer/Inhibitor

See page 82 for all footnotes; see page 3 for abbreviations

TABLE 9A (5) (Footnotes at the end of table)

| DRUG | DOSE, ROUTE OF ADMINIS-TRATION | FOR PO DOSING—Take Drug[7] | | | % AB[1] | PEAK SERUM LEVEL mcg per mL[6] | PROTEIN BINDING, % | INTRACELLULAR T½, HOURS[2] | SERUM T½, HOURS[2] | CYTOCHROME P450 |
		WITH FOOD	WITHOUT FOOD[8]	WITH OR WITHOUT FOOD						
ANTI-HIV VIRAL DRUGS *(continued)*										
Emtricitabine	200 mg po			X	93	1.8	<4	39	10	
Enfuvirtide	90 mg sc				84	5	92		4	
Etravirine	200 mg po	X			No data		99.9		41	
Fosamprenavir	1400 mg po+RTV			X	65	6	90	No data	7.7	Inducer/inhibitor
Indinavir	800 mg po		X		65	12.6 mcM[14]	60		1.2-2	Inhibitor
Lamivudine	300 mg po			X	86	2.6	<36	18-22	5-7	
Lopinavir	400 mg po			X	No data	9.6	98-99		5-6	Inhibitor
Maraviroc	300 mg po			X	33	3-9	76		14-18	
Nelfinavir	1250 mg po	X			20-80	3-4	98		3.5-5	Inhibitor
Nevirapine	200 mg po			X	>90	2	60		25-30	Inducer
Raltegravir	400 mg po			X	?	2	83	alpha 1/beta 9	7-12	
Ritonavir	300 mg po	X			65	7.8	98-99		3-5	Potent inhibitor
Saquinavir	1000 mg po (with 100 mg ritonavir)	X			4	3.1	97		1-2	Inhibitor
Stavudine	40 mg			X	86	1.4	<5	7.5	1	
Tenofovir	300 mg po	X			25	0.3	<1-7	>60	17	
Tipranavir	500 mg + 200 mg ritonavir	X				78-95 mcM[14]	99.9		5.5-6	
Zalcitabine	0.75 mg po			X	85	0.03	<4	Unknown	1.2	
Zidovudine	300 mg po			X	60	1-2	<38	11	0.5-3	

FOOTNOTES:

1 % absorbed under optimal conditions
2 Assumes CrCl >80 mL per min.
3 Peak concentration in bile/peak concentration in serum x 100. If blank, no data.
4 CSF levels with inflammation
5 Judgment based on drug dose & organ susceptibility. CSF concentration ideally ≥10 above MIC.

6 Total drug; adjust for protein binding to determine free drug concentration.
7 For adult oral preps; not applicable for peds suspensions.
8 Food decreases rate and/or extent of absorption.
9 Concern over seizure potential; see Table 10

10 Take all po FQs 2–4 hours before sucralfate or any multivalent cations: Ca++, Fe++, Zn++
11 Given with atovaquone as Malarone for malaria prophylaxis.
12 Oseltamivir/oseltamivir carboxylate
13 EC = enteric coated
14 mcM=micromolar

TABLE 9B – PHARMACODYNAMICS OF ANTIBACTERIALS*

BACTERIAL KILLING/PERSISTENT EFFECT	DRUGS	THERAPY GOAL	PK/PD MEASUREMENT
Concentration-dependent/Prolonged persistent effect	Aminoglycosides; daptomycin; ketolides; quinolones; metro	High peak serum concentration	24-hr AUC*/MIC
Time-dependent/No persistent effect	Penicillins; cephalosporins; carbapenems; monobactams	Long duration of exposure	Time above MIC
Time-dependent/Moderate to long persistent effect	Clindamycin; erythro/azithro/clarithro; linezolid; tetracyclines; vancomycin	Enhanced amount of drug	24-hr AUC*/MIC

* Adapted from Craig, WA: IDC No. Amer 17:479, 2003 & Drusano, G.L.:CID 44:79, 2007   ¹ **AUC** = area under drug concentration curve

See page 82 for all footnotes; see page 3 for abbreviations

TABLE 10A – SELECTED ANTIBACTERIAL AGENTS—ADVERSE REACTIONS—OVERVIEW

Adverse reactions in individual patients represent all-or-none occurrences, even if rare. After selection of an agent, the physician should read the manufacturer's package insert [statements in the product labeling (package insert) must be approved by the FDA].

Numbers = **frequency of occurrence (%); + = occurs, incidence not available; ++ = significant adverse reaction; 0 = not reported; R = rare, defined as <1%.**

NOTE: Important reactions in bold print. A blank means no data found.

Drug groups: PENICILLINS (Penicillin G,V) · PENICILLINASE-RESISTANT ANTI-STAPH. PENICILLINS (Dicloxacillin, Nafcillin, Oxacillin) · AMINOPENICILLINS (Amoxicillin, Amox-Clav, Ampicillin, Amp-Sulb) · AP PENS (Piperacillin, Pip-Taz, Ticarcillin, Ticar-Clav) · CARBAPENEMS (Doripenem, Ertapenem, Imipenem, Meropenem) · MONOBACTAMS (Aztreonam) · AMINOGLYCOSIDES (Amikacin, Gentamicin, Kanamycin, Netilmicin[NUS], Tobramycin) · MISC. (Linezolid, Telithromycin)

ADVERSE REACTIONS	Pen G,V	Diclox	Nafcillin	Oxacillin	Amoxicillin	Amox-Clav	Ampicillin	Amp-Sulb	Piperacillin	Pip-Taz	Ticarcillin	Ticar-Clav	Doripenem	Ertapenem	Imipenem	Meropenem	Aztreonam	Aminoglycosides	Linezolid	Telithromycin
Rx stopped due to AE	+				2-4.4				3.2	3.2			3.4			1.2	<1		3/1	7/2
Local: phlebitis	+		++	+		3		3	4	1	3		+	4	3	1	4		4	10
Hypersensitivity																				
Fever	+	+	+	+	+	+	+	+	+	2	+	+		+	3	3			+	
Rash	**3**	**4**	**4**	**4**	**5**	**3**	**5**	**2**	**1**	**4**	**3**	**2**	**+**	**+**	**+**	**+**	**2**	**+**		
Photosensitivity	0	0	0	0	0	0	0	0	0	0	0	0			0		+			
Anaphylaxis	R	0	R	0	R	R	R	+	0	0	+	R		+	+	+	+			
Serum sickness	4			R	+	+	+	0	+	+	+	+		+	+	+	+			
Hematologic																				
+ Coombs	3	0	R	R	+	0	+	0	+	+	0	+		1	2	2	R			
Neutropenia	R	0	+	R	6		+	+	6	+	0	0	+	+	+	+	+		1.1	
Eosinophilia	+	+	22	22	2	+	22	22	+	+	R	R	+	+	+	+	8			
Thrombocytopenia	R	0	R	R	R	R	R	R	+	+	R	R			+	+	+		3-10 (see 10C)	3-10 (see 10C)
↑ PT/PTT	R	0	+	0	+	0	+	0	+	+	+	+			R		R			
GI																				
Nausea/vomiting		+	0	0	2	3	2	+	+	7	+	1	+	3	2	4	R		3/1	7/2
Diarrhea		+	0	0	**5**	**9**	**10**	**2**	2	11	3	1	+	6	2	5	R		4	10
C. difficile colitis		R	R	R	R	+	R	+	+	+	+	+	+	+	+	+	+		+	+
Hepatic: LFTs	R	R	0	+	R	+	R	6	0	+	0	0	+	6	4	4	2		1.3	
Hepatic failure	0	0	0	0	0	0	0	0	0	0	0	0		0	0	0	0		+	+
Renal: ↑BUN, Cr	R	0	0	R	R	0	R	R	R	R	R	0	*See footnote[2]*				0	**5–25[1]**	0	
CNS																				
Headache	R	0	R	R	0	+	R	R	R	8	R	R	+	2	2	3	+	+	2	2
Confusion	R	0	R	R	0	0	R	R	R	R	R	R	+	+	+	2	+	+	+	2
Seizures	R	0	0	+	0	R	R	0	R	R	R	+	+	+	+	3	+			

[1] Varies with criteria used

[2] **All β-lactams in high concentration can cause seizures** (JAC 45:5, 2000). In rabbit, IMP 10x more neurotoxic than benzylpenicillin (JAC 22:687, 1988). In clinical trial of IMP for ped meningitis, trial stopped due to seizures in 7/25 IMP recipients; hard to interpret as purulent meningitis causes seizures (PIDJ 10:122, 1991). Risk with IMP ↓ with careful attention to dosage (Epilepsia 42:1590, 2001).
Postulated mechanism: Drug binding to $GABA_A$ receptor. IMP binds with greater affinity than MER.
Package insert, percent seizures: ERTA 0.5, IMP 0.4, MER 0.7. However, in 3 clinical trials of MER for bacterial meningitis, no drug-related seizures (Scand J Inf Dis 31:3, 1999; Drug Safety 22:191, 2000).
In febrile neutropenic cancer pts, IMP-related seizures reported at 2% (CID 32:381, 2001; Peds Hem Onc 17:585, 2000).

TABLE 10A (2)

PENICILLINS, CARBAPENEMS, MONOBACTAMS, AMINOGLYCOSIDES

ADVERSE REACTIONS	Penicillin G,V	Dicloxacillin	Nafcillin	Oxacillin	Amoxicillin	Amox-Clav	Ampicillin	Amp-Sulb	Piperacillin	Pip-Taz	Ticarcillin	Ticar-Clav	Doripenem	Ertapenem	Imipenem	Meropenem	Aztreonam	Aminoglycosides (Amikacin, Gentamicin, Kanamycin, Netilmicin^NUS, Tobramycin)	Linezolid	Telithromycin
Special Senses																				
Ototoxicity	0	0	0	0	0	0	0	0	0	0	0	0			R		0	3–14[1]		
Vestibular	0	0	0	0	0	0	0	0	0	0	0	0			0		0	4–6[1]		
Cardiac																				
Dysrhythmias	R	0		0	0		0		0		0	0			0		+			++
Miscellaneous, Unique (Table 10C)	+	+	+	+	+	+	+	+		+				+	+		+		+	++
Drug/drug interactions, common (Table 22)	0	0	0	0	0	0	0	0	0	0	0	0			0		0	+	+	+

Column groupings: Penicillin G,V | PENICILLINASE-RESISTANT ANTI-STAPH. PENICILLINS (Dicloxacillin, Nafcillin, Oxacillin) | AMINOPENICILLINS (Amoxicillin, Amox-Clav, Ampicillin, Amp-Sulb) | AP PENS (Piperacillin, Pip-Taz, Ticarcillin, Ticar-Clav) | CARBAPENEMS (Doripenem, Ertapenem, Imipenem, Meropenem) | Aztreonam | AMINOGLYCOSIDES | MISC. (Linezolid, Telithromycin)

CEPHALOSPORINS/CEPHAMYCINS

ADVERSE REACTIONS	Cefazolin	Cefotetan	Cefoxitin	Cefuroxime	Cefotaxime	Ceftazidime	Ceftizoxime	Ceftriaxone	Cefepime	Ceftobiprole	Cefaclor/Cef.ER[1]/Loracarb	Cefadroxil	Cefdinir	Cefixime	Cefpodoxime	Cefprozil	Ceftibuten	Cefditoren pivoxil	Cefuroxime axetil	Cephalexin
Rx stopped due to AE	+	R	R	2	5	1	4	2	1.5	4			3		2.7	2	2	2	2.2	
Local, phlebitis	5	1	1			2			1		2									
Hypersensitivity																				
Fever	+	+	+			R	+	R	+	+	+	+		R	R	+		R	R	
Rash	+	2	2	R	2	2	2	2	2	+	1	+	R	1	1	1	R	R	R	1
Photosensitivity	0	0	0	0	0	R	0	0												
Anaphylaxis	R	+				R					R				R			R	R	
Serum sickness											≤0.5[2]	+								+

[1] Cefaclor extended release tablets

[2] Serum sickness requires biotransformation of parent drug plus inherited defect in metabolism of reactive intermediates (*Ped Pharm & Therap 125:805, 1994*)

* *See note at head of table, page 83*

TABLE 10A (3)

CEPHALOSPORINS/CEPHAMYCINS

ADVERSE REACTIONS	Cephalexin	Cefuroxime axetil	Cefditoren pivoxil	Ceftibuten	Cefprozil	Cefpodoxime	Cefixime	Cefdinir	Cefadroxil	Cefaclor/Cef.ER[1]/Loracarb	Ceftobiprole	Cefepime	Ceftriaxone	Ceftizoxime	Ceftazidime	Cefotaxime	Cefuroxime	Cefoxitin	Cefotetan	Cefazolin
Hematologic																				
+ Coombs	+	R	R		R	R	R	R		R	+	14			4	6	R	2	+	3
Neutropenia	3	R	R		R	R	R		+	+	+	1	2	+	1	+	R	2		+
Eosinophilia	9	1	R	5	2	3	R	R	+		+	1	6	4	8	1	7	3	+	
Thrombocytopenia				R	+	R				2		+								
↑ PT/PTT												+	+	+	+	+		+	++	+
GI																				
Nausea/vomiting	2	3	6/1	6/2	4	4	13/7	3		3/2	+	1	R		R	R	R	2	1	
Diarrhea		4	1.4	3	3	7	16	15	+	1-4	+	1	3		1	1	R		4	
C. difficile colitis	+	+	+	+	+	+	+	+		+	+	+	+	+	+	+	+	+	+	+
Hepatic: ↑ LFTs		2	R	R	2	4	R	1	+	3	+	+	3	4	6	1	4	3	1	+
Hepatic failure	+											0	0	0	0	0	0	0	0	0
Renal: ↑ BUN, Cr	+	+	R	R	R	4	+	R		+	+	+	1		R	+		3		+
CNS																				
Headache	+	R	2	R	R	1	R	2		3	+	2	R		1					0
Confusion	+				R					+										0
Seizures																				0
Special Senses																				
Ototoxicity	0	0	0	0	0	0	0	0	0	0			0	0	0	0	0	0	0	0
Vestibular	0	0	0	0	0	0	0	0	0	0			0	0	0	0	0	0	0	0
Cardiac																				
Dysrhythmias	0	0	0	0	0	0	0	0	0	0			0	0	0	0	0	0	0	0
Miscellaneous, Unique (Table 10C)			+							+[2]	+		+							
Drug/drug interactions, common (Table 22)	0	0	0	0	0	0	0	0	0	0			0	0	0	0	0	0	0	0

[1] Cefaclor extended release tablets

[2] Serum sickness requires biotransformation of parent drug plus inherited defect in metabolism of reactive intermediates (Ped Pharm & Therap 125:805, 1994)

* See note at head of table, page 83

TABLE 10A (4)

ADVERSE REACTIONS (AE)	MACROLIDES			QUINOLONES						OTHER AGENTS										
	Azithromycin, Reg. & ER[1]	Clarithromycin, Reg. & ER[1]	Erythromycin	Ciprofloxacin/Cipro XR	Gatifloxacin[NUS]	Gemifloxacin	Levofloxacin	Moxifloxacin	Ofloxacin	Chloramphenicol	Clindamycin	Colistimethate (Colistin)	Daptomycin	Metronidazole	Quinupristin-dalfopristin	Rifampin	Tetracycline/Doxy/Mino	Tigecycline	TMP-SMX	Vancomycin
Rx stopped due to AE	1	3		3.5	2.9	2.2	4	3.8	4				2.8					5		
Local, phlebitis			++		5								6		++			2		13
Hypersensitivity																				
Fever				R	R		R			+	+	+	2			1	R	7	++	**8**
Rash	R		+	3	R	1-22[2]	1.7	R		+	+	+	4	+		+	+	2.4	+	1
Photosensitivity	R			R	R	R	R	R	2		4				R		+		+	3
Anaphylaxis			+	R	R	R	R	R	R	+	+						+	+	+	0
Serum sickness							R				+									R
Hematologic																				
Neutropenia	R	1		R	R				1	+	+			+		R	R	R	+	2
Eosinophilia	R			R	R				1		+						+	+	+	+
Thrombocytopenia	R	R		R			R			+	+			R			+	+	+	+
↑ PT/PTT		1	++	R						+							+	4		0
GI																				
Nausea/vomiting	3	3[3]	**25**	5	8/<3	2.7	7/2	7/2	7	+	+	+	6.3	**12**		+		30/20	3	
Diarrhea	5	3–6	**8**	2	4	3.6	5	5	4		7		5	+		+		13	3	
C. difficile colitis	R	+	+	**R**	**R**	**R**	**R**	**R**	**R**		++		+			R	+			+
Hepatic, LFTs	R	R	+	2	R	1.5	R	R	2		+				2	+	+	4		0
Hepatic failure	0	0														+	+			0
Renal																				
↑ BUN, Cr	+			1	R				R		0	+	R			+	+		+	5
CNS																				
Dizziness, light headedness	R			R	3	0.8	3.5	**2**	**3**					++				2		
Headache		2		1	4	1.2	6	2		+	+	+	5	+		+	+	3.5	+	
Confusion			+	+	R		R	R	2	+		+		+					+	
Seizures	+	+	+	+	R		R	R	R			+		+					+	

[1] Regular and extended-release formulations
[2] **Highest frequency:** females <40 years of age after 14 days of rx; with 5 days or less of Gemi, incidence of rash <1.5%
[3] Less GI upset/abnormal taste with ER formulation

* See note at head of table, page 83

TABLE 10A (5)

ADVERSE REACTIONS (AE)	MACROLIDES			QUINOLONES						OTHER AGENTS										
	Azithromycin, Reg. & ER[1]	Clarithromycin, Reg. & ER[1]	Erythromycin	Ciprofloxacin/Cipro XR	Gatifloxacin[NUS]	Gemifloxacin	Levofloxacin	Moxifloxacin	Ofloxacin	Chloramphenicol	Clindamycin	Colistimethate (Colistin)	Daptomycin	Metronidazole	Quinupristin-dalfopristin	Rifampin	Tetracycline/Doxy/Mino	Tigecycline	TMP-SMX	Vancomycin
Special senses																				
Ototoxicity	+		+	0					0											R
Vestibular																	21[1]			
Cardiac																				
Dysrhythmias			+	R	+[2]	+[2]	+[2]	+[2]	+[2]		R									0
Miscellaneous, Unique (Table 10C)	+	+	+	+	+	+	+	+	+	+	+	+	+	+	+	+	+	+	+	+
Drug/drug interactions, common (Table 22)	+	+	+	+	+	+	+	+	+						++		+	+	+	+

[1] Minocycline has 21% vestibular toxicity
[2] Fluoroquinolones as class assoc. **with QT$_c$ prolongation.** Ref.: CID 34:861, 2002.

TABLE 10B – ANTIMICROBIAL AGENTS ASSOCIATED WITH PHOTOSENSITIVITY

The following drugs are known to cause photosensitivity in some individuals. There is no intent to indicate relative frequency or severity of reactions.
Source: 2007 Red Book, Thomson Healthcare, Inc. Listed in alphabetical order:

Azithromycin, benznidazole, ciprofloxacin, dapsone, doxycycline, erythromycin ethyl succinate, flucytosine, erythromycin ethyl succinate, flucytosine, ganciclovir,gatifloxacin, gemifloxacin, griseofulvin, interferons, lomefloxacin, ofloxacin, pyrazinamide, saquinavir, sulfonamides, tetracyclines, tigecycline, tretinoins, voriconazole

* See note at head of table, page 83

TABLE 10C –ANTIBIOTIC DOSAGE* AND SIDE-EFFECTS

CLASS, AGENT, GENERIC NAME (TRADE NAME)	USUAL ADULT DOSAGE*	ADVERSE REACTIONS, COMMENTS (See Table 10A for Summary)
NATURAL PENICILLINS		
Benzathine penicillin G (Bicillin L-A)	600,000–1.2 million units IM q2–4 wks	**Allergic reactions a major issue.** 10% of all hospital admissions give history of pen allergy; but only 10% have allergic reaction if given penicillin. Why? Possible reasons: inaccurate history, waning immunity with age, aberrant response during viral illness, reaction to concomitant procaine.
Penicillin G	**Low:** 600,000–1.2 million units IM per day **High:** ≥20 million units IV q24h(=12 gm)	**Most serious reaction is immediate IgE-mediated anaphylaxis;** incidence only 0.05% but 5-10% fatal. Other IgE-mediated reactions: urticaria, angioedema, laryngeal edema, bronchospasm. Morbilliform rash after 72 hrs is not IgE-mediated and not serious.
Penicillin V	0.25–0.5 gm po bid, tid, qid before meals & at bedtime	**Serious late allergic reactions:** Coombs-positive hemolytic anemia, neutropenia, thrombocytopenia, serum sickness, interstitial nephritis, hepatitis, eosinophilia, drug fever. **Cross-allergy to cephalosporins and carbapenems** roughly 10%. **For pen desensitization, see Table 7.** For skin testing, suggest referral to allergist. High **CSF** concentrations cause seizures. Reduce dosage with renal impairment; see Table 17. Allergy reference: AJM 121:572, 2008.
PENICILLINASE-RESISTANT PENICILLINS		
Dicloxacillin (Dynapen)	0.125–0.5 gm po q6h ac.	Blood levels ~2 times greater than cloxacillin. Acute hemorrhagic cystitis reported. Acute abdominal pain with GI bleeding without antibiotic-associated colitis also reported.
Flucloxacillin[NUS] (Floxapen, Lutropin, Staphcil)	0.25–0.5 gm po q6h 1–2 gm IV q4h	In Australia, cholestatic hepatitis [women predominate, age >65, rx mean 2 weeks, onset 3 weeks from starting rx (Ln 339:679, 1992)] 16 deaths since 1980; recommendation: use only in severe infection (Ln 344:676, 1994).
Nafcillin (Unipen, Nafcil)	1–2 gm IV/IM q4h.	Extravasation can result in tissue necrosis. With dosages of 200–300 mg per kg per day hypokalemia may occur. **Reversible neutropenia (over 10% with ≥21-day rx, occasionally WBC <1000 per mm³).**
Oxacillin (Prostaphlin)	1–2 gm IV/IM q4h.	**Hepatic dysfunction with ≥12 gm per day.** LFTs usually ↑ 2–24 days after start of rx, reversible. In children, more rash and liver toxicity with oxacillin as compared to nafcillin (CID 34:50, 2002)
AMINOPENICILLINS		
Amoxicillin (Amoxil, Polymox)	250 mg–1 gm po tid	IV available in UK, Europe. IV amoxicillin rapidly converted to ampicillin. Rash with infectious mono—see Ampicillin.
Amoxicillin-clavulanate (Augmentin)	See Comment for adult products	500–875 mg po bid listed in past; may be inadequate due to ↑ in resistance. With bid regimen, less clavulanate & less diarrhea. Clavulanate assoc. with rare reversible cholestatic hepatitis, esp. men >60 yrs, on rx >2 weeks (ArIM 156:1327, 1996). 2 cases anaphylactic reaction to clavulanic acid (J All Clin Immun 95:748, 1995). **Comparison adult Augmentin product dosage regimens:**
AM-CL extra-strength peds suspension (ES-600)	**Peds Extra-Strength susp.:** 600/42.9 per 5 mL. **Dose:** 90/6.4 mg/kg div bid.	Augmentin 500/125 1 tab po tid
AM-CL-ER—extended release adult tabs	For adult formulations, see Comments IV amox-clav available in Europe	Augmentin 875/125 1 tab po bid Augmentin-XR 1000/62.5 2 tabs po bid
Ampicillin (Principen)	0.25–0.5 gm po q6h. 150–200 mg/kg IV/day.	A maculopapular rash occurs (not urticarial), **not true penicillin allergy**, in 65–100% pts with infectious mono, 90% with chronic lymphocytic leukemia, and 15–20% with allopurinol therapy.
Ampicillin-sulbactam (Unasyn)	1.5–3 gm IV q6h.	Supplied in vials: ampicillin 1 gm, sulbactam 0.5 gm or amp 2 gm, sulbactam 1 gm. AM-SB is not active vs pseudomonas. Total daily dose sulbactam ≤4 gm.
ANTIPSEUDOMONAL PENICILLINS NOTE: Platelet dysfunction may occur with any of the antipseudomonal penicillins, esp. in renal failure patients.		
Piperacillin (Pipracil) (Canada only)	3–4 gm IV q4–6h (200–300 mg per kg per day up to 500 mg per kg per day). For urinary tract infection: 2 gm IV q6h. See Comment	1.85 mEq Na+ per gm. See PIP-TZ comment on extended infusion. For P. aeruginosa infections: 3 gm IV q4h.

* NOTE: all dosage recommendations are for adults (unless otherwise indicated) & assume normal renal function. (See page 3 for abbreviations)

TABLE 10C (2)

CLASS, AGENT, GENERIC NAME (TRADE NAME)	USUAL ADULT DOSAGE*	ADVERSE REACTIONS, COMMENTS (See Table 10A for Summary)
ANTIPSEUDOMONAL PENICILLINS (continued)		
Piperacillin-tazobactam (Zosyn)	3.375 gm IV q6h. 4.5 gm q8h available For P. aeruginosa: see Comment for dosage.	Supplied as: piperacillin 3 gm + tazobactam (TZ) 0.375 gm. TZ more active than sulbactam as β-lactamase inhibitor. PIP-TZ 3.375 gm q6h as monotherapy **not adequate for serious pseudomonas infections. For empiric or specific treatment of P. aeruginosa dose is 4.5 gm IV q6h or 3.375 gm IV q4h.** For P. aeruginosa, **PIP-TZ can also be given as an extended infusion of 3.375 gm IV for 4 hrs & then repeated every 8 hrs** (CID 44:357, 2007). For severe P. aeruginosa infection, **tobra** or **CIP** is added to the **PIP-TZ.** In patients with ventilator-assoc pneumonia & no/mild renal impairment, alveolar PIP-TZ concentration optimized with 2 doses of 4.5 gm then continuos infusion of 18 gm/day (CCM 36:1500 & 1663, 2008). Piperacillin can cause false-pos. serum antigen test for galactomannan—a test for invasive aspergillosis.
Ticarcillin disodium (Ticar)	3 gm IV q4–6h.	Coagulation abnormalities common with large doses, interferes with platelet function, ↑ bleeding times; may be clinically significant in pts with renal failure. (4.5 mEq Na⁺ per gm)
Ticarcillin-clavulanate (Timentin)	3.1 gm IV q4–6h.	Supplied in vials: ticarcillin 3 gm, clavulanate 0.1 gm per vial. 4.5–5 mEq Na⁺ per gm. Diarrhea due to clavulanate. Rare reversible cholestatic hepatitis secondary to clavulanate (ArIM 156:1327, 1996).
CARBAPENEMS. NOTE: In pts with pen allergy, 11% had allergic reaction after imipenem or meropenem (CID 38:1102, 2004); 9% in a 2ⁿᵈ study (JAC 54:1155, 2004); and 0% in 2 other studies (NEJM 354:2835, 2006; AnIM 146:266, 2007).		
Doripenem	500 mg IV q8h (infusion duration varies with indication)	Most common adverse reactions (≥5%): Headache, nausea, diarrhea, rash & phlebitis. Can lower serum valproic acid levels. Adjust dose if renal impairment. More stable in solution than **IMP** or **MER.**
Ertapenem (Invanz)	1 gm IV/IM q24h.	**Lidocaine** diluent for IM use; ask about lidocaine allergy. Standard dosage may be inadequate in obesity (BMI ≥40) (AAC 50:1222, 2006).
Imipenem + cilastatin (Primaxin) Ref: JAC 58:916, 2006	0.5–1 gm IV q6h; for P. aeruginosa: 1 gm q6–8h (see Comment).	For infection due to P. aeruginosa, increase dosage to 3 or 4 gm per day div. q8h or q6h. Continuous infusion of carbapenems may be more efficacious & safer (AAC 49:1881, 2005). Seizure comment, see footnote 2, Table 10A, page 83. Clastatin decreases risk of prox. tubule toxicity.
Meropenem (Merrem)	0.5–1 gm IV q8h. Up to 2 gm IV q8h for meningitis.	For seizure incidence comment, see Table 10A, page 83. Comments: Does not require a dehydropeptidase inhibitor (cilastatin). Activity vs aerobic gm-neg. slightly ↑ over IMP, activity vs staph & strep slightly ↓; anaerobes = to IMP. B. ovatus, B. distasonis more resistant to meropenem.
MONOBACTAMS		
Aztreonam (Azactam)	1 gm q8h–2 gm IV q6h.	Can be used in pts with allergy to penicillins/cephalosporins. Animal data and a letter raise concern about cross-reactivity with ceftazidime (Rev Inf Dis 7:613, 1985); side-chains of aztreonam and ceftazidime are identical.
CEPHALOSPORINS (1st parenteral, then oral drugs).	**NOTE:** Prospective data demonstrate correlation between use of cephalosporins (esp. 3ʳᵈ generation) and ↑ risk of C. difficile toxin-induced diarrhea. May also ↑ risk of colonization with vancomycin-resistant enterococci. **For cross-allergenicity, see Oral, on page 90.**	
1ˢᵗ Generation, Parenteral		
Cefazolin (Ancef, Kefzol)	0.25 gm q8h–1.5 gm IV/IM q6h.	Do not give into lateral ventricles—seizures! No activity vs. community-associated MRSA.
2ⁿᵈ Generation, Parenteral		
Cefotetan (Cefotan)	1–3 gm IV/IM q12h. (Max. dose not >6 gm q24h).	Increasing resistance of B. fragilis, Prevotella bivius, Prevotella disiens (most common in pelvic infections). Ref.: CID 35 (Suppl.1):S126, 2002. Methylthiotetrazole (MTT) side chain can inhibit vitamin K activation.
Cefoxitin (Mefoxin)	1 gm q8h–2 gm IV/IM q4h.	In vitro may induce ↑ β-lactamase, esp. in Enterobacter sp.
Cefuroxime (Kefurox, Ceftin, Zinacef)	0.75–1.5 gm IV/IM q8h.	More stable vs staphylococcal β-lactamase than cefazolin.
3ʳᵈ Generation, Parenteral—Use of P Ceph 3 drugs correlates with incidence of C. difficile toxin diarrhea; perhaps due to cephalosporin resistance of C. difficile (CID 38:646, 2004).		
Cefoperazone-sulbactamⁿᵘˢ (Sulperazon)	Usual dose 1–2 gm IV q12h; if larger doses, do not exceed 4 gm/day of sulbactam.	Investigational in U.S. In SE Asia & elsewhere, used to treat intra-abdominal, biliary, & gyn. infections. Other uses due to broad spectrum of activity. Possible clotting problem due to side-chain. For dose logic: JAC 15:136, 1985.
Cefotaxime (Claforan)	1 gm q8–12h to 2 gm IV q4h.	Maximum daily dose: 12 gm.
Ceftazidime (Fortaz, Tazicef)	1–2 gm IV/IM q8–12h.	Excessive use may result in ↑ incidence of C. difficile-assoc. diarrhea and/or selection of vancomycin-resistant E. faecium. Ceftaz is susceptible to extended-spectrum cephalosporinases (CID 27:76 & 81, 1998).

* NOTE: all dosage recommendations are for adults (unless otherwise indicated) & assume normal renal function. (See page 3 for abbreviations)

TABLE 10C (3)

CLASS, AGENT, GENERIC NAME (TRADE NAME)	USUAL ADULT DOSAGE*	ADVERSE REACTIONS, COMMENTS (See Table 10A for Summary)
CEPHALOSPORINS/3ʳᵈ Generation, Parenteral (continued)		
Ceftizoxime (Cefizox)	1 gm q8–12h to 4 gm IV q8h.	Maximum daily dose: 12 gm.
Ceftriaxone (Rocephin)	**Commonly used IV dosage in adults:** 1 gm once daily **Purulent meningitis: 2 gm q12h.** Can give **IM** in 1% lidocaine.	"**Pseudocholelithiasis**," 2° to sludge in gallbladder by ultrasound (50%), symptomatic (9%) (NEJM 322:1821, 1990). More likely with ≥2 gm per day with pt on total parenteral nutrition and not eating (AnIM 115:712, 1991). Clinical significance still unclear but has led to cholecystectomy (JID 17:356, 1995) and gallstone pancreatitis (Ln 17:662, 1998). In pilot study: 2 gm once daily by continuous infusion superior to 2 gm bolus once daily (JAC 59:285, 2007).
Other Generation, Parenteral		
Cefepime (Maxipime)	1–2 gm IV q12h.	Active vs P. aeruginosa and many strains of Enterobacter, serratia, C. freundii resistant to ceftazidime, cefotaxime, aztreonam (LnID 7:338, 2007). More active vs S. aureus than 3ʳᵈ generation cephalosporins.
Cefpirome^MDS (HR 810)	1–2 gm IV q12h	Similar to cefepime; ↑ activity vs enterobacteriaceae, P. aeruginosa, Gm + organisms. Anaerobes: less active than cefoxitin, more active than cefotax or ceftaz.
Ceftobiprole	0.5 gm IV q8h for mixed gm- neg & gm-pos infections. 0.5 gm IV q12h for gm-pos infections	Infuse over 2 hrs for q8h dosing, over 1 hr for q12h dosing. Associated with caramel-like taste disturbance. Ref.: Clin Microbiol Infections 13(Suppl 2):17 & 25, 2007. First cephalosporin active vs. MRSA.
Oral Cephalosporins **1st Generation, Oral**		**Cross-Allergenicity: Patients with a history of IgE-mediated allergic reactions to a penicillin (e.g., anaphylaxis, angioneurotic edema, immediate urticaria) should not receive a cephalosporin.** If the history is a
Cefadroxil (Duricef)	0.5–1 gm po q12h.	"measles-like "rash to a penicillin, available data suggest a 5–10% risk of rash in such patients; there is no enhanced risk of anaphylaxis. Cephalosporin skin tests, if available, predictive of reaction (AnIM 141:16, 2004; AJM 121:572, 2008).
Cephalexin (Keflex, Keftab generic)	0.25–0.5 gm po q6h.	Any of the cephalosporins can result in **C. difficile toxin-**mediated diarrhea/enterocolitis. The reported frequency of nausea/vomiting and non-C. difficile toxin diarrhea is summarized in Table 10A.
2nd Generation, Oral		There are **few drug-specific adverse effects, e.g.:**
Cefaclor (Ceclor)	0.25–0.5 gm po q8h.	**Cefaclor:** Serum sickness-like reaction 0.1–0.5%—arthralgia, rash, erythema multiforme but no adenopathy, protein-uria or demonstrable immune complexes. Appear due to mixture of drug biotransformation and genetic susceptibility (Ped Pharm & Therap 125:805, 1994).
Cefaclor-ER (Ceclor CD)	0.375–0.5 gm po q12h.	**Cefdinir:** Drug-iron complex causes red stools in roughly 1% of pts.
Cefprozil (Cefzil)	0.25–0.5 gm po q12h.	**Cefditoren pivoxil:** Hydrolysis yields pivalate. Pivalate absorbed (70%) & becomes pivaloylcarnitine which is renally excreted; 39–63% ↓ **in serum carnitine concentrations** Carnitine involved in fatty acid (FA) metabolism & FA
Cefuroxime axetil po (Ceftin)	0.125–0.5 gm po q12h.	transport into mitochondria. Effect transient & reversible. No clinical events documented to date (Med Lett 44:5, 2002). Also contains caseinate (milk protein); **avoid if milk allergy** (not same as lactose intolerance). Need gastric acid for optimal absorption.
3rd Generation, Oral		**Cefpodoxime:** There are rare reports of acute liver injury, bloody diarrhea, pulmonary infiltrates with eosinophilia.
Cefdinir (Omnicef)	300 mg po q12h or 600 mg q24h.	**Cefixime:** Now available from Lupin Pharmaceuticals.
Cefditoren pivoxil (Spectracef)	200–400 mg po bid.	**Cephalexin:** Can cause false-neg. urine dipstick test for leukocytes.
Cefixime (Suprax)	0.4 gm po q12–24h.	
Cefpodoxime proxetil (Vantin)	0.1–0.2 gm po q12h.	
Ceftibuten (Cedax)	0.4 gm po q24h.	

---

* NOTE: all dosage recommendations are for adults (unless otherwise indicated) & assume normal renal function.
(See page 3 for abbreviations)

TABLE 10C (4)

CLASS, AGENT, GENERIC NAME (TRADE NAME)	USUAL ADULT DOSAGE*	ADVERSE REACTIONS, COMMENTS (See Table 10A for Summary)
AMINOGLYCOSIDES AND RELATED ANTIBIOTICS—See Table 10D, page 96, and Table 17A, page 179		
GLYCOPEPTIDES		
Teicoplanin[NUS] (Targocid)	**For septic arthritis—maintenance dose 12 mg/kg per day; S. aureus endocarditis— trough serum levels >20 mcg/mL required (12 mg/kg q12h times 3 loading dose, then 12 mg/kg q24h)**	Hypersensitivity: fever (at 3 mg/kg 2.2%, at 24 mg per kg 8.2%), skin reactions 2.4%. Marked ↓ platelets (high dose ≥15 mg per kg per day). Red neck syndrome less common than with vancomycin.
Vancomycin (Vancocin) Ref. on obesity: *Pharmacotherapy 27:108, 2007.*	**Normal weight patient:** 15 mg/kg IV q12h. If in ICU, first dose 25 mg/kg IV. **Morbidly obese:** 15 mg/kg IV q12h based on actual body weight. **Check serum levels:** *see Comment* **PO dosage for C. difficile colitis:** 125 mo po q6h. Commercial product very expensive. Can compound po preparation from IV vanco: 5 gm vanco + 47.5 mL sterile H₂O. 0.2 gm saccharin, 0.05 gm stevia powder, 40 mL glycerin and then enough cherry syrup to yield 100 mL. Final concentration: 50 mg vanco/mL. Dose = 2.5 mL q6h.	Vanco dosage currently in flux due to rising vanco MICs for S. aureus; as a result, some authorities suggest higher vanco doses to achieve trough vanco levels of 15-20 g/mL (*AJRCCM 171:388, 2005*). Result is higher q12h doses or continuous infusion regimens; however, both approaches associated with reports of nephrotoxicity (*AAC 52:1330, 2008; JAC 62:168, 2008*). No reports of greater clinical efficacy with higher trough levels. Hence, at present, **editors suggest** trough levels no higher than 15-20 mcg/mL. If MIC of vanco vs. pts S. aureus is ≥2 mcg/mL consider alternative therapy. **Intrathecal vanco dose:** 5-10 mg/day (infants) & 10-20 mg/day (children/adults); target CSF concentration of 10-20 g/mL. **"Red Neck" syndrome:** consequence of rapid infusion with non-specific histamine release. Other adverse effects: rash, fever, neutropenia, IgA bullous dermatitis (*CID 38:442, 2004*).
CHLORAMPHENICOL, CLINDAMYCIN(S), ERYTHROMYCIN GROUP, KETOLIDES, OXAZOLIDINONES, QUINUPRISTIN-DALFOPRISTIN (SYNERCID)		
Chloramphenicol (Chloromycetin)	0.25–1 gm po/IV q6h to max. of 4 gm per day.	No oral drug distrib in U.S. Hematologic (↓ RBC ~1/3 pts, aplastic anemia 1:21,600 courses). Gray baby syndrome in premature infants, anaphylactoid reactions, optic atrophy or neuropathy (very rare), digital paresthesias, minor disulfiram-like reactions.
Clindamycin (Cleocin) Lincomycin (Lincocin)	0.15–0.45 gm po q6h. 600–900 mg IV/IM q8h. 0.6 gm IV/IM q8h.	Based on number of exposed pts, these drugs are the most frequent cause of **C. difficile toxin-mediated diarrhea.** In most severe form can cause pseudomembranous colitis/toxic megacolon.
Erythromycin Group (Review drug interactions before use)		Motilin is gastric hormone that activates duodenal/jejunal receptors to initiate peristalsis. Erythro (E) and E esters, both po and IV, activate motilin receptors and cause uncoordinated peristalsis with resultant 20–25% incidence of anorexia,
Azithromycin (Zithromax) Azithromycin ER (ZMax)	**po preps:** Tabs 250 & 600 mg. Peds suspension: 100 & 200 mg per 5 mL. Adult ER suspension: 2 gm. Dose varies with indication, *see Table 1A,* Acute otitis media (*page 10*), acute exac. chronic bronchitis (*page 33*), Comm.-acq. pneumonia (*pages 36–37*) & sinusitis (*page 46*). IV: 0.5 gm per day.	nausea or vomiting (*Gut 33:397, 1992*). Less binding and GI distress with azithromycin/clarithromycin. Systemic erythro in 1st 2 wks of life associated with **infantile hypertrophic pyloric stenosis** (*J Ped 139:380, 2001*). **Frequent drug-drug interactions:** *see Table 22, page 193.* Major concern is prolonged QT₀ interval on EKG. **Prolonged QTc:** Mutations in 6 genes (LQT 1–3) produce abnormal cardiac K⁺/Na⁺ channels. Variable penetrance: no symptoms, repeated syncope, to sudden death (*NEJM 358:169, 2008*). ↑ **risk if female & QTc >500 msec! Risk amplified by other drugs** [macrolides, antiarrhythmics, & drug-drug interactions **(see FQs page 93 for list)**]. Can
Base and esters (Erythrocin, Ilosone) IV name: E. lactobionate	0.25 gm q6h–0.5 gm po/IV q6h: 15–20 mg/kg up to 4 gm q24h. Infuse over 30+ min.	result in torsades de pointes (ventricular tachycardia) and/or cardiac arrest. Refs: *CID 43:1603, 2006; www.qtdrugs.org & www.torsades.org.* Cholestatic hepatitis in approx. 1:1000 adults (not children) given E estolate.
Clarithromycin (Biaxin) or clarithro extended release (Biaxin XL)	0.5 gm po q12h. **Extended release: Two 0.5 gm tabs po per day.**	**Transient reversible tinnitus or deafness** with ≥4 gm per day of erythro IV in pts with renal or hepatic impairment. Reported with ≥600 mg per day of azithro (*CID 24:76, 1997*). Dosages of oral erythro preparations expressed as base equivalents. With differences in absorption/biotransformation, variable amounts of erythro esters required to achieve same free erythro serum level, e.g., 400 mg E ethyl succinate = 250 mg E base.
Ketolide **Telithromycin** (Ketek) (*Med Lett 46:66, 2004; Drug Safety 31:561, 2008*)	**Two 400 mg tabs po q24h.** 300 mg tabs available.	As of 9/06, 2 cases acute liver failure & 23 cases serious liver injury reported, or 23 cases per 10 million prescriptions. Occurred during or immediately after treatment. (*AnIM 144:415, 447, 2006*). **Uncommon: blurred vision** 2° slow accommodation; may cause exacerbation of **myasthenia gravis (Black Box Warning)**. Potential QT₀ prolongation. Several **drug-drug interactions** (*Table 22, pages 193–194*) (*NEJM 355:2260, 2006*).

* NOTE: all dosage recommendations are for adults (unless otherwise indicated) & assume normal renal function.
(*See page 3 for abbreviations*)

TABLE 10C (5)

CLASS, AGENT, GENERIC NAME (TRADE NAME)	USUAL ADULT DOSAGE*	ADVERSE REACTIONS, COMMENTS (See Table 10A for Summary)
CHLORAMPHENICOL, CLINDAMYCIN(S), ERYTHROMYCIN GROUP, KETOLIDES, OXAZOLIDINONES, QUINUPRISTIN-DALFOPRISTIN (continued)		
Linezolid (Zyvox)	**PO or IV dose: 600 mg q12h.** Available as 600 mg tabs, oral suspension (100 mg per 5 mL), & IV solution.	**Reversible myelosuppression:** thrombocytopenia, anemia, & neutropenia reported. Most often after >2 wks of therapy. Incidence of thrombocytopenia after 2 wks of rx: 7/20 osteomyelitic pts; 5/7 pts treated with vanco & then linezolid. Refs.: *CID 37:1609, 2003 & 38:1058 & 1065, 2004.* 6-fold increased risk in pts with ESRD *(CID 42:66, 2006).* **Lactic acidosis; peripheral neuropathy, optic neuropathy:** After 4 or more wks of therapy. Data consistent with time and dose-dependent inhibition of intramitochondrial protein synthesis *(CID 42:1111,2006; AAC 50:2042, 2006; Pharmacotherapy 27:771, 2007).* **Inhibitor of monoamine oxidase:** risk of severe hypertension if taken with foods rich in tyramine. Avoid concomitant pseudoephedrine, phenylpropanolamine, and caution with SSRIs[1] **Serotonin syndrome** (fever, agitation, mental status changes, tremors). Risk with concomitant SSRIs: *(CID 42:1578 and 43:180, 2006).*
Quinupristin + dalfopristin (Synercid) *(CID 36:473, 2003)*	7.5 mg per kg IV q8h via central line	Venous irritation (5%): none with central venous line. Asymptomatic ↑ in unconjugated bilirubin. **Arthralgia** 2%–50% *(CID 36:476, 2003).* **Drug-drug interactions:** Cyclosporine, nifedipine, midazolam, many more—see Table 22.
TETRACYCLINES *(Mayo Clin Proc 74:727, 1999)*		
Doxycycline (Vibramycin, Doryx, Monodox, Adoxa, Periostat)	0.1 gm po/IV q12h.	Similar to other tetracyclines. ↑ nausea on empty stomach. Erosive esophagitis. esp. if taken at bedtime. Phototoxicity + but less than with tetracycline. Deposition in teeth less. Can be used in patients with renal failure. *Comments:* Effective in treatment and prophylaxis for malaria, leptospirosis, typhus fevers.
Minocycline (Minocin, Dynacin)	0.1 gm po q12h IV minocycline no longer available.	**Vestibular symptoms** (30–90% in some groups, none in others): vertigo 33%, ataxia 43%, nausea 50%, vomiting 3%, women more frequently than men. Hypersensitivity pneumonitis, reversible. ~34 cases reported *(BMJ 310:1520, 1995).* Can increase **pigmentation** of the skin. *Comments:* More effective than other tetracyclines vs staph and in prophylaxis of meningococcal disease. P. acnes: many resistant to other tetracyclines, not to mino. Induced autoimmunity reported in children treated for acne *(J Ped 153:314, 2008).* Active vs Nocardia asteroides, Mycobacterium marinum.
Tetracycline, Oxytetracycline (Sumycin) *(CID 36:462, 2003)*	0.25–0.5 gm po q6h, 0.5–1 gm IV q12h.	GI (oxy 19%, tetra 4), anaphylactoid reaction (rare), deposition in teeth, negative N balance, hepatotoxicity, enamel agenesis, pseudotumor cerebri/encephalopathy. Outdated drug; Fanconi syndrome. *See drug-drug interactions, Table 22.* **Contraindicated in pregnancy, hepatotoxicity in mother, transplacental to fetus.** *Comments:* IV dosage over 2.0 gm per day may be associated with fatal hepatotoxicity. False-neg. urine dipstick for leukocytes.
Tigecycline (Tygacil)	100 mg IV initially, then 50 mg IV q12h with po food, if possible to decrease risk of nausea.	**If severe liver dis. (Child Pugh C):** 100 mg IV initially, then 25 mg IV q12h	Derivative of tetracycline. High incidence of nausea (25%) & vomiting (20%) but only 1% of pts discontinued therapy due to an adverse event. Details on AEs in *JAC 62 (Suppl 1):i17, 2008.* Pregnancy Category D. Do not use in children under age 18. Like other tetracyclines, may cause photosensitivity, pseudotumor cerebri, pancreatitis, a catabolic state (elevated BUN) and maybe hyperpigmentation *(CID 45:136, 2007).*

[1] **SSRI** = selective serotonin reuptake inhibitors, e.g., fluoxetine (Prozac).

* NOTE: all dosage recommendations are for adults (unless otherwise indicated) & assume normal renal function.
(See page 3 for abbreviations)

TABLE 10C (6)

CLASS, AGENT, GENERIC NAME (TRADE NAME)	USUAL ADULT DOSAGE*	ADVERSE REACTIONS, COMMENTS (See Table 10A for Summary)
FLUOROQUINOLONES (FQs): All can cause false-positive urine drug screen for opiates *(Pharmacother 26:435, 2006)*		
Ciprofloxacin (Cipro) and Ciprofloxacin-extended release (Cipro XR, Proquin XR)	**Urinary tract infection:** 500-750 mg po bid. 250 mg bid po or Cipro XR 500 mg q24h **Cipro IV:** 400 mg IV q12h; for P. aeruginosa 400 mg IV q8h *(AAC 49:4009, 2005).* **Ophthalmic solution**	**Children:** No FQ approved for use under age 16 based on joint cartilage injury in immature animals. Articular SEs in children est. at 2–3% *(LnID 3:537, 2003).* The exception is anthrax. **CNS toxicity:** Poorly understood. Varies from mild (lightheadedness) to moderate (confusion) to severe (seizures). May be aggravated by NSAIDs.
Gatifloxacin (Tequin)^NUS See comments	200–400 mg IV/po q24h. *(See comment)* Ophthalmic solution (Zymar)	**Gemi skin rash:** Macular rash after 8–10 days of rx. Incidence of rash with ≤5 days of therapy only 1.5%. Frequency highest females, < age 40, treated 14 days (22.6%). In men, < age 40, treated 14 days, frequency 7.7%. Mechanism unclear. Indication to DC therapy.
Gemifloxacin (Factive)	320 mg po q24h.	**Hypoglycemia/hyperglycemia** Due to documented hypo and hyperglycemic reactions *(NEJM 354:1352, 2006),* US distribution of Gati in US ceased in 6/2006. Gati ophthalmic solution remains available. **Opiate screen false-positives:** FQs can cause false-positive urine assay for opiates *(JAMA 286:3115, 2001; AnPharmacotherapy 38:1525, 2004).* **Photosensitivity:** See Table 10B, page 87
		QTc (corrected QT) interval prolongation: ↑ QTc (>500msec or >60msec from baseline) is considered possible with any FQ. ↑ QTc can lead to torsades de pointes and ventricular fibrillation. Risk low with current marketed drugs). Risk ↑ in women, ↓ K⁺, ↓ mg⁺⁺, bradycardia. (Refs.: *CID 43:1603, 2006).* Major problem is ↑ risk with concomitant drugs.
Levofloxacin (Levaquin)	250–750 mg po/IV q24h.	**Avoid concomitant drugs with potential to prolong QTc:**

Antiarrhythmics:	Anti-Infectives:	CNS Drugs	Misc.
Amiodarone	Azoles (not posa)	Fluoxetine	Dolasetron
Disopyramide	Clarithro/erythro	Haloperidol	Droperidol
Dofetilide	FQs (not CIP)	Phenothiazines	Fosphenytoin
Flecainide	Halofantrine	Pimozide	Indapamide
Ibutilide	NNRTIs	Quetiapine	Methadone
Procainamide	Protease Inhibitors	Risperidone	Naratriptan
Quinidine	Pentamidine	Sertraline	Salmeterol
Sotalol	Telithromycin	Tricyclics	Sumatriptan
	Anti-Hypertensives:	Venlafaxine	Tamoxifen
	Bepridil	Ziprasidone	Tizanidine
	Isradipine		
	Nicardipine		
	Moexipril		

		Updates online: www.qtdrugs.org; www.torsades.org
Moxifloxacin (Avelox)	400 mg po/IV q24h Ophthalmic solution (Vigamox)	**Tendinopathy:** Over age 60, approx. 2–6% of all Achilles tendon ruptures attributable to use of FQ *(ArIM 163:1801, 2003).* ↑ risk with concomitant steroid or renal disease *(CID 36:1404, 2003).* Overall incidence is low *(Eur J Clin Pharm*
Ofloxacin (Floxin)	200–400 mg po bid. Ophthalmic solution (Oculfox)	*63:499, 2007).*

* NOTE: all dosage recommendations are for adults (unless otherwise indicated) & assume normal renal function. *(See page 3 for abbreviations)*

TABLE 10C (7)

CLASS, AGENT, GENERIC NAME (TRADE NAME)	USUAL ADULT DOSAGE*	ADVERSE REACTIONS, COMMENTS (See Table 10A for Summary)
POLYMYXINS Ref: *CID 40:1333, 2005.* **Polymyxin B** (Poly-Rx)	15,000–25,000 units/kg/day divided q12h	Also used as/for: bladder irrigation, intrathecal, ophthalmic preps. Source: Bedford Labs, Bedford, OH. Differs from colistin by one amino acid.
Colistin (=Polymyxin E) (*LnID 6:589, 2006*) Don't confuse dose calc for the "base" vs the "salt": 10,000 units = 1 mg base. 1 mg colistin base = 2.4 mg colisthimethate sodium salt. In US, label refers to mgs of base. See AAC 50:2274 & 4231, 2006.	**Parenterals:** **In US: Colymycin-M** 2.5-5 mg/kg per day of base divided into 2-4 doses = 6.7–13.3 mg/kg per day of colistimethate sodium (max 800 mg/day). **Elsewhere: Colomycin** and **Promixin** **≤60 kg**, 50,000–75,000 IU/kg per day IV in 3 divided doses (=4-6 mg/kg per day of colisthimethate sodium). **>60kg**, 1-2 mill IU IV tid (= 80–160 mg IV tid) NOTE: Can give IM, but need to combine with "caine" anesthetic due to pain.	**Intrathecal** 10 mg/day and reported **Intraventricular** doses range from 1 6-20 mg/day. **Inhalation:** Colisthimethate 80 mg bid with cystic fibrosis and others (*CID 41:754, 2005).* **Combination therapy:** Few studies – 1) some reports of efficacy of colistin & rifampin vs A. baumannii and P. aeruginosa VAP. 2) In cystic fibrosis pts, attempts at eradication of P. aeruginosa combining p.o cipro + nebulized colisthimethate sodium. **Topical & oral:** Colistin sulfate used. **Nephrotoxicity:** Reversible tubular necrosis. Exact frequency unclear **Neurotoxicity:** Frequency Vertigo, facial paresthesia, abnormal vision, confusion, ataxia, & neuromuscular blockade → respiratory failure. Dose-dependent. In cystic fibrosis pts, 29% experienced paresthesia, ataxia or both. **Other:** Maybe hyperpigmentation (*CID 45:136, 2007).*
MISCELLANEOUS AGENTS **Daptomycin** (Cubicin) (Ref on resistance: *CID 45:601, 2007*)	**Skin/soft tissue: 4 mg per kg IV q24h** **Bacteremia/right-sided endocarditis: 6 mg per kg IV q24h** **Morbid obesity:** base dose on total body weight (*J Clin Pharm 45:48, 2005*)	**Potential muscle toxicity:** At 4 mg per kg per day., ↑ CPK in 2.8% dapto pts & 1.8% comparator-treated pts. Suggest weekly CPK; DC dapto if CPK exceeds 10x normal level or if symptoms of myopathy and CPK > 1,000. Manufacturer suggests stopping statins during dapto rx). Selected reagents (HemosIL Recombiplastin, Hemoliance Recombiplastin,) can falsely prolong PT & INR (*Blood Coag & Fibrinolysis 19:32, 2008).* NOTE: Dapto well-tolerated in healthy volunteers at doses up to 12 mg/kg q24h x 14d (*AAC 50:3245, 2006).* *Resitance of S. aureus reported during dapto therapy, post-vanco therapy & de novo.*
Fosfomycin (Monurol)	**3 gm with water po times 1 dose.**	Diarrhea in 9% compared to 6% of pts given nitrofurantoin and 2.3% given TMP-SMX. Available outside U.S., IV & PO, for treatment of multi-drug resistant bacteria (*CID 46:1069, 2008).*
Fusidic acid[NUS] (Fucidin)	**500 mg po/IV tid (Denmark & Canada)**	Jaundice (17% with IV use; 6% with po) (*CID 42:394, 2006).*
Methenamine hippurate (Hiprex, Urex)	**1 gm po q6h** 1 gm = 480 mg methenamine	Nausea and vomiting, skin rash or dysuria. Overall ~3%. Methenamine requires (pH ≤5) urine to liberate formaldehyde. Useful in suppressive therapy after infecting organisms cleared; do not use for pyelonephritis. *Comment:* Do not force fluids; may dilute formaldehyde. Of no value in pts with chronic Foley. If urine pH >5.0, co-administer ascorbic acid (1–2 gm q4h) to acidify the urine: cranberry juice (1200–4000 mL per day) has been used, results ±
Methenamine mandelate (Mandelamine)	**1 gm po q6h (480 mg methenamine).**	
Metronidazole (Flagyl) Ref.: *Activity vs. B. fragilis AAC 51:1649, 2007.*	**Anaerobic infections:** usually IV, 7.5 mg per kg (~500 mg) q6h (not to exceed 4 gm q24h). With long T½, can use IV at 15 mg per kg q12h. If life-threatening, use loading dose of IV 15 mg per kg. Oral dose: 500 mg qid; extended release tabs available 750 mg	Can be given rectally (enema or suppository). In pts with **decompensated liver disease** (manifest by ≥2 L of ascites, encephalopathy, ↑ prothrombin time, ↓ serum albumin) **t½ prolonged; unless dose ↓ by approx. ½ , side-effects ↑**. Absorbed into serum from vaginal gel. **Neurol.:** headache, rare paresthesias or peripheral neuropathy, ataxia, seizures, aseptic meningitis; report of reversible metro-induced cerebellar lesions (*NEJM 346:68, 2002).* **Avoid alcohol during & 48 hrs after (disulfiram-like reaction).** Very dark urine (common but harmless) Skin: urticaria. Mutagenic in Ames test. Tumorigenic in animals (high dose over lifetime). No evidence of risk in man. No teratogenicity.
Nitrofurantoin macrocrystals (Macrodantin, Furadantin)	**100 mg po q6h** Dose for long-term UTI suppression: 50–100 mg at bedtime	Absorption ↑ with meals. Increased activity in acid urine, much reduced at pH 8 or over. Not effective in endstage renal disease (*JAC 33(Suppl. A):121, 1994*). Nausea and vomiting, hypersensitivity, peripheral neuropathy. Pulmonary reactions (with chronic rx): acute ARDS type, **chronic desquamative interstitial pneumonia with fibrosis**. Intrahepatic cholestasis & **hepatitis** similar to chronic active hepatitis. Hemolytic anemia in G6PD deficiency. **Contraindicated in renal failure.** Should not be used in infants <1 month of age.
monohydrate/macrocrystals (Macrobid)	**100 mg po bid**	Efficacy of Macrobid 100 mg po bid = Macrodantin 50 mg qid. Adverse effects 5.6%, less nausea than with Macrodantin.

* NOTE: all dosage recommendations are for adults (unless otherwise indicated) & assume normal renal function.
(*See page 3 for abbreviations*)

TABLE 10C (8)

CLASS, AGENT, GENERIC NAME (TRADE NAME)	USUAL ADULT DOSAGE*	ADVERSE REACTIONS, COMMENTS (See Table 10A for Summary)
MISCELLANEOUS AGENTS (continued)		
Rifampin (Rimactane, Rifadin)	300 mg po bid or 600 mg po once daily	Causes orange-brown discoloration of sweat, urine, tears, contact lens. Many important drug-drug interactions, see Table 22.
Rifaximin (Xifaxan)	200 mg tab po tid times 3 days.	For traveler's diarrhea. In general, adverse events equal to or less than placebo.
Sulfonamides [e.g., sulfisoxazole (Gantrisin), sulfamethoxazole (Gantanol), (Truxazole)]	Dose varies with indications.	**Short-acting are best:** high urine concentration and good solubility at acid pH. More active in alkaline urine. **Allergic reactions:** skin rash, drug fever, pruritus, photosensitization. Periarteritis nodosa & SLE, Stevens-Johnson syndrome, serum sickness syndrome, myocarditis. Neurotoxicity (psychosis, neuritis). Blood dyscrasias, usually agranulocytosis. Crystalluria. Nausea & vomiting, headache, dizziness, lassitude, mental depression, acidosis, sulf-hemoglobin. Hemolytic anemia in G6PD deficient & unstable hemoglobins (Hb Zurich). Do not use in newborn infants or in women near term, ↑ frequency of kernicterus (binds to albumin, blocking binding of bilirubin to albumin).
Tinidazole (Tindamax)	Tabs 250, 500 mg. Dose for giardiasis: 2 gm po times 1 with food.	**Adverse reactions:** metallic taste 3.7%, nausea 3.2%, anorexia/vomiting 1.5%. All higher with multi-day dosing.
Trimethoprim (Trimpex, Proloprim, and others)	100 mg po q12h or 200 mg po q24h.	Frequent side-effects are rash and pruritus. Rash in 3% pts at 100 mg bid; 6.7% at 200 mg q24h. Rare reports of photosensitivity, exfoliative dermatitis, Stevens-Johnson syndrome, toxic epidermal necrosis, and aseptic meningitis (CID 19:431, 1994). Check drug interaction with phenytoin. Increases serum K+ (see TMP-SMX Comments). TMP can ↑ homocysteine blood levels (Ln 352:1827, 1998).
Trimethoprim (TMP)-Sulfamethoxazole (SMX) (Bactrim, Septra, Sulfatrim, Clotrimoxazole) Single-strength (SS) is 80 TMP/400 SMX, double-strength (DS) 160 TMP/800 SMX Ref.: ArIM 163:402, 2003	Standard po rx (UTI, otitis media): 1 DS tab bid. P. carinii: see Table 13, page 128. IV rx (base on TMP component): standard 8–10 mg per kg per day divided q6h, q8h, or q12h. For shigellosis: 2.5 mg per kg IV q6h.	Adverse reactions in 10%: GI: nausea, vomiting, anorexia. Skin: Rash, urticaria, photosensitivity. More serious (1–10%): Stevens-Johnson syndrome & toxic epidermal necrolysis. Skin reactions may represent toxic metabolites of SMX rather than allergy (AnPharmacotherapy 32:381, 1998). Daily ascorbic acid 0.5–1.0 gm may promote detoxification (JAIDS 36:1041, 2004). Rare hypoglycwemia, esp AIDS pts: (LnID 6:178, 2006). TMP competes with creatinine for tubular secretion: serum creatinine can ↑; TMP also blocks distal renal tubule secretion of K+: ↑ serum K+ in 21% of pts (AnIM 124:316, 1996). TMP one etiology of aseptic meningitis (CID 19:431, 1994). TMP-SMX contains sulfites and may trigger asthma in sulfite-sensitive pts. Frequent drug cause of thrombocytopenia (AnIM 129:886, 1998). No cross allergenicity with other sulfonamide non-antibiotic drugs (NEJM 349:1628, 2003). **Rapid Oral TMP-SMX Desensitization:** <table><tr><th>Hour</th><th>Dose TMP/SMX (mg)</th><th>Hour</th><th>Dose TMP/SMX (mg)</th></tr><tr><td>0</td><td>0.004/0.02</td><td>3</td><td>4/20</td></tr><tr><td>1</td><td>0.04/0.2</td><td>4</td><td>40/200</td></tr><tr><td>2</td><td>0.4/2</td><td>5</td><td>160/800</td></tr></table>
Topical Antimicrobial Agents Active vs. S. aureus & Strep. pyogenes		
Bacitracin (Baciguent)	20% bacitracin zinc ointment, apply bid, 3.5 gm	Active vs. staph, strep & clostridium. Contact dermatitis incidence 9.2% (IDC No Amer 18:717, 2004).
Fusidic acid[US] ointment	2% ointment, apply tid	CID 42:394, 2006. Available in Canada and Europe (Leo Laboratories).
Mupirocin (Bactroban)	Skin cream or ointment 2%: Apply tid times 10 days. Nasal ointment 2%: apply bid times 5 days.	Skin cream: itch, burning, stinging 1–1.5%; Nasal: headache 9%, rhinitis 6%, respiratory congestion 5%. Not active vs. enterococci or gm-neg bacteria.
Polymyxin B—Bacitracin (Polysporin)	5000 units/gm; 400 units/gm	Apply 1-3 times/day. Polymyxin active vs. gm-neg bacteria but not Proteus sp. Serratia sp. or gm-pos bacteria. See Bacitracin comment above.
Polymyxin B—Bacitracin—Neomycin (Neosporin, triple antibiotic ointment (TAO))	5000 units/gm; 400 units/gm; 3.5 mg/gm.	Apply 1-3 times/day. See Bacitracin and polymyxin B comments above. Neomycin active vs. gm-neg bacteria and staphylococci; not active vs. streptococci. Contact dermatitis incidence 1%; risk of nephro- & oto-toxicity if absorbed. TAO spectrum broader than mupirocin and active mupirocin-resistant strains (DMD 54:63, 2006).
Retapamulin (Altabax)	1% ointment; apply bid. 5, 10 & 15 gm tubes.	Microbiologic success in 90% S. aureus infections and 97% of S. pyogenes infections (J Am Acd Derm 55:1003, 2006). Package insert says **do not use for MRSA** (not enough pts in clinical trials).

Also for Trimethoprim-Sulfamethoxazole row, under ADVERSE REACTIONS:

Comment: Perform in hospital or clinic. Use oral suspension [40 mg TMP/ 200 mg SMX per 5 mL (tsp)]. Take 6 oz water after each dose. Cortico-steroids, anti-histaminics NOT used. Refs.: CID 20:849, 1995; AIDS 5:311, 1991

* NOTE: all dosage recommendations are for adults (unless otherwise indicated) & assume normal renal function.
(See page 3 for abbreviations)

TABLE 10D – AMINOGLYCOSIDE ONCE-DAILY AND MULTIPLE DAILY DOSING REGIMENS
(See Table 17, page 179, if estimated creatinine clearance <90 mL per min.)

General: Dosage given as both once-daily (OD) and multiple daily dose (MDD) regimens.

Pertinent formulae: (1) **Estimated creatinine clearance** (CrCl): $\frac{(140 - age)(ideal\ body\ weight\ in\ kg)}{(72)(serum\ creatinine)}$[1] = CrCl for men in mL per min; multiply answer times 0.85 for CrCl of women

Alternative method to calculate CrCl, see *NEJM 354:2473, 2006*

(2) **Ideal body weight (IBW)**– Females: 45.5 kg + 2.3 kg per inch over 5' = weight in kg

Males: 50 kg + 2.3 kg per inch over 5' = weight in kg

(3) **Obesity adjustment:** use if actual body weight (ABW) is ≥30% above IBW. To calculate adj dosing weight in kg: IBW + 0.4 (ABW–IBW) = adjusted weight *(Pharmacotherapy 27:1081, 2007; CID 25:112, 1997)*

DRUG	MDD AND OD IV REGIMENS/ TARGETED PEAK (P) AND TROUGH (T) SERUM LEVELS	COMMENTS For more data on once-daily dosing, see *AJM 105:182, 1998, and Table 17, page 179*
Gentamicin (Garamycin), **Tobramycin** (Nebcin)	MDD: 2 mg per kg load, then 1.7 mg per kg q8h P 4–10 mcg/mL, T 1–2 mcg per mL ————————————————— OD: 5.1 (7 if critically ill) mg per kg q24h P 16–24 mcg per mL, T <1 mcg per mL	**All aminoglycosides have potential to cause tubular necrosis and renal failure, deafness due to cochlear toxicity, vertigo due to damage to vestibular organs, and rarely neuromuscular blockade.** Risk minimal with oral or topical application due to small % absorption unless tissues altered by disease.
Kanamycin (Kantrex), **Amikacin** (Amikin), **Streptomycin**	MDD: 7.5 mg per kg q12h P 15–30 mcg per mL, T 5–10 mcg per mL ————————————————— OD: 15 mg per kg q24h P 56–64 mcg per mL, T <1 mcg per mL	Risk of nephrotoxicity ↑ with concomitant administration of cyclosporine, vancomycin, ampho B, radiocontrast. Risk of nephrotoxicity ↓ by concomitant AP Pen and perhaps by once-daily dosing method (especially if baseline renal function normal).
Netilmicin[NUS]	MDD: 2 mg per kg q8h P 4–10 mcg per mL, T 1–2 mcg per mL ————————————————— OD: 6.5 mg per kg q24h P 22–30 mcg per mL, T <1 mcg per mL	In general, same factors influence risk of ototoxicity. **NOTE: There is no known method to eliminate risk of aminoglycoside nephro/ototoxicity. Proper rx attempts to ↓ the % risk.** The clinical trial data of OD aminoglycosides have been reviewed extensively by meta-analysis *(CID 24:816, 1997)*.
Isepamicin[NUS]	Only OD: Severe infections 15 mg per kg q24h, less severe 8 mg per kg q24h	**Serum levels:** Collect serum for a peak serum level (PSL) exactly 1 hr after the start of the infusion of the 3rd dose. In critically ill pts, it is reasonable to measure the PSL after the 1st dose as well as later doses as volume of distribution and renal function may change rapidly.
Spectinomycin (Trobicin)[NUS]	2 gm IM times 1–gonococcal infections	
Neomycin—oral	Prophylaxis GI surgery: 1 gm po times 3 with erythro, see *Table 15B, page 169* For hepatic coma: 4–12 gm per day po	Other dosing methods and references: For once-daily 7 mg per kg per day of gentamicin—Hartford Hospital method, see *AAC 39:650, 1995.*
Tobramycin—inhaled (Tobi): See *Cystic fibrosis, Table 1A, page 41.* Adverse effects few: transient voice alteration (13%) and transient tinnitus (3%).		
Paromomycin—oral: *See Entamoeba and Cryptosporidia, Table 13, page 125.*		

[1] Estimated CrCl invalid if serum creatinine <0.6 mg per dL. Consultation suggested.

TABLE 11A – TREATMENT OF FUNGAL INFECTIONS—ANTIMICROBIAL AGENTS OF CHOICE*

TYPE OF INFECTION/ORGANISM/ SITE OF INFECTION	ANTIMICROBIAL AGENTS OF CHOICE		COMMENTS
	PRIMARY	ALTERNATIVE	
Aspergillosis (A. fumigatus most common, also A. flavus and others)			
Allergic bronchopulmonary aspergillosis (ABPA) (See Am J Respir Crit Care Med. 27:185, 2006. Clinical manifestations: wheezing, pulmonary infiltrates, bronchiectasis & fibrosis. Airway colonization assoc. with ↑ blood eosinophils, ↑ serum IgE, ↑ specific serum antibodies.	Acute asthma attacks associated with ABPA: **Corticosteroids**	Rx of ABPA: **Itraconazole[1]** 200 mg po q24h times 16 wks or longer (Allergy 60:1004, 2005)	Itra decreases number of exacerbations requiring corticosteroids with improved immunological markers improved lung function & exercise tolerance (Cochrane Database Syst Rev 3:CD001108, 2004; IDSA Guidelines updated CID vol 46, 2008).
Allergic fungal sinusitis: relapsing chronic sinusitis; nasal polyps without bony invasion; asthma, eczema or allergic rhinitis; ↑ IgE levels and isolation of Aspergillus sp. or other dematiaceous sp. (Alternaria, Cladosporium, etc.)	**Rx controversial:** systemic corticosteroids + surgical debridement (relapse common).	For failures try **Itra[1]** 200 mg po bid times 12 mo or flucon nasal spray.	Controversial area.
Aspergilloma (fungus ball)	No therapy or surgical resection.	Efficacy of antimicrobial agents not proven.	Aspergillus may complicate pulmonary sequestration (Eur J Cardio Thor Surg 27:28, 2005). Paranasal fungus balls respond to surgery; 172 of 175 cases (Med Mycol 44:61, 2006).
Invasive, pulmonary (IPA) or extrapulmonary: (See CID 46:327, 2008). Post-transplantation and post-chemotherapy in neutropenic pts (PMN < 500 per mm³) but may also present with neutrophil recovery. Most common pneumonia in transplant recipients. Usually a late (≥100 days) complication in allogeneic bone marrow & liver transplantation: High mortality (CID 44:531, 2007). (continued on next page)	**Primary therapy** (See CID 46:327, 2008): **Voriconazole 6 mg/kg IV q12h on day 1; then either (4 mg/kg/day IV q12h) or (200 mg po q12h for body weight ≥40kg, but 100 mg po q12h for body weight <40kg)** **Alternative therapies:** **Liposomal ampho B** (L-AmB) 3-5 mg/kg/day IV OR **Ampho B lipid complex** (ABLC) 5 mg/kg/d IV OR **Caspofungin** 70 mg/day then 50 mg/day thereafter OR **Micafungin**[NFDA-I] 100-150 mg/day OR **Posaconazole**[NFDA-I] 200 mg qid, then 400 mg bid after stabilization of disease.		**Voriconazole** more effective than ampho B. Vori, both a substrate and an inhibitor of CYP2C19, CYP2C9, and CYP3A4, has potential for deleterious drug interactions (e.g., with protease inhibitors) and careful review of concomitant medications is mandatory. Measurement of serum concentrations advisable with prolonged therapy or for patients with possible drug-drug interactions. **Ampho B: not recommended except as a lipid formulation,** either L-AMB or ABLC. 10 mg/kg and 3 mg/kg doses of L-AMB are equally efficacious with greater toxicity of higher dose (CID 2007; 44:1289–97). One comparative trial found much greater toxicity with ABLC than with L-AMB: 34.6% vs 9.4% adverse events and 21.2% vs 2.8% nephrotoxicity (Cancer; 2008 Jan 25; Epub ahead of print). Vori preferred as primary therapy. **Caspo:** ~ 50% response rate in IPA. Licensed for salvage therapy. Efavirenz, nelfinavir, nevirapine, phenytoin, rifampin, dexamethasone, and carbamazepine, may reduce caspofungin concentrations. **Micafungin:** Favorable responses to micafungin as a single agent in 6/12 patients in primary therapy group and 9/22 in the salvage therapy group of an open-label, non-comparative trial (J Infect 53: 337, 2006). Outcomes no better with combination therapy. **Posaconazole:** In a prospective controlled trial of IPA immunocompromised pts refractory or intolerant to other agents, 42% of 107 pts receiving posa vs 26% controls were successful (CID 44:2, 2007). Posa inhibits CYP3A with potential for drug-drug interactions. Do not use for treatment of azole-non-responders as there is a potential for cross-resistance. Measurement of serum concentrations advisable to document these are within the therapeutic range. (continued on next page)

[1] **Oral solution preferred to tablets because of ↑ absorption** (see Table 11B, page 108).

See page 3 for abbreviations. All dosage recommendations are for adults (unless otherwise indicated) and assume normal renal function

TABLE 11A (2)

TYPE OF INFECTION/ORGANISM/ SITE OF INFECTION	ANTIMICROBIAL AGENTS OF CHOICE		COMMENTS
	PRIMARY	ALTERNATIVE	
(continued from previous page)			(continued from previous page)
Typical x-ray/CT lung lesions (halo sign, cavitation, or macronodules) (CID 44:373, 2007). Initiation of antifungal Rx based on halo signs on CT associated with better response to Rx & improved outcome. An immunologic test that detects circulating **galactomannan** is available for dx of invasive aspergillosis (Lancet ID 4:349, 2005). Galactomannan detection in the blood relatively insensitive; antifungal rx may decrease sensitivity (CID 40:1762.2005). One study suggests improved sensitivity when performed on BAL fluid. (Am J Respir Crit Care Med 177:27, 2008). **False-pos. tests occur with serum from pts receiving PIP-TZ & AM-CL.** Numerous other causes of false positive galactomannan tests reported. For strengths & weaknesses of the test see CID 42:1417, 2006. Posaconazole superior to Flu or Itra with fewer invasive fungal infections and improved survival in patients with hematologic malignancies undergoing induction chemotherapy (NEJM 356:348, 2007).			**Itraconazole: Licensed for treatment of invasive aspergillosis in patients refractory to or intolerant of standard antifungal therapy.** Itraconazole formulated as capsules, oral solution in hydroxypropyl-beta-cyclodextrin (HPCD), and parenteral solution with HPCD as a solubilizer; oral solution and parenteral formulation not licensed for treatment of invasive aspergillosis. 2.5 mg/kg oral solution provides dose equivalent to 400 mg capsules. Parenteral HPCD formulation dosage is 200 mg every 12h IV for 2 days, followed by 200 mg daily thereafter. Oral absorption of capsules enhanced by low gastric pH, erratic in fasting state and with hypochlorhydria; measurements of plasma concentrations recommended during oral therapy of invasive aspergillosis. Itraconazole is a substrate of CYP3A4 and non-competitive inhibitor of CYP3A4 with potential for significant drug-drug interactions. Do not use for azole-non-responders. **Combo therapy:** Uncertain role and not routinely recommended for primary therapy; consider for treatment of refractory disease, although benefit unproven. A typical combo regimen would be an echinocandin in combination with either an azole or a lipid formulation of ampho B.
Blastomycosis (CID 46: 1902, 2008) (Blastomyces dermatitidis) Cutaneous, pulmonary or extrapulmonary.	**LAB**, 3 -5 mg/kg per day, OR **Ampho B**[1], 0.7 -1 mg/kg per day, for 1 -2 weeks, **then itra**[1] 200 mg tid for 3 days followed by itra 200 mg bid for 6 -12 months	**Itra** 200 mg tid for 3 days then once or twice per day for 6 -12 months for mild to moderate disease OR **Flu** 400-800 mg per day for those intolerant to itra	Serum levels of **itra** should be determined after 2 weeks to ensure adequate drug exposure. Flu less effective than itra; role of vori or posa unclear but active in vitro.
Blastomycosis: CNS disease	**LAB** 5 mg/kg per day for 4–6 weeks, followed by **Flu** 800 mg per day OR **Itra** 200 mg bid or tid OR **Vori** 200–400 mg bid		Flu and vori have excellent CNS penetration, perhaps counterbalance their slightly reduced activity compared to itra. Treat for at least 12 months and until CSF has normalized. Document serum itra levels to assure adequate drug concentrations.

[1] **Oral solution preferred to tablets because of ↑ absorption** (see Table 11B, page 108).

See page 3 for abbreviations. All dosage recommendations are for adults (unless otherwise indicated) and assume normal renal function

TABLE 11A (3)

TYPE OF INFECTION/ORGANISM/ SITE OF INFECTION	ANTIMICROBIAL AGENTS OF CHOICE		COMMENTS
	PRIMARY	ALTERNATIVE	
Candidiasis: Candidemia in US is 4th most common nosocomial blood stream infection with significant morbidity and up to 30% mortality. Increasing prevalence of non-albicans species which are less susceptible to antifungal agents (esp. fluconazole). Pts who develop disseminated candidiasis while receiving fluconazole are likely to be infected with an azole resistant C. glabrata or C. krusei. (CID 42;249, 2006). In vitro susceptibility profiles help select empirical antifungal rx.			
Bloodstream: clinically stable with or without venous catheter & C. glabrata or C. krusei unlikely (no flu with in 30 days) (IDSA Guidelines): CID 38:161, 2004, CID 42:244, 2006). • **All positive blood cultures require therapy!** • **Remove & replace venous catheter** ("not over a wire") (J Clin Micro 43:1829, 2005), esp. in non-neutropenic: mortality 21% vs 4% if catheter not removed. • Treat for 2 wk after last pos. blood culture & resolution of signs & symptoms of infection	**Fluconazole** ≥6 mg/kg per day or 400 mg q24h IV or po times 7 days then po for 14 days after last + blood culture	Echinocandin (see caspofungin, anidulafungin & micafungin below)	Fluconazole still preferred here because of impressive efficacy in randomized studies, favorable safety profile and very low cost (CID 42:249, 2006. JAC 57;384, 2006). In centers with relatively higher rates of non-albicans candida species, an echinocandin may be preferred empirical therapy. A double-blind randomized trial comparing anidulafungin to fluconazole for invasive candiasis showed an 88% response rate in patients (n= 135) treated with anidulafungin vs a 76% response rate (n= 130) treated with fluconazole (p= 0.02) (NEJM 356:2472, 2007). Fluconazole not recommended for treatment of documented C. glabrata or C. krusei: use an echinocandin or voriconazole or posaconazole (note: echinocandins have better in vitro activity than either vori or posa against C. glabrata).
Bloodstream: unstable • Failure to respond to fluconazole or deteriorating • (Critical to remove intravenous catheter) • Hemodynamic instability (sepsis) • C. glabrata or C. krusei likely (immunosuppressed/flu prophylaxis) • Neutropenia (controversial) **Mortality rates inc with delay in initiation of therapy:** 15% day 0, 24% day 1, 37% day 2 & 41% > day 4- p>.0009. (CID 43:25, 2006)	**Caspofungin** 70 mg IV on day 1 followed by 50 mg IV q24h (reduce to 35 mg IV q24h with moderate hepatic insufficiency). **OR** **Micafungin** 100 mg IV q24h **OR** **Anidulafungin** 200 mg IV times 1, then 100 mg q24h (no dosage adjustments for renal or hepatic insufficiency)	**Ampho B** 0.7 mg/kg IV q24h, (> 0.7 mg/kg/d IV for C. glabrata, 1 mg/kg/d for C. krusei) **OR** **Lipid-based Amphotericin** 3-5 mg/kg/d **OR** **Voriconazole:** 6 mg per kg IV q12h times 2 doses, then maintenance doses of 3 mg per kg IV q12h (if > 40 kg), or 200 mg po q12h, after at least 3 days of IV therapy	**Echinocandins** have efficacy similar to and perhaps better than ampho B and are less toxic: response rates of ~ 70% for candins vs ~ 60% for **ampho B**. One comparative study suggests that anidulafungin may be superior to fluconazole (see above) (NEJM 356:2472, 2007). MICs of candins are higher for C. parapsilosis than for other candidal species and clinical response rates may be less. **Micafungin** and **anidulafungin** have no known important drug-drug interactions. Cross-resistance can occur between **voriconazole** and **fluc**, especially with C. glabrata (J Clin Micro 44:529, 2006); vori still active vs C. krusei (J Clin Micro 44:1740, 2006). Vori not preferred for initial Rx in those with extensive azole exposure.
Cutaneous (including paronychia, Table 1A, page 25)	Apply topical **ampho B, clotrimazole, econazole, miconazole,** or **nystatin** 3-4 x daily for 7–14 days or **ketoconazole** 400 mg po once daily x 14 days. **Ciclopirox olamine** 1% cream/lotion. Apply topically bid x 7–14 days.		Ciclopirox lotion, 30 mL; cream 30 gm.

See page 3 for abbreviations. All dosage recommendations are for adults (unless otherwise indicated) and assume normal renal function

TABLE 11A (4)

TYPE OF INFECTION/ORGANISM/ SITE OF INFECTION	ANTIMICROBIAL AGENTS OF CHOICE		COMMENTS
	PRIMARY	ALTERNATIVE	
Candidiasis/Bloodstream: clinically stable with or without venous catheter (continued)			
Endocarditis See Eur J Clin Microbiol Infect Dis 27:519, 2008 Causes of fungal endocarditis: C. albicans 24%, other Candida sp. 24%, Aspergillus sp. 24%, others 27%	**Ampho B** 0.6 mg/kg per day IV for 7 days, then 0.8 mg/kg IV every other day or **lipid-based ampho B** 3–5 mg/kg per day. Continue 6–8 wks after surgery + **flucytosine** 25–37.5 mg/kg po qid + surgical resection	**Caspofungin** 50-100 mg qd **Flu** 200-400 mg per day for chronic suppression may be of value when valve cannot be replaced	**Adjust flucyt dose and interval to produce serum levels; peak 70–80 mg per L, trough 30–40 mg per L. Caspofungin** cidal vs candida; several reports of cure.
Endophthalmitis (IDSA Guidelines: CID 38:161,2004) • Occurs in 10% of candidemia, thus ophthalmological consult for all pts • Diagnosis: typical white exudates on retinal exam and/or isolation by vitrectomy	**Ampho B** (0.7-1 mg/kg/d) or LAB 5 mg/kg/d **OR fluconazole** 400 mg/day IV or po either as initial rx or follow-up after ampho B. Role of intravitreal ampho B not well defined but commonly used in pts with substantial vision loss. Treat 6–12 wk		Patients with chorioretinitis only generally respond to systemically administered antifungals. Intravitreal amphotericin and/or vitrectomy may be necessary for those with vitritis or endophthalmitis (Br J Ophthalmol 92:466, 2008; Pharmacotherapy 27:1711, 2007)
Oral (thrush)—not AIDS patient (See below for vaginitis)	**Fluconazole** 200 mg single dose or 100 mg/day po x 14 days **OR** Itraconazole oral solution 200 mg (20 mL) q24h without food x 7 days.	**Nystatin pastilles** (200,000 units) lozenge qid, 500,000 units (swish & swallow) qid or 2 (500,000 units) tabs tid for 14 days **OR** **Clotrimazole** 1 troche (10 mg) 5x/day x 14 days.	Maintenance not required in non-AIDS pts. Usually improves in 3–4 days, longer rx ↓ relapse.
AIDS patients **Stomatitis, esophagitis** An AIDS-defining illness: correlates with HIV RNA levels in plasma & with CD4 counts. HAART has resulted in dramatic ↓ in prevalence of oropharyngeal & esophageal candidiasis & ↓ in refractory disease.	**Oropharyngeal**, initial episodes (7–14d rx): • **Fluconazole** 100 mg po q24h; OR • **itraconazole** oral solution 200 mg po q24h; OR • **clotrimazole** troches 10 mg po 5x/day; OR • **nystatin** suspension 4–6 mL q6h or 1–2 flavored pastilles 4–5x/day **Esophageal** (14–21d): • **Flucon** 100 mg (up to 400 mg) po or IV q24h; OR • **itra** oral solution 200 mg po q24h; OR • **caspofungin** 50 mg IV q24h; OR • **micafungin** 150 mg/d IV or anidulafungin 100 mg IV day 1 followed by 50 mg per day	**Fluconazole-refractory oropharyngeal:** • **Itra** oral solution ≥200 mg po q24h; or • **Posaconazole** 200 mg qd x 1 followed by 100 mg qd x 13d; or • **Ampho B** suspension 100 mg/mL[NUS] 1 mL po q6h; or • **Ampho B** 0.3 mg/kg IV q24h **Fluconazole-refractory esophageal:** • **Caspofungin** 50 mg IV q24h; or • **Vori** 200 mg po or IV q12h; or • **Posaconazole** 400 mg po bid x 3 d followed by 400 mg po qd; or • **Micafungin** 150 mg IV per day; or • **Ampho B** 0.3–0.7 mg/kg IV q24h; or • **Ampho liposomal or lipid complex** 3–5 mg/kg IV q24h	**Fluconazole-refractory disease remains uncommon** & is seen in pts with low CD4 counts (< 50/ mm³). MICs > 4 mcg/ml predictive of failure (Antimicrob Agents Chemother 51:3599, 2007). **Flu** superior to oral suspension of **nystatin. Itra** 100 mg po q12h x 14d may be effective in pts unresponsive to flu. **Ampho B oral suspension** may be effective for pts refractory to **flu**, but relapse is common. Posa equivalent to Flu for oropharyngeal candidiasis (CID 42:1179, 2006). For esophagitis, **caspofungin** as effective as **ampho B IV** but less toxic. **Voriconazole** as effective as **fluconazole** for esophagitis. **Micafungin** 100 mg or 150 mg IV per day equal to flu 200 mg per day. **Anidulafungin** 100 mg IV day 1 followed by 50 mg per day = to flu 200 mg on day 1 followed by 100 mg per day in cure rates (98-99%) but higher relapse rates in HIV-infected patients.

See page 3 for abbreviations. All dosage recommendations are for adults (unless otherwise indicated) and assume normal renal function

TABLE 11A (5)

TYPE OF INFECTION/ORGANISM/ SITE OF INFECTION	ANTIMICROBIAL AGENTS OF CHOICE		COMMENTS
	PRIMARY	ALTERNATIVE	
Candidiasis/AIDS patient (continued)			
Vulvovaginitis Common among healthy young females & unrelated to HIV status.	• **Topical azoles** (clotrimazole, buto, mico, tico, or tercon) x 3–7d; or • **topical nystatin** 100,000units/day as vaginal tablet x 14d; or • oral **itra** 200 mg q12h x 1d or 200 mg q24h x 3d; or • oral **flu** 150 mg x 1 dose		
Peritonitis (Chronic Ambulatory Peritoneal Dialysis) See Table 19, page 186	**Fluconazole** 400 mg po q24h x 2–3 wks or **caspofungin** 70 mg IV on day 1 followed by 50 mg IV q24h for 14 days or **micafungin** 100 mg q24h for 14 days.	**Ampho B**, continuous IP dosing at 1.5 mg/L of dialysis fluid times 4–6 wk	Remove cath immediately or if no clinical improvement in 4–7 days. In 1 study, all 8 pts with candida peritonitis who received caspo responded favorably (as compared to 7/8 pts on ampho B) (NEJM 347:2020, 2002).
Urinary: Candiduria • Usually colonization of urinary catheter, a benign event • Rarely may be source of dissemination if pt has obstructive uropathy or marker of acute hematogenous dissemination Persistent candiduria in immunocompromised pt warrants ultrasound or CT of kidneys	**Remove urinary catheter or stent** Antifungal rx not indicated unless pt has symptoms of UTI, neutropenic, low birth-weight infant, has renal allograft or is undergoing urologic manipulation. Then: **fluconazole** 200 mg per day po or IV times 7–14 days OR **ampho B** 0.5 mg per kg per day IV times 7–14 days.		**Fluconazole:** candiduria cleared in pts treated with flu 200 mg/day x 14 days but recurrences are common. **Bladder washout** with ampho B not recommended. **Caspofungin** may be effective in clearing candiduria. **NOTE: Vori** not in urine in active form.
Vaginitis—Non-AIDS patients Sporadic/Infrequent	**Oral: Fluconazole** 150 mg po x 1 **OR** itraconazole 200 mg po bid x 1 day ** For over-the-counter preparations, see below in footnote[1]	**Intravaginal:** Multiple **imidazoles** with 85–95% cure rates. See footnote[1]	**In general, oral & vaginal rx are similarly effective.** Rx aided by avoiding tight clothing, e.g., pantyhose. Oral drugs ↓ rectal candida & may ↓ relapses. **Ampho B** vaginal 50 mg suppository effective in non-albicans candida infec when other rx failed (Am J Ob Gyn 192:2009 & 2012, 2005).
Chronic recurrent (5–8%) ≥4 episodes/yr Ref.: NEJM 351:876, 2004	**Fluconazole** 150 mg po q12h times 3 & then 150 mg po q wk	Relapse or recurrence is common.	
Chromoblastomycosis (J Am Acad Derm 44:585, 2001) (Cladosporium or Fonsecaea); Cutaneous (usually feet, legs): raised scaly lesions, most common in tropical areas	If lesions small & few, **surgical excision or cryosurgery with liquid nitrogen** (Int J Dermatol 42:408, 2003). If lesions chronic, extensive, burrowing: **itraconazole.**	**Itraconazole:** 100 mg po q24h times 18 months (or until response)[NFDA-I]. Fluconazole experience disappointing.	**Terbinafine**[NFDA-I] (800 mg per day) and **posaconazole** (400–800 mg/d) also may be effective (Drugs 65:1560, 2005, Rev Inst Med Trop Sao Paulo 47:339, 2005).

[1] Intravaginal products for candidiasis: **Butoconazole** 2% cream (5 gm) q24h at bedtime x 3 days or 2% cream SR 5 gm x 1; or **clotrimazole** 100 mg vaginal tabs (2 at bedtime x 3 days) or 1% cream (5 gm) at bedtime times 7 days (14 days may ↑ cure rate) or 100 mg vaginal tab x 7 days or 500 mg vaginal tab x 1; or **miconazole** 200 mg vaginal suppos. (1 at bedtime x 3 days**) or 100 mg vaginal suppos. q24h x 7 days or 2% cream (5 gm) at bedtime x 7 days; or **terconazole** 80 mg vaginal tab (1 at bedtime x 3 days) or 0.4% cream (5 gm) or 0.8% cream x 7 days or 0.8% cream 5 gm intravaginal q24h x 3 days; or **tioconazole** 6.5% vag. ointment x 1 dose**. ** = over-the-counter product

See page 3 for abbreviations. All dosage recommendations are for adults (unless otherwise indicated) and assume normal renal function

TABLE 11A (6)

TYPE OF INFECTION/ORGANISM/ SITE OF INFECTION	ANTIMICROBIAL AGENTS OF CHOICE		COMMENTS
	PRIMARY	ALTERNATIVE	

Coccidioidomycosis (Coccidioides immitis) (IDSA Guidelines 2005: CID 41:1217, 2005; see also Mayo Clin Proc 83:343, 2008)

Primary pulmonary (San Joaquin or Valley Fever): **Antifungal rx not generally recommended.** Treat if fever, wt loss and/or fatigue do not resolve within several wks to 2 mo (see below). — Uncomplicated pulmonary in normal host common in endemic areas (Emerg Infect Dis 12:958, 2006) Influenza -like illness of 1–2 wk duration.

Pts low risk persistence/complication

Primary pulmonary in pts with ↑ risk for complications or dissemination. Rx indicated:
- Immunosuppressive disease. AIDS (CID 41:1174, 2005), post-transplantation (Am J Transp 6:340, 2006), hematological malignancies (ArIM 165:113, 2005), or therapies (steroids, TNF-α antagonists) (Arth Rheum 50:1959, 2004).
- Pregnancy in 3rd trimester.
- Diabetes
- CF antibody > 1:16
- Pulmonary Infiltrates
- Dissemination (identification of spherules or culture of organism from ulcer, joint effusion, pus from subcutaneous abscess or bone biopsy, etc.)

	Mild to moderate severity:		**Ampho B cure rate 50–70%. Responses to azoles are similar. Itra** may have slight advantage esp. in soft tissue infection. Relapse rates after rx 40%: Relapse rate ↑ if ↑ CF titer ≥1:256. Following CF titers after completion of rx important; rising titers warrant retreatment. **Posaconazole** reported successful in 73% of pts with refractory non-meningeal cocci (Chest 132:952, 2007). Not frontline therapy.
	Itraconazole solution 200 mg po or IV bid OR		
	Fluconazole 400 mg po q24h for 3–12 mo		
	Locally severe or disseminated disease		
	Ampho B 0.6–1 mg/kg per day x 7 days then 0.8 mg/kg every other day or **liposomal ampho B** 3–5 mg/kg/d IV or **ABLC** 5 mg/kg/d IV, until clinical improvement (usually several wks or longer in disseminated disease), followed by **itra** or **flu** for at least 1 year. Some use combination of Ampho B & Flu for progressive severe disease; controlled series lacking (CID 41:1177, 2005) **Consultation with specialist recommended:** surgery may be required.		
	Lifetime suppression in HIV+ patients or until CD4 > 250 & infection controlled: flu 200 mg po q24h or itra 200 mg po bid (Mycosis 46:42, 2003).		

Meningitis: occurs in 1/3 to 1/2 of pts with disseminated coccidioidomycosis

| Adult (CID 42:103, 2006) | **Fluconazole** 400–1,000 mg po q24h indefinitely | **Ampho B** IV as for pulmonary (above) + 0.1–0.3 mg daily intra-thecal (intraventricular) via reservoir device. **OR itra** 400–800 mg q24h **OR voriconazole** (see Comment) | **80% relapse rate, continue flucon indefinitely, Voriconazole** successful in high doses (6 mg/kg IV q12h) followed by oral suppression (400 mg po q12h) (CID 36:1619, 2003; AAC 48: 2341, 2004). |
| Child | **Fluconazole** (po) (Pediatric dose not established, 6 mg per kg q24h used) | | |

Cryptococcosis (IDSA Guideline: CID 30:710, 2000). New Guidelines due in Spring 2009. Excellent review: Brit Med Bull 72:99, 2005

Non-meningeal (non-AIDS)
Risk 57% in organ transplant (Transpl Inf Dis 4:183, 2002 & 7:26, 2005) & those receiving other forms of immunosuppressive agents (alemtuzumab—Transplant Proc 37:934, 2005 & adalimumab; EID 13:953, 2007).

	Fluconazole 400 mg/day IV or po for 8 wk to 6 mo	**Itraconazole** 200–400 mg solution q24h for 6-12 mo OR	**Flucon alone 90% effective for meningeal and non-meningeal forms.** Fluconazole as effective as ampho B (CID 32:E145, 2001). Addition of **interferon-γ** (IFN-γ-lb 50 mcg per M² subcut. 3x per wk x 9 wk) to liposomal ampho B assoc. with response in pt failing antifungal rx (CID 38: 910, 2004).
	For more severe disease:	**Ampho B** 0.3 mg/kg per day IV + **flucytosine** 37.5 mg/kg¹ po qid times 6 wk	Posaconazole 400-800 mg also effective in a small series of patients (CID 45:562, 2007; Chest 132:952, 2007)
	Ampho B 0.5–0.8 mg/kg per day IV till response then change to **fluconazole** 400 mg po q24h for 8–10 wk course		

| **Meningitis (non-AIDS)** | **Ampho B** 0.5–0.8 mg/kg per day IV + **flucytosine** 37.5 mg/kg¹ po q6h until pt afebrile & cultures neg (~ 6 wk) (NEJM 301:126, 1979), then stop ampho B/flucyt, start **fluconazole** 200 mg po q24h (AnIM 113:183, 1990)   OR | **Ampho B** 0.3 mg/kg per day IV + **flucytosine** 37.5 mg/kg¹ po qid times 6 wk | If CSF opening pressure > 25cm H₂O, repeat LP to drain fluid to control pressure. Outbreaks of C. gattii meningitis have been reported in the Pacific Northwest (EID 13:42, 2007); severity of disease and prognosis appear to be worse than with C. neoformans; initial therapy with ampho B + flucytosine recommended. C. gattii less susceptible to flucon than C. neoformans (Clin Microbiol Inf 14:727, 2008). Outcomes in both AIDS and non-AIDS cryptococcal meningitis improved with Ampho B + 5-FC induction therapy for 14 days in those with neurological abnormalities or high organism burden (PLoS ONE 3:e2870, 2008). |
| | **Fluconazole** 400 mg po q24h x 8–10 wk (less severely ill pt). Some recommend flu for 2 yr to reduce relapse rate (CID 28:297, 1999). Some recommend AMB plus fluconazole as induction Rx. Studies underway. | | |

¹ Some experts would reduce to 25 mg per kg q6h

See page 3 for abbreviations. All dosage recommendations are for adults (unless otherwise indicated) and assume normal renal function

TABLE 11A (7)

TYPE OF INFECTION/ORGANISM/ SITE OF INFECTION	ANTIMICROBIAL AGENTS OF CHOICE		COMMENTS
	PRIMARY	ALTERNATIVE	

Cryptococcosis (continued)

HIV+/AIDS: Cryptococcemia and/or Meningitis

Treatment
↓ with ARV but still common presenting OI in newly diagnosed AIDS pts. Cryptococcal infection may be manifested by positive blood culture or positive serum cryptococcal antigen (CRAG; > 95% sens). CRAG no help in monitoring response to therapy.
With ARV, symptoms of acute meningitis may return: immune reconstitution inflammatory syndrome (IRIS).
↑ CSF pressure (> **25cm H₂O**) associated with high mortality: lower with CSF removal. If frequent LPs not possible, ventriculoperitoneal shunts an option (Surg Neurol 63:529 & 531, 2005).
	[**Ampho B** 0.7 mg/kg IV q24h + **flucytosine**[1] 25 mg/kg po q6h x 2 wks
	or
	Liposomal amphotericin B 4 mg/kg IV q24h + **flucytosine** 25 mg/kg po q6h x 2 wks]
	See Comment.
	
	Then
	Consolidation therapy: Fluconazole 400 mg po q24h to complete a 10-wk course or until CSF culture sterile, then suppression (see below).
	
	Start Antiretroviral Therapy (ARV) if possible.
		[**Fluconazole** 400–800 mg/day po or IV for less severe disease
		or
		Fluconazole 400–800 mg/day po or IV + **flucytosine** 25 mg/kg po q6h x 4–6 wks]
			Ampho B + 5FC treatment ↓ crypto CFUs more rapidly than ampho + flu or ampho + 5FC + flu. Ampho B 1 mg/kg/d alone much more rapidly fungical in vivo than flu 400 mg/d (CID 45:76&81, 2007).
			   Monitor 5-FC levels: peak 70 -80 mg/L, trough 30 -40 mg/L. Higher levels assoc. with bone marrow toxicity. No difference in outcome if given IV or po (AAC Dec 28, 2006).
			If normal mental status, > 20 cells/mm³ CSF, & CSF CRAG < 1:1024, flu alone may be reasonable.
			Failure of flu may rarely be due to resistant organism, especially if burden of organism high at initiation of Rx. Although 200 mg qd = 400 mg qd of flu: median survival 76 & 82 days respectively, authors prefer 400 mg po qd (BMC Infect Dis 18:118, 2006).
			   Role of other azoles uncertain: successful outcomes were observed in 14/29 (48%) subjects with cryptococcal meningitis treated with posaconazole (JAC 56:745, 2005). Voriconazole also may be effective.
			   Survival probably improved with ARV, but IRIS may complicate its use. Of 52 patients treated with ARV initiated at a median time of 2.6 mo after dx of crypto meningitis, 10 (19%) developed IRIS; median time to onset of IRIS 9.9 months after initiation of ARV (J Acquir Immune Defic Syndr 45:595, 2007). Presentation: aseptic meningitis, high CSF opening pressure, positive CSF CRAG, negative culture; prognosis good. Short course corticosteroids may be beneficial in severe disease (Expert Rev Anti Infect Ther. 4:469, 2006).

Suppression (chronic maintenance therapy) Discontinuation of antifungal rx can be considered among pts who remain asymptomatic, with CD4 > 100–200/mm³ for ≥6 months. Some perform a lumbar puncture before discontinuation of maintenance rx. Reappearance of pos. serum CRAG may predict relapse	**Fluconazole** 200 mg/day po [If CD4 count rises to > 100/mm³ with effective antiretroviral rx, some authorities recommend dc suppressive rx. See www.hivatis.org. Authors would only dc if CSF culture negative.]	**Itraconazole** 200 mg po q12h if flu intolerant or failure. No data on Vori for maintenance.	Itraconazole less effective than fluconazole & not recommended because of higher relapse rate (23% vs 4%). Recurrence rate of 0.4 to 3.9 per 100 patient-years with discontinuation of suppressive therapy in 100 patients on ARV with CD4 > 100 cells/mm³.

[1] Flucytosine = 5-FC

See page 3 for abbreviations. All dosage recommendations are for adults (unless otherwise indicated) and assume normal renal function

TABLE 11A (8)

TYPE OF INFECTION/ORGANISM/ SITE OF INFECTION	ANTIMICROBIAL AGENTS OF CHOICE		COMMENTS
	PRIMARY	ALTERNATIVE	
Dermatophytosis (See Superficial fungal infections, Ln 364:1173, 2004)			
Onychomycosis (Tinea unguium) (Derm Ther 17:517, 2004; Cutis 74:516, 2004) Topical nail lacquer (**ciclopirox**) approved but cure in only 5–9% after 48 wks (Med Lett 42:51, 2000) but ↑ to 50% cure in another study (Cutis 73:81, 2004). May enhance oral rx (Cutis 74:55, 2004). **Terbinafine** appears to be most cost-effective rx (Manag Care Interface 18:55, 2005). Overall cure rate from 18 randomized control trials, 76% (J DrugsDerm 4:302, 2005).	**Fingernail Rx Options:** **Terbinafine**[1] 250 mg po q24h [children < 20 kg: 67.5 mg/day, 20–40 kg: 125 mg/day, > 40 kg: 250 mg/day] x 6 wk (79% effective) OR **Itraconazole**[2] 200 mg po q24h x 3 mo.[NFDA-I] or **Itraconazole** 200 mg po bid x 1 wk/mo x 2 mo.[NFDA-I] or **Fluconazole** 150–300 mg po q wk x 3–6 mo.[NFDA-I] **NOTE:** For side-effects, see footnotes 1 & 2 & meta analysis in AJM 120:791, 2007: risk of stopping therapy due to adverse event varied between 2–6% with specific drug & drug regimen.		**Toenail Rx Options:** **Terbinafine**[2] 250 mg po q24h [children < 20kg: 67.5 mg/day, 125 mg/day, > 40 kg: 250 mg/day] x 12 wks (76% effective) OR **Itraconazole**[3] 200 mg po q24h x 3 mo (59% effective) OR **Itraconazole** 200 mg po bid x 1 wk/mo. x 3–4 mo (63% effective)[NFDA-I] OR **Fluconazole** 150–300 mg po q wk x 6–12 mo (48% effective)[NFDA-I] [Data reflect cure rate from meta-analysis of all randomized controlled trials (Brit J Derm 150:537, 2004).]
Tinea capitis ("ringworm") (Trichophyton tonsurans, Microsporum canis; N. America; other sp. elsewhere) (PIDJ 18:191, 1999)	**Terbinafine**[2] 250 mg po q24h x 4 wk for T. tonsurans, 4–8 wk for Micro-sporum canis[NFDA-I] Children 125 mg (or 6–12 mg/kg per day) po q24h. (COID 17:97, 2004; Exp Opin Pharm Ther 5:219, 2004).	**Itraconazole**[2] 3–5 mg/kg per day for 30 days[NFDA-I] **Fluconazole** 8 mg/kg q wk x 8–12 wk.[NFDA-I] Cap at 150 mg po q wk for adults **Griseofulvin:** adults 500 mg po q24h x 4–6 wks, children 10–20 mg/kg per day until hair regrows. 6–8 wk.	All agents with similar cure rates (60-100%) in clinical studies (Ped Derm 17:304, 2000). Addition of topical ketoconazole or selenium sulfate shampoo reduces transmissibility (Int J Dermatol 39:261, 2000)
Tinea corporis, cruris, or pedis (Trichophyton rubrum, T. mentagrophytes, Epidermophyton floccosum) "Athlete's foot, jock itch," and ringworm	**Topical rx:** Generally applied 2x/day. Available as creams, ointments, sprays, by prescription & "over the counter." Apply 2x/day for 2–3 wks. Recommend: Lotrimin Ultra or Lamisil AT; contain butenafine & terbinafine—both are fungicidal	**Terbinafine** 250 mg po q24h x 2 wks[NFDA-I] OR **ketoconazole** 200 mg po q24h x 4 wks OR **fluconazole** 150 mg po 1x/wk for 2–4 wks[NFDA-I] **Griseofulvin:** adults 500 mg po q24h times 4–6 wks, children 10–20 mg/kg per day. Duration: 2-4 wks for corporis, 4–8 wks for pedis.	**Keto** po often effective in severe recalcitrant infection. Follow for hepatotoxicity; many drug-drug interactions. **Terbinafine:** 87% achieved mycological cure in double-blind study (32 pts) (J Med Assn Thai 76:388, 1993; Brit J Derm 130(S43):22, 1994) and fluconazole 78% (J Am Acad Derm 40:S31, 1999). **Itra** likely effective but no data.
Tinea versicolor (Malassezia furfur or Pityrosporum orbiculare) Rule out erythrasma—see Table 1A, page 51	**Ketoconazole** (400 mg po single dose)[NFDA-I] or (200 mg q24h x 7 days) or (2% cream 1x q24h x 2 wks)	**Fluconazole** 400 mg po single dose or **Itraconazole** 400 mg po q24h x 3–7 days	**Keto** (po) times 1 dose was 97% effective in 1 study. Another alternative: **Selenium sulfide** (Selsun), 2.5% lotion, apply as lather, leave on 10 min then wash off, 1/day x 7 day or 3–5/wk times 2–4 wks

[1] **Serious but rare cases of hepatic failure** have been reported in pts receiving terbinafine & should not be used in those with chronic or active liver disease (see Table 11B, page 108).

[2] Use of itraconazole has been associated with myocardial dysfunction and with onset of congestive heart failure (see Ln 357:1766, 2001).

See page 3 for abbreviations. All dosage recommendations are for adults (unless otherwise indicated) and assume normal renal function

TABLE 11A (9)

TYPE OF INFECTION/ORGANISM/ SITE OF INFECTION	ANTIMICROBIAL AGENTS OF CHOICE		COMMENTS
	PRIMARY	ALTERNATIVE	
Histoplasmosis (Histoplasma capsulatum): See IDSA Guideline: CID 45:807, 2007. Best diagnostic test is urinary, serum, or CSF histoplasma antigen: MiraVista Diagnostics (1-866-647-2847)			
Acute pulmonary histoplasmosis	**Mild to moderate disease, symptoms <4 wk:** No rx; If symptoms last over one month: Itraconazole 200 mg po tid for 3 days then once or twice daily for 6-12 wk. **Moderately severe or severe: Liposomal ampho B,** 3-5 mg/kg/d or **ABLC** 5 mg/kg/d IV or ampho B 0.7-1.0 mg/kg/d for 1-2 wk, then itra 200 mg tid for 3 days, then bid for 12 wk. + **methylprednisolone** 0.5-1.0 mg/kg/d for 1-2 wk.		Ampho B for patients at low risk of nephrotoxicity.
Chronic cavitary pulmonary histoplasmosis	Itra 200 mg po tid for 3 days then once or twice daily for at least 12 mo (some prefer 18-24 mo)		Document therapeutic itraconazole blood levels at 2 wk. Relapses occur in 9-15% of patients.
Mediastinal lymphadenitis, mediastinal granuloma, pericarditis; and rheumatologic syndromes	**Mild cases:** Antifungal therapy not indicated. Nonsteroidal anti-inflammatory drug for pericarditis or rheumatologic syndromes. If no response to non-steroidals, **Prednisone** 0.5-1.0 mg/kg/d tapered over 1-2 weeks for 1) pericarditis with hemodynamic compromise, 2) lymphadenitis with obstruction or compression syndromes, or 3) severe rheumatologic syndromes. **Itra** 200 mg po once or twice daily for 6-12 wk for moderately severe to severe cases, or if prednisone is administered.		Check itra blood levels to document therapeutic concentrations.
Progressive disseminated histoplasmosis	**Mild to moderate disease:** itra 200 mg po tid for 3 days then bid for at least 12 mo **Moderately severe to severe disease: Liposomal ampho B,** 3 mg/kg/d or **ABLC** 5 mg/kg/d for 1-2 weeks then **itra** 200 mg tid for 3 days, then bid for at least 12 mo.		**Ampho B** 0.7-1.0 mg/kg/d may be used for patients at low risk of nephrotoxicity. Confirm therapeutic itra blood levels. Azoles are teratogenic; itra should be avoided in pregnancy; use a lipid ampho formulation. Urinary antigen levels useful for monitoring response to therapy and relapse
CNS histoplasmosis	**Liposomal ampho B,** 5 mg/kg/d, for a total of 175 mg/kg over 4-6 wk, then **itra** 200 mg 2-3x a day for at least 12 mo. Vori likely effective for CNS disease or itra failures. (Arch Neurology 65: 666, 2008; J Antimicro Chemo 57:1235, 2006).		Monitor CNS histo antigen, monitor itra blood levels. PCR may be better for Dx than histo antigen.
Prophylaxis (immunocompromised patients)	Itra 200 mg po daily		Consider primary **prophylaxis in HIV-infected** patients with < 150 CD4 cells/mm³ in high prevalence areas. Secondary prophylaxis (i.e., suppressive therapy) indicated in HIV-infected patients with < 150 CD4 cells/mm³ and other immunocompromised patients in who immunosuppression cannot be reversed
Madura foot (See Nocardia & Scedosporium, below)			

See page 3 for abbreviations. All dosage recommendations are for adults (unless otherwise indicated) and assume normal renal function

TABLE 11A (10)

TYPE OF INFECTION/ORGANISM/ SITE OF INFECTION	ANTIMICROBIAL AGENTS OF CHOICE		COMMENTS
	PRIMARY	ALTERNATIVE	
Mucormycosis & other **Zygomycosis**—Rhizopus, Rhizomucor, Absidia. (CID 41:521, 2005) Rhinocerebral, pulmonary, Invasive; Eur J Clin Microbiol Infect Dis 25:215, 2006. Key to successful rx: early dx with symptoms suggestive of sinusitis (or lateral facial pain or numbness): think mucor with palatal ulcers, &/or black eschars, onset unilateral blindness in immunocompromised or diabetic pt (J Otolaryn 34:166, 2005). Rapidly fatal without rx. Dx by culture of tissue or stain: wide ribbon-like, non-septated with variation in diameter & right angle branching (ClinMicro&Infect 12:7, 2006).	**Lipid-based Ampho B OR Ampho B:** Increase rapidly to 0.8–1.5 mg/kg per day IV: when improving, then every other day. Total dose usually 2.5–3 gm.	**Posaconazole** 400 mg po bid with meals (if not taking meals, 200 mg po qid)[NFDA-I] .	Cure dependent on: (1) surgical debridement, (2) rx of hyperglycemia, correction of neutropenia, or reduction in immunosuppression; (3) antifungal rx: liposomal amphotericin (J Clin Micro 43:2012, 2005) longterm or **posaconazole**. Complete or partial response rates or 60-80% in posaconazole salvage protocols (JAC 61, Suppl. 1, i35, 2008). Resistant to voriconazole: prolonged use of voriconazole prophylaxis predisposes to zygomycetes infections (Lancet ID 5:594, 2005).
Paracoccidioidomycosis (South American blastomycosis) /P. brasiliensis (Dermatol Clin 26:257, 2008; Expert Rev Anti Infect Ther 6:251, 2008).	**TMP/SMX** 800/160 mg every bid-tid for 30 days, then 400/80 mg/day indefinitely (up to 3-5 years) **Itraconazole** (100 or 200 mg orally daily)	**Ketoconazole** 200-400 mg daily for 6-18 mo **Ampho B** total dose > 30 mg/kg	Improvement in > 90% pts on itra or keto.[NFDA-I] **Ampho B** reserved for severe cases and for those intolerant to other agents. TMP-SMX suppression life-long in HIV+ .
Lobomycosis (keloidal blastomycosis)/ P. loboi	**Surgical excision, clofazimine** or **itraconazole.**		
Penicilliosis (Penicillium marneffei): Common disseminated fungal infection in AIDS pts in SE Asia (esp. Thailand & Vietnam).	**Ampho B** 0.5–1 mg/kg per day times 2 wks followed by **itraconazole** 400 mg/day for 10 wks followed by 200 mg/day po indefinitely for HIV-infected pts.	For less sick patients **Itra** 200 mg. po tid x 3 days, then 200 mg po bid x 12 wks, then 200 mg po q24h.[1] (IV if unable to take po)	3rd most common OI in AIDS pts in SE Asia following TBc and cryptococcal meningitis. Prolonged fever, lymphadenopathy, hepatomegaly. Skin nodules are umbilicated (mimic cryptococcal infection or molluscum contagiosum). Preliminary data suggests vori effective: CID 43:1060, 2006.
Phaeohyphomycosis, Black molds, Dematiaceous fungi (See CID 41:521, 2005, CID 43:S3, 2006) Sinuses, skin, bone & joint, brain abscess, endocarditis, emerging especially in HSCT pts with disseminated disease. **Scedosporium prolificans,** Bipolaris, Wangiella, Curvularia, Exophiala, Phialemonium, Scytalidium, Alternaria	**Surgery + itraconazole** 400 mg/day po, duration not defined, probably 6 mo[NFDA-I]	Case report of success with **voriconazole + terbinafine** (Scand J Infect Dis 39:87, 2007). OR **Itraconazole + terbinafine** synergistic against S. prolificans. No clinical data & combination could show ↑ toxicity (see Table 11B, page 108).	**Posaconazole** successful in case of brain abscess (CID 34:1648, 2002) and refractory infection (Mycosis:519, 2006). **Notoriously resistant to antifungal rx including amphotericin & azoles.** 44% of patients in compassionate use/salvage therapy study responded to voriconazole (AAC 52:1743, 2008). > 80% mortality in immunocompromised hosts.

[1] **Oral solution preferred to tablets because of ↑ absorption** (see Table 11B, page 108).

See page 3 for abbreviations. All dosage recommendations are for adults (unless otherwise indicated) and assume normal renal function

TABLE 11A (11)

TYPE OF INFECTION/ORGANISM/ SITE OF INFECTION	ANTIMICROBIAL AGENTS OF CHOICE		COMMENTS
	PRIMARY	ALTERNATIVE	
Scedosporium apiospermum (Pseudallescheria boydii) (not considered a true dematiaceous mold) (Medicine 81:333, 2002) Skin, subcut (Madura foot), brain abscess, recurrent meningitis. May appear after near-drowning incidents. Also emerging especially in hematopoietic stem cell transplant (HSCT) pts with disseminated disease	**Voriconazole** 6 mg/kg IV q12h on day 1, then either (4 mg/kg IV q12h) or (200 mg po q12h for body weight ≥40 kg, but 100 mg po q12h for body weight < 40 kg) (AAC 52:1743, 2008). 300 mg bid if serum concentrations are subtherapeutic, i.e., < 1 mcg/mL (CID 46:201, 2008).	Surgery + **itraconazole** 200 mg po bid until clinically well.[NFDA-I] (Many species now resistant or refractory to itra) OR **Posa** 400 mg po bid with meals (if not taking meals, 200 mg po qid).	**Resistant to many antifungal drugs including amphotericin.** In vitro voriconazole more active than itra and posaconazole in vitro (Clin Microbiol Rev 21:157, 2008). Case reports of successful rx of disseminated and CNS disease with voriconazole (AAC 52:1743, 2008). Posaconazole active in vitro and successful in several case reports
Sporotrichosis IDSA Guideline: CID 45:1255, 2007. **Cutaneous/Lymphocutaneous**	**Itraconazole** po 200 mg/day for 2-4 wks after all lesions resolved, usually 3-6 mos.	If no response, **itra** 200 mg po bid or **terbinafine** 500 mg po bid or **SSKI** 5 drops (eye drops) tid & increase to 40-50 drops tid	Fluconazole 400-800 mg daily only if no response to primary or alternative suggestions. Pregnancy or nursing: local hyperthermia (see below).
Osteoarticular	**Itra** 200 mg po bid x 12 mos.	**Liposomal ampho B** 3-5 mg/kg/d IV or **ABLC** 5 mg/kg/d IV or **ampho B deoxycholate** 0.7-1 mg/kg IV daily; if response, change to **itra** 200 mg po bid x total 12 mos.	After 2 wks of therapy, document adequate serum levels of itraconazole.
Pulmonary	If severe, **lipid ampho B** 3-5 mg/kg IV or **standard ampho B** 0.7-1 mg/kg IV once daily until response, then **itra** 200 mg po bid. Total of 12 mos.	Less severe: **itraconazole** 200 mg po bid x 12 mos.	After 2 weeks of therapy document adequate serum levels of itra. Surgical resection plus ampho B for localized pulmonary disease.
Meningeal or Disseminated	**Lipid ampho B** 5 mg/kg IV once daily x 4-6 wks, then—if better—**itra** 200 mg po bid for total of 12 mos.	AIDS/Other immunosuppressed pts: chronic therapy with **itra** 200 mg po once daily.	After 2 weeks, document adequate serum levels of itra.
Pregnancy and children	**Pregnancy:** Cutaneous—local hyperthermia. Severe: **lipid ampho B** 3-5 mg/kg IV once daily. **Avoid itraconazole.**	**Children:** Cutaneous: **Itra** 6-10 mg/kg (max of 400 mg) daily. Alternative is **SSKI** 1 drop tid increasing to max of 1 drop/kg or 40-50 drops tid/day, whichever is lowest.	For children with disseminated sporatrichosis: Standard ampho B 0.7 mg/kg IV once daily & after response, itra 6-10 mg/kg (max 400 mg) once daily.

See page 3 for abbreviations. All dosage recommendations are for adults (unless otherwise indicated) and assume normal renal function

108

TABLE 11B – ANTIFUNGAL DRUGS: DOSAGE, ADVERSE EFFECTS, COMMENTS

DRUG NAME, GENERIC (TRADE)/USUAL DOSAGE	ADVERSE EFFECTS/COMMENTS
Non-lipid amphotericin B deoxycholate (Fungizone); 0.3–1 mg/kg per day as single infusion **Ampho B predictably not active vs. Scedosporium, Candida lusitaniae & Aspergillus terreus** (Table 11C, page 111)	**Admin:** Ampho B is a colloidal suspension that must be prepared in electrolyte-free D5W at 0.1 mg/mL to avoid precipitation. No need to protect suspensions from light. Infusions cause chills/fever, myalgia, anorexia, nausea, rarely hemodynamic collapse/hypotension. Postulated due to proinflammatory cytokines, doesn't appear to be histamine release (Pharmacol 23:966, 2003). Infusion duration usu. 4+ hrs. No difference found in 1 vs 4 hr infus. except chills/fever occurred sooner with 1hr infus. Febrile reactions ↓ with repeat doses. Rare pulmonary reactions (severe dyspnea & focal infiltrates suggest pulmonary edema) assoc with rapid infus. **Severe rigors respond to meperidine (25–50 mg IV).** Premedication with acetaminophen, diphenhydramine, hydrocortisone (25–50 mg) and heparin (1000 units) had no influence on rigors/fever. NSAIDs or high-dose steroids may prove efficacious but their use may risk worsening infection under rx or increased risk of **nephrotoxicity** (i.e., NSAIDs). Clinical side effects ↓ with ↑ age. **Toxicity:** Major concern is nephrotoxicity. Manifest initially by kaliuresis and hypokalemia, then fall in serum bicarbonate (may proceed to renal tubular acidosis), ↓ in renal erythropoietin and anemia, and rising BUN/serum creatinine. Hypomagnesemia may occur. Can reduce risk of renal injury by **(a) pre- & post-infusion hydration with 500mL saline (if clinical status allows salt load), (b)** avoidance of other nephrotoxins, eg, radiocontrast, aminoglycosides, cis-platinum, **(c)** use of lipid prep of ampho B.
Lipid-based ampho B products[†]: Amphotericin B lipid complex (ABLC) (Abelcet): 5 mg/kg per day as single infusion	**Admin:** Consists of ampho B complexed with 2 lipid bilayer ribbons. Compared to standard ampho B, larger volume of distribution, rapid blood clearance and high tissue concentrations (liver, spleen, lung). Dosage: **5 mg/kg once daily;** infuse at 2.5 mg/kg per hr; adult and ped. dose the same. Do NOT use an in-line filter. Do not dilute with saline or mix with other drugs or electrolytes.[2] **Toxicity:** Fever and chills in 14–18%; nausea 9%, vomiting 8%; serum creatinine ↑ in 11%; renal failure 5%; anemia 4%; ↓ K 5%; rash 4%. A fatal case of fat embolism reported following ABLC infusion (Exp Mol Path 177:246, 2004).
Liposomal amphotericin B (LAB, AmBisome): 1–5 mg/kg per day as single infusion.	**Admin:** Consists of vesicular bilayer liposome with ampho B intercalated within the membrane. Dosage: **3–5 mg/kg per day** IV as single dose infused over a period of approx. 120min. If well tolerated, infusion time can be reduced to 60 min. (see footnote 2). Tolerated well in elderly pts (J Inf 50:277, 2005). **Major toxicity:** Gen less than ampho B. Nephrotoxicity 18.7% vs 33.7% for ampho B, chills 47% vs 75%, nausea 39.7% vs 38.7%, vomiting 31.8% vs 43.9%, rash 24% for both, ↓ Ca 18.4% vs 20.9%, ↓ K 20.4% vs 25.6%, ↓ mg 20.4% vs 25.6%. Acute infusion-related reactions common with liposomal ampho B, 20–40%. 86% occur within 5 min of infusion, incl chest pain, dyspnea, hypoxia or severe abdom, flank or leg pain; 14% dev flushing & urticaria near end of 4hr infusion. All responded to diphenhydramine (1 mg/kg) & interruption of infusion. Reactions may be due to complement activation by liposome (CID 36:1213, 2003).
Caspofungin (Cancidas) 70 mg IV on day 1 followed by 50 mg IV q24h (reduce to 35 mg IV q24h with moderate hepatic insufficiency)	An echinocandin which inhibits synthesis of β-(1,3)-D-glucan. Fungicidal against candida (MIC < 2mcg/mL) including those resistant to other antifungals & active against aspergillus (MIC 0.4–2.7mcg/mL). Approved indications for caspo incl: empirical rx for febrile, neutropenic pts; rx of candidemia, candida intraabdominal abscesses, peritonitis, & pleural space infections; esophageal candidiasis; & invasive aspergillosis in pts refractory to or intolerant of other therapies. Serum levels on rec. dosages = peak 12, trough 1.3 (24hrs) mcg/mL. **Toxicity:** remarkably non-toxic. Most common adverse effect: pruritus at infusion site & headache, fever, chills, vomiting, & diarrhea assoc with infusion. ↑ serum creatinine in 8% on caspo vs 21% short-course ampho B in 422 pts with candidemia (Ln, Oct. 12, 2005, online). Drug metab in liver & dosage ↓ to 35 mg in moderate to severe hepatic failure. Class C for preg (embryotoxic in rats & rabbits). See Table 22, page 193 for drug-drug interactions, esp. cyclosporine (hepatic toxicity) & tacrolimus (drug level monitoring recommended). Reversible thrombocytopenia reported (Pharmacother 24:1408, 2004). **No drug in CSF or urine.**
Micafungin (Mycamine) 50 mg/day for prophylaxis post-bone marrow stem cell trans; 100 mg candidemia, 150 mg candida esophagitis.	The 2nd echinocandin approved by FDA for rx of esophageal candidiasis & prophylaxis against candida infections in HSCT[3] recipients. Active against most strains of candida sp. & aspergillus sp. incl those resist to fluconazole such as C. glabrata & C. krusei. No antagonism seen when combo with other antifungal drugs. No dosage adjust for severe renal failure or moderate hepatic impairment. Watch for drug-drug interactions with sirolimus or nifedipine. Micafungin well tolerated & common adverse events incl nausea 2.8%, vomiting 2.4%, & headache 2.4%. Transient ↑ LFTs, BUN, creatinine reported; rare cases of significant hepatitis & renal insufficiency. See CID 42:1171, 2006. **No drug in CSF or urine.**

---

1   Published data from patients intolerant of or refractory to conventional ampho B deoxycholate (Amp B d). **None of the lipid ampho B preps has shown superior efficacy compared to ampho B in prospective trials (except liposomal ampho B was more effective vs ampho B in rx of disseminated histoplasmosis at 2 wks). Dosage equivalency has not been established** (CID 36:1500, 2003). Nephrotoxicity ↓ with all lipid ampho B preps.

2   Comparisons between Abelcet & AmBisome suggest higher infusion-assoc. toxicity (rigors) & febrile episodes with Abelcet (70% vs 36%) but higher frequency of mild hepatic toxicity with AmBisome (59% vs 38%, p= 0.05). Mild elevations in serum creatinine were observed in 1/3 of both (BJ Hemat 103:198, 1998; Focus on Fungal Inf # 9, 1999; Bone Marrow Tx 20:39, 1997; CID 26:1383, 1998).

3   HSCT = hematopoietic stem cell transplant.

See page 3 for abbreviations. All dosage recommendations are for adults (unless otherwise indicated) and assume normal renal function

TABLE 11B (2)

DRUG NAME, GENERIC (TRADE)/USUAL DOSAGE	ADVERSE EFFECTS/COMMENTS
Anidulafungin (Eraxis) For Candidemia; 200 mg IV on day 1 followed by 100 mg/day IV). Rx for EC; 100 mg IV x 1, then 50 mg IV once/d.	An echinocandin with antifungal activity (cidal) against candida sp. & aspergillus sp. including ampho B- & triazole-resistant strains. FDA approved for treatment of esophageal candidiasis (EC), candidemia, and other complicated Candida infections. Effective in clinical trials of esophageal candidiasis & in 1 trial was superior to fluconazole in rx of invasive candidiasis/candidemia in 245 pts (75.6% vs 60.2%). Like other echinocandins, remarkably non-toxic; most common side-effects: nausea, vomiting, ↓ mg, ↓ K & headache in 11–13% of pts. No dose adjustments for renal or hepatic insufficiency. See CID 43:215, 2006. **No drug in CSF or urine.**
Fluconazole (Diflucan) 100 mg tabs 150 mg tabs 200 mg tabs 400 mg IV Oral suspension: 50 mg per 5 mL.	IV= oral dose because of excellent bioavailability. **Pharmacology:** absorbed po, water solubility enables IV. For peak serum levels (see Table 9, page 80). T½ 30hr (range 20–50hr). 12% protein bound. **CSF levels 50–90% of serum in normals**, ↑ in meningitis. No effect on mammalian steroid metabolism. **Drug-drug interactions common**, see Table 22. Side-effects overall 16% [more common in HIV+ pts (21%)]. Nausea 3.7%, headache 1.9%, skin rash 1.8%, abdominal pain 1.7%, vomiting 1.7%, diarrhea 1.5%, ↑ SGOT 20%. Alopecia (scalp; pubic crest) in 12–20% pts on ≥400 mg po q24h after median of 3mo (reversible in approx. 6mo). Rare: severe hepatotoxicity (CID 41:301, 2005), exfoliative dermatitis. **Note: Candida krusei and Candida glabrata resistant to Flu.**
Flucytosine (Ancobon) 500 mg cap	AEs: Overall 30%. GI 6% (diarrhea, anorexia, nausea, vomiting); hematologic 22% [leukopenia, thrombocytopenia, when serum level > 100mcg/mL (esp. in azotemic pts)]; hepatotoxicity (asymptomatic ↑ SGOT, reversible); skin rash 7%; aplastic anemia (rare—2 or 3 cases). False ↑ in serum creatinine on EKTACHEM analyzer.
Griseofulvin (Fulvicin, Grifulvin, Grisactin) 500 mg, susp 125 mg/mL.	Photosensitivity, urticaria, GI upset, fatigue, leukopenia (rare). Interferes with warfarin drugs. Increases blood and urine porphyrins, should not be used in patients with porphyria. Minor disulfiram-like reactions. Exacerbation of systemic lupus erythematosus.
Imidazoles, topical For vaginal and/or skin use	Not recommended in 1st trimester of pregnancy. Local reactions: 0.5-1.5%: dyspareunia, mild vaginal or vulvar erythema, burning, pruritus, urticaria, rash. Rarely similar symptoms in sexual partner.
Itraconazole (Sporanox) 100 mg cap - - - - - - - - - - - - - - - - 10 mg/mL oral solution - - - - - - - - - - - - - - - - IV usual dose 200 mg bid x 4 doses followed by 200 mg q24h for a max of 14 days	**Itraconazole tablet & solution forms not interchangeable, solution preferred.** Many authorities recommend measuring drug serum concentration after 2 wk to ensure satisfactory absorption. To obtain highest plasma concentration, tablet is given with food & acidic drinks (e.g., cola) while solution is taken in fasted state; under these conditions, the peak conc. of capsule is approx. 3mcg/mL & of solution 5.4mcg/mL. Peak levels reached faster (2.2 vs 5hrs) with solution. **Peak plasma concentrations after IV injection (200 mg) compared to oral capsule (200 mg): 2.8mcg/mL (on day 7 of rx) vs 2mcg/mL (on day 36 of rx).** Protein-binding for both preparations is over 99%, which explains virtual absence of penetration into CSF **(do not use to treat meningitis).** Most common adverse effects are dose-related nausea 10%, diarrhea 8%, vomiting 6%, & abdominal discomfort 5.7%. Allergic rash 8.6%, ↑ bilirubin 6%, edema 3.5%, & hepatitis 2.7% reported. ↑ doses may produce hypokalemia 8% & ↑ blood pressure 3.2%. Delirium & peripheral neuropathy reported. **Reported to produce impairment in cardiac function** (see footnote 2 page 83). Severe liver failure req transplant in pts receiving pulse rx for onychomycosis: FDA reports 24 cases with 11 deaths out of 50mill people who received the drug prior to 2001. Other concern, as with fluconazole and ketoconazole, is **drug-drug interactions;** see Table 22. Some can be life-threatening.
Ketoconazole (Nizoral) 200 mg tab	Gastric acid required for absorption—cimetidine, omeprazole, antacids block absorption. In achlorhydria, dissolve tablet in 4 mL 0.2N HCl, drink with a straw. Coca-Cola ↑ absorption by 65%. CSF levels "none." **Drug-drug interactions important**, see Table 22. **Some interactions can be life-threatening. Dose- dependent nausea and vomiting.** Liver toxicity of hepatocellular type reported in about 1:10,000 exposed pts—usually after several days to weeks of exposure. At doses of ≥800 mg per day serum testosterone and plasma cortisol levels fall. With high doses, adrenal (Addisonian) crisis reported.
Miconazole (Monistat IV) 200 mg—not available in U.S.	IV miconazole indicated in patient critically ill with Scedosporium (Pseudallescheria boydii) infection. Very toxic due to vehicle needed to get drug into solution.
Nystatin (Mycostatin) 30 gm cream 500,000 units oral tab	Topical: virtually no adverse effects. Less effective than imidazoles and triazoles. PO: large doses give occasional GI distress and diarrhea.

See page 3 for abbreviations. All dosage recommendations are for adults (unless otherwise indicated) and assume normal renal function

TABLE 11B (3)

DRUG NAME, GENERIC (TRADE)/USUAL DOSAGE	ADVERSE EFFECTS/COMMENTS
Posaconazole (Noxafil) 400 mg po bid with meals (if not taking meals, 200 mg qid). 200 mg po TID (with food) for prophylaxis. 40 mg/mL suspension. **Takes 7–10 days to achieve steady state.** No IV formulation.	An oral triazole with activity against a wide range of fungi refractory to other antifungal rx including: aspergillosis, zygomycosis, fusariosis, Scedosporium (Pseudallescheria), phaeohyphomycosis, histoplasmosis, refractory candidiasis, refractory coccidioidomycosis, refractory cryptococcosis, & refractory chromoblastomycosis. **Should be taken with high fat meal for maximum absorption.** Approved for prophylaxis (NEJM 356:348, 2007). Clinical response in 75% of 176 AIDS pts with azole-refractory oral/esophageal candidiasis. Posaconazole has similar toxicities as other triazoles: nausea 9%, vomiting 6%, abd. pain 5%, headache 5%, diarrhea, ↑ ALT, AST, & rash (3% each). In pts rx for > 6 mos., serious side-effects have included adrenal insufficiency, nephrotoxicity, & QTc interval prolongation. Significant drug-drug interactions; inhibits CYP3A4 (see Table 22). (See Drugs 65:1552, 2005)
Terbinafine (Lamisil) 250 mg tab	In pts given terbinafine for onychomycosis, rare cases (8) of idiosyncratic & symptomatic hepatic injury & more rarely liver failure leading to death or liver transplant. The drug is **not recommended** for pts with **chronic or active liver disease;** hepatotoxicity may occur in pts with or without pre-existing disease. Pretreatment serum transaminases (ALT & AST) advised & alternate rx used for those with abnormal levels. Pts started on terbinafine should be warned about symptoms suggesting liver dysfunction (persistent nausea, anorexia, fatigue, vomiting, RUQ pain, jaundice, dark urine or pale stools). If symptoms develop, drug should be discontinued & liver function immediately evaluated. In controlled trials, changes in ocular lens and retina reported—clinical significance unknown. Major drug-drug interaction is 100% ↑ in rate of clearance by rifampin. AEs: usually mild, transient and rarely caused discontinuation of rx. % with AE, terbinafine vs placebo: nausea/diarrhea 2.6–5.6 vs 2.9; rash 5.6 vs 2.2; taste abnormality 2.8 vs 0.7. Inhibits CYP2D6 enzymes (see Table 22). An acute generalized exanthematous pustulosis and subacute cutaneous lupus erythematosus reported.
Voriconazole (Vfend) IV: Loading dose 6 mg per kg q12h times 1 day, then 4 mg per kg q12h IV for invasive aspergillus & serious mold infections; **3 mg per kg IV q12h** for serious candida infections. **Oral: >40 kg body weight:** 400 mg po q12h, then 200 mg po q12h. **<40 kg body weight:** 200 mg po q12h, then 100 mg po q12h **Take oral dose 1 hour before or 1 hour after eating.** Oral suspension (40 mg per mL). Oral suspension dosing: Same as for oral tabs. Reduce to ½ maintenance dose for moderate hepatic insufficiency	A triazole with activity against Aspergillus sp., **including Ampho resistant strains of A. terreus.** Active vs Candida sp. (including krusei), Fusarium sp., & various molds. Steady state serum levels reach 2.5–4 mcg per mL. Up to 20% of patients with subtherapeutic levels with oral administration: check levels for suspected treatment failure, life threatening infections. 300 mg bid oral dose or 8 mg/kg/d IV dose may be required to achieve target steady-state drug concentrations of 1–6 mcg/mL. Toxicity similar to other azoles/triazoles including uncommon serious hepatic toxicity (hepatitis, cholestasis & fulminant hepatic failure. Liver function tests should be monitored during rx & drug dc'd if abnormalities develop. Rash reported in up to 20%; occ. photosensitivity & rare Stevens-Johnson, hallucinations & anaphylactoid infusion reactions with fever and hypertension. 1 case of QT prolongation with ventricular tachycardia in a 15 y/o pt with ALL reported. **Approx. 21% experience a transient visual disturbance** following IV or po ("altered/enhanced visual perception", blurred or colored visual change or photophobia) within 30–60 minutes. Visual changes resolve within 30–60 min. after administration & are attenuated with repeated doses **(do not drive at night for outpatient rx).** Persistent visual changes occur rarely. Cause unknown. In patients with ClCr < 50 mL per min., the drug should be given orally, not IV, since the intravenous vehicle (SBECD-sulfobutylether-B cyclodextrin) may accumulate. Hallucinations, hypoglycemia, electrolyte disturbance & pneumonitis attributed to ↑ drug concentrations. Potential for drug-drug interactions high—see Table 22. **NOTE: Not in urine in active form. No activity vs. zygomycetes, e.g., mucor.**

See page 3 for abbreviations. All dosage recommendations are for adults (unless otherwise indicated) and assume normal renal function

Table 11C – AT A GLANCE SUMMARY OF SUGGESTED ANTIFUNGAL DRUGS AGAINST TREATABLE PATHOGENIC FUNGI

Microorganism	Antifungal[1-4]					
	Fluconazole[5]	Itraconazole	Voriconazole	Posaconazole	Echinocandin	Polyenes
Candida albicans	+++	+++	+++	+++	+++	++
Candida dubliniensis	+++	+++	+++	+++	+++	++
Candida glabrata	±	±	+	+	+++	++
Candida tropicalis	+++	+++	+++	+++	+++	+++
Candida parapsilosis[6]	+++	+++	+++	+++	++ (higher MIC)	+++
Candida krusei	-	+	++	++	+++	++
Candida guilliermondii	+++	+++	+++	+++	++ (higher MIC)	++
Candida lusitaniae	+	+	++	++	++	++
Cryptococcus neoformans	+++	+	+++	+++	-	+++
Aspergillus fumigatus[7]	-	++	+++	+++	++	++
Aspergillus flavus[7]	-	++	+++	+++	++	++ (higher MIC)
Aspergillus terreus	-	++	+++	+++	++	-
Fusarium sp.	-	±	++	++	-	++ (lipid formulations)
Scedosporium apiospermum (*Pseudoallescheria boydii*)[8]	-	-	+++	+++	±	±
Scedosporium prolificans[8]	-	-	±	±	-	-
Trichosporon spp.	±	+	++	++	-	+
Zygomycetes (e.g., *Absidia, Mucor, Rhizopus*)	-	±	-	+++	-	+++ (lipid formulations)
Dematiaceous molds[9] (e.g., *Alternaria, Bipolaris, Curvularia, Exophiala*)	±	++	+++	+++	+	+
Dimorphic Fungi						
Blastomyces dermatitidis	+++	+++	++	++	-	+++
Coccidioides immitis/posadasii	+++	++	++	++	-	+++
Histoplasma capsulatum	+++	+++	++	++	-	+++
Sporothrix schenckii	±	++	-		-	+++

- = no activity; ± = possibly activity; + = active, 3rd line therapy (least active clinically)
++ = Active, 2nd line therapy (less active clinically); +++ = Active, 1st line therapy (usually active clinically)

1. Minimum inhibitory concentration values do not always predict clinical outcome.
2. Echinocandins, voriconazole, posaconazole and polyenes have poor urine penetration.
3. During severe immune suppression, success requires immune reconstitution.
4. **Flucytosine** has activity against *Candida* sp., *Cryptococcus* sp., and dematiaceous molds, but is primarily used in combination therapy.
5. For infections secondary to *Candida* sp., patients with prior triazole therapy have higher likelihood of triazole resistance.
6. Successful treatment of infections from *Candida parapsilosis* requires removal of foreign body or intravascular device.
7. Lipid formulations of amphotericin may have greater activity against *A. fumigatus* and *A. flavus* (+++).
8. *Scedosporium prolificans* is poorly susceptible to single agents and may require combination therapy (e.g., addition of terbinafine).
9. Infections from zygomycetes, some *Aspergillus* spp., and dematiaceous molds often require surgical debridement.

TABLE 12A – TREATMENT OF MYCOBACTERIAL INFECTIONS*

Tuberculin skin test (TST). Same as PPD *[MMWR 52(RR-2):15, 2003]*.

Criteria for positive TST after 5 tuberculin units (intermediate PPD) read at 48–72 hours:

≥5 mm induration: + HIV, immunosuppressed, ≥15 mg prednisone per day, healed TBc on chest x-ray, recent close contact

≥10 mm induration: foreign-born, countries with high prevalence; IVDUsers; low income; NH residents; chronic illness; silicosis

≥15 mm induration: otherwise healthy

Two-stage to detect sluggish positivity: If 1st PPD + but <10 mm, repeat intermediate PPD in 1wk. Response to 2nd PPD can also happen if pt received BCG in childhood.

BCG vaccine as child: if ≥10 mm induration, & from country with TBc, should be attributed to M. tuberculosis. In areas of low TB prevalence, TST reactions of ≤18mm more likely from BCG than TB *(CID 40:211, 2005)*. Prior BCG may result in booster effect in 2-stage TST *(AnIM 161:1760, 2001; Clin Micro Inf 10:980, 2005)*.

Routine anergy testing no longer recommended in HIV+ or HIV-negative patients *(JAMA 283:2003, 2000)*.

Whole blood interferon-gamma release assay [QuantiFERON-TB (QFT)] approved by U.S. FDA as diagnostic test for TB *(JAMA 286:1740, 2001; CID 34:1449 & 1457, 2002)*. CDC recommends TST for TB suspects & pts at ↑ risk for progression to active TB & suggests either TST or QFT for individuals at ↑ risk for latent TB (LTBI) & for persons who warrant testing but are deemed at low risk for LTBI *[MMWR 52(RR-2):15, 2003]*. IFN-γ assay is better indicator of TBc risk than TST in BCG-vaccinated population *(JAMA 293:2756, 2005)*. A more sensitive assay based on M. tbc-specific antigens (QuantiFERON-TB GOLD) was approved by the USFDA 5/2/05 and an enzyme-linked immunospot method (ELISpot) using antigens specific for MTB (do not cross-react with BCG) is under evaluation & looks promising *(Thorax 58:916, 2003; Ln 361:1168, 2003; AnIM 140:709, 2004; LnID 4:761, 2005; CID 40:246, 2005; JAMA 293:2756, 2005; MMWR 54:49, 2005)*. However, none of these tests can distinguish latent from active TB and none is 100% sensitive (ELISpot slightly higher sensitivity than Quantiferon-TB Gold and ELISpotPLUS, which is not yet commercially available, is more sensitive than ELISpot.)*(AnIM 146:340, 2007; CID 44:74, 2007; AIM 148:325, 2008)*. None of these tests can be used to exclude tuberculosis in persons with suggestive signs or symptoms *(CID 45:837, 2007)*.

CAUSATIVE AGENT/DISEASE	MODIFYING CIRCUMSTANCES	INITIAL THERAPY	SUGGESTED REGIMENS
			CONTINUATION PHASE OF THERAPY
I. Mycobacterium tuberculosis exposure but TST negative (household members & other close contacts of potentially infectious cases)	Neonate—Rx essential	INH (10 mg/kg/day for 3 mo)	Repeat tuberculin skin test (TST) in 3 mo. If mother's smear neg & infant's TST neg & chest x-ray (CXR) normal, stop INH. In UK, BCG is then given *(Ln 2:1479, 1990)*, unless mother HIV+. If infant's repeat TST +&/or CXR abnormal (hilar adenopathy &/or infiltrate), INH + RIF (10–20 mg/kg/day) (or SM). Total rx 6 mo. If mother is being rx, separation of infant from mother not indicated.
	Children <5 years of age—Rx indicated	As for neonate for 1st 3 mos	**if + rx** with INH for total of 9 mos. *(see Category II below)*. If repeat TST at 3 mo is negative, stop. If repeat TST +, continue INH for total of 9 mos. If INH not given initially, repeat TST at 3 mo.
	Older children & adults— Risk 2–4% 1st 1st yr		No rx

(Continued on next page)

See page 3 for abbreviations, page 118 for footnotes   * *Dosages are for adults (unless otherwise indicated) and assume normal renal function*   † **DOT** = directly observed therapy

TABLE 12A (2)

CAUSATIVE AGENT/DISEASE	MODIFYING CIRCUMSTANCES	SUGGESTED REGIMENS	
		INITIAL THERAPY	ALTERNATIVE
II. Treatment of latent infection with M. tuberculosis (formerly known as "prophylaxis) (*NEJM 347:1860, 2002; NEJM 350:2060, 2004; JAMA 293:2776, 2005*) **A. INH indicated due to high-risk** Assumes INH susceptibility likely. INH 54–88% effective in preventing active TB for ≥20 yr.	(1) + tuberculin reactor & HIV+ (risk of active disease 10% per yr. AIDS 170 times ↑, HIV+ 113 times ↑). Development of active TBc in HIV+ pts after INH usually due to reinfection, not INH failure (*CID 34:386, 2002*). (2) Newly infected persons (TST conversion in past 2 yrs— risk 3.3% 1st yr). (3) Past tuberculosis, not rx with adequate chemotherapy (INH, RIF, or alternatives). (4) + tuberculin reactors with CXR consistent with non-progressive tuberculous disease (risk 0.5–5.0% per yr). (5) + tuberculin reactors with specific predisposing conditions: illicit IV drug use (*MMWR 38:236, 1989*), silicosis, diabetes mellitus, prolonged adrenocorticoid rx (>15 mg prednisone/day), immunosuppressive rx, hematologic diseases (Hodgkin's, leukemia), endstage renal disease, clinical condition with rapid substantial weight loss or chronic under-nutrition, previous gastrectomy (*CID 45:428, 2007*). (6) + tuberculin reactors due to start anti-TNF-(alpha) therapy (*CID 46:1738, 2008*). For management algorithm see Thorax 60:800, 2005. **NOTE: For HIV, see Sanford Guide to HIV/AIDS Therapy &/or JID 196:S35, 2007**	**INH** (5 mg/kg/day, max 300 mg/ day for adults: 10 mg/kg/day not to exceed 300 mg/day for children). May use 2x/wk INH with DOT (*MMWR 52:735, 2003*). Optimal duration 9 mos. (includes children, HIV–, HIV+, old fibrotic lesions on chest x-ray). In some cases, 6 mos. may be given for cost-effectiveness (*AJRCCM 161:S221, 2000*). Do not use 6 mo. regimen in HIV+ persons <18yr, or those with fibrotic lesions on chest film (*NEJM 345:189, 2001*).	If compliance problem: **INH** by DOT† 15 mg/kg 2x/wk times 9 mo. 2 mo **RIF + PZA** regimen effective in HIV– and HIV+ for adults (*AJRCCM 161:S221, 2000; JAMA 283:1445, 2000*). **However, there are descriptions of severe & fatal hepatitis in immunocompetent pts on RIF + PZA** (*MMWR 50:289, 2001*). Monitoring for cofactors did not seem to allow prediction of fatalities (*CID 42:346, 2006*). Therefore, regimen is no longer recommended by CDC for LTBI (*MMWR 52:735, 2003; CID 39:488, 2004*). Not all agree with CDC recommendation and recent study suggests short course therapy is safe with monitoring and more likely to be completed than longer therapy (*CID 43:271, 2006*). **RIF** 600 mg/day po for 4 mo. (HIV– and HIV+). Meta-analysis suggests 3 mo of INH + RIF may be equiv to "standard" (6–12 mo) INH therapy (*CID 40:670, 2005*). 3-4 month INH + RIF regimens also as safe and effective as 9 months INH in children (*CID 45:715, 2007*).
B. TST positive (organisms likely to be INH-susceptible)	Age no longer considered modifying factor (see *Comments*)	**INH** (5 mg per kg per day for adults; 10 mg per kg per day for children). Results with 6 mos. rx not quite as effective as 12 mos. (65% vs 75% reduction in disease). 9 mos. is current recommendation. See *II.A above for details and alternate rx.*	Reanalysis of earlier studies favors **INH** prophylaxis (if INH related, hepatitis case fatality rate <1% and TB case fatality ≥6.7%, which appears to be the case) (*ArIM 150:2517, 1990*). Recent data suggest INH prophylaxis has positive risk-benefit ratio in pts ≥35 if monitored for hepatotoxicity (*AnIM 127:1051, 1997*). Overall risk of hepatotoxicity 0.1–0.15% (*JAMA 281:1014, 1999*).
	Pregnancy—Any risk factors (*II.A above*)	Treat with **INH** as above. For women at risk for progression of latent to active disease, esp. those who are HIV+ or who have been recently infected, rx should not be delayed even during the first trimester.	Risk of INH hepatitis may be ↑ (*Ln 346:199, 1995*)
	Pregnancy—No risk factors	No initial rx (see *Comment*)	Delay rx until after delivery (*AJRCCM 149:1359, 1994*)
C. TST positive & drug resistance likely (For data on worldwide prevalence of drug resistance, see *NEJM 344:1294, 2001; JID 185:1197, 2002; JID 194:479, 2006; EID 13:380, 2007*)	INH-resistant (or adverse reaction to INH), RIF-sensitive organisms likely	**RIF** 600 mg per day po for 4 mos. (HIV+ or HIV–)	IDSA guideline lists rifabutin in 600 mg per day dose as another alternative; however, current recommended max. dose of rifabutin is 300 mg per day. Estimate RIF alone has protective effect of 56%; 26% of pts reported adverse effects (only 2/157 did not complete 6 mos. rx) (*AJRCCM 155:1735, 1997*).
	INH- and RIF-resistant organisms likely	Efficacy of all regimens unproven. (**PZA** 25–30 mg per kg per day to max. of 2 gm per day) + **ETB** 15–25 mg per kg per day po) times 6–12 mos.	[(**PZA** 25 mg per kg per day to max. of 2 gm per day) + (**levo** 500 mg per day or **oflox** 400 mg bid)], all po, times 6–12 mos. PZA + oflox has been associated with asymptomatic hepatitis (*CID 24:1264, 1997*).

See page 3 for abbreviations, page 118 for footnotes   * Dosages are for adults (unless otherwise indicated) and assume normal renal function   † **DOT** = directly observed therapy

TABLE 12A (3)

CAUSATIVE AGENT/DISEASE

III. Mycobacterium tuberculosis
A. Pulmonary TB
[General reference on rx in adults & children: Ln 362: 887, 2003; MMWR 52(RR-11):1, 2003; CID 40(Suppl.1): S1, 2005]

Isolation essential! Pts with active TB should be isolated in single rooms, not cohorted (MMWR 54(RR-17), 2005). Older observations on infectivity of suscepti-ble & resistant M. tbc before and after rx (ARRD 85:5111, 1962) may not be applicable to MDR M. tbc or to the HIV+ individual. Extended isolation may be appropriate.

See footnotes, page 118

USE DOT REGIMENS IF POSSIBLE

(continued on next page)

MODIFYING CIRCUMSTANCES

Rate of INH resistance known to be <4% (drug-susceptible organisms) [Modified from MMWR 52 (RR-11):1, 2003]

SUGGESTED REGIMENS

SEE COMMENTS FOR DOSAGE AND DIRECTLY OBSERVED THERAPY (DOT) REGIMENS

INITIAL PHASE[8]

Regimen: in order of preference	Drugs	Interval/Doses[1] (min. duration)
1 (See Figure 1, page 117)	INH RIF PZA ETB	7 days per wk times 56 doses (8 wk) or 5 days per wk times 40 doses (8 wk)[3]
2 (See Figure 1, page 117)	INH RIF PZA ETB	7 days per wk times 14 doses (2 wk), then 2 times per wk times 12 doses (6 wk) or 5 days per wk times 10 doses (2 wk) then 2 times per wk times 12 doses (6 wk)[3]
3 (See Figure 1, page 117)	INH RIF PZA ETB	3 times per wk times 24 doses (8 wk)
4 (See Figure 1, page 117)	INH RIF ETB	7 days per wk times 56 doses (8 wk) or 5 days per wk times 40 doses (8 wk)[3]

CONTINUATION PHASE OF THERAPY[7] (in vitro susceptibility known)

Regimen	Drugs	Interval/Doses[1,2] (min. duration)	Range of Total Doses (min. duration)
1a	INH/RIF[9]	7 days per wk times 126 doses (18 wk) or 5 days per wk times 90 doses (18 wk)[3]	182–130 (26 wk)
1b	INH/RIF	2 times per wk times 36 doses (18 wk)	92–76 (26 wk)[4]
1c[5]	INH/RFP	1 time per wk times 18 doses (18 wk)	74–58 (26 wk)
2a	INH/RIF	2 times per wk times 36 doses (18 wk)	62–58 (26 wk)[4]
2b[5]	INH/RFP	1 time per wk times 18 doses (18 wk)	44–40 (26 wk)
3a	INH/RIF	3 times per wk times 54 doses (18 wk)	78 (26 wk)
4a	INH/RIF[6]	7 days per wk times 217 doses (31 wk) or 5 days per wk times 155 doses (31 wk)[3]	273–195 (39 wk)
4b	INH/RIF[6]	2 times per wk times 62 doses (31 wk)	118–102 (39 wk)

COMMENTS

Dose in mg per kg (max. q24h dose)

Regimen*	INH	RIF	PZA	ETB	SM	RFB
Q24h:						
Child	10–20 (300)	10–20 (600)	15–30 (2000)	15–25	20–40 (1000)	10–20 (300)
Adult	5 (300)	10 (600)	15–30 (2000)	15–25	15 (1000)	5 (300)
2 times per wk (DOT):						
Child	20–40 (900)	10–20 (600)	50–70 (4000)	50	25–30 (1500)	10–20 (300)
Adult	15 (900)	10 (600)	50–70 (4000)	50	25–30 (1500)	5 (300)
3 times per wk (DOT):						
Child	20–40 (900)	10–20 (600)	50–70 (3000)	25–30	25–30 (1500)	NA
Adult	15 (900)	10 (600)	50–70 (3000)	25–30	25–30 (1500)	NA

Second-line anti-TB agents can be dosed as follows to facilitate DOT: Cycloserine 500–750 mg po q24h (5 times per wk) Ethionamide 500–750 mg po q24h (5 times per wk) Kanamycin or capreomycin 15 mg per kg IM/IV q24h (3–5 times per wk) Ciprofloxacin 750 mg po q24h (5 times per wk) Ofloxacin 600–800 mg po q24h (5 times per wk) Levofloxacin 750 mg po q24h (5 times per wk) (CID 21:1245, 1995)

Risk factors for drug-resistant TB: Recent immigration from Latin America or Asia or living in area of ↑ resistance (≥4%) or previous rx without RIF; exposure to known MDR TB. Incidence of MDR TB in U.S. **appears** to have stabilized and may be slightly decreasing in early 1990s (JAMA 278:833, 1997). Incidence of primary drug resistance is particularly high (>25%) in parts of China, Thailand, Russia, Estonia & Latvia (NEJM 344:1294, 2001; NEJM 347:1850, 2002). (continued on next page)

See page 3 for abbreviations, page 118 for footnotes   * Dosages are for adults (unless otherwise indicated) and assume normal renal function   † DOT = directly observed therapy

TABLE 12A (4)

CAUSATIVE AGENT/DISEASE	MODIFYING CIRCUM-STANCES	SUGGESTED REGIMEN[8]	DURATION OF TREATMENT (mo.)[8]	SPECIFIC COMMENTS[8]	COMMENTS
III. Mycobacterium tuberculosis A. Pulmonary TB (continued from previous page) REFERENCES: CID 22:683, 1996; Clin Micro Rev 19:658, 2006; Med Lett 5(55):15, 2007	INH (± SM) resistance	RIF, PZA, ETB (an FQ may strengthen the regimen for pts with extensive disease). Emergence of FQ resistance a concern (LnID 3:432, 2003; AAC 49:3178, 2005)	6	(continued from previous page) In British Medical Research Council trials, 6-mo. regimens have yielded ≥95% success rates despite resistance to INH if 4 drugs were used in the initial phase & RIF + ETB or SM was used throughout (ARRD 133: 423, 1986). Additional studies suggested that results were best if PZA was also used throughout the 6 mos (ARRD 136:1339, 1987). FQs were not employed in BMRC studies, but may strengthen the regimen for pts with more extensive disease. INH should be stopped in cases of INH resistance [see MMWR 52(RR-11):1, 2003 for additional discussion].	(continued from previous page) For MDR TB, consider rifabutin (~30% RIF-resistant strains are rifabutin-susceptible). Note that CIP not as effective as PZA + ETB in multidrug regimen for susceptible TB (CID 22:287, 1996). Moxifloxacin, and levofloxacin have enhanced activity compared with CIP against M. tuberculosis (AAC 46: 1022, 2002; AAC 47:2442, 2003; AAC 47:3117, 2003; JAC 53:441, 2004; AAC 48:780, 2004). FQ resistance may be seen in pts previously treated with FQ (CID 37:1448, 2003). Linezolid has excellent in vitro activity, including MDR strains (AAC 47: 416, 2003). Mortality reviewed: Ln 349:71, 1997. Rapid (24-hr) diagnostic tests for M. tuberculosis: (1) the Amplified Mycobacterium tuberculosis Direct Test amplifies and detects M. tuberculosis ribosomal RNA; (2) the AMPLICOR Mycobacterium tuberculosis Test amplifies and detects M. tuberculosis DNA. Both tests have sensitivities & specificities >95% in sputum samples that are AFB-positive. In negative smears, specificity remains >95% but sensitivity is 40–77% (AJRCCM 155:1497, 1997). Note that MTB may grow out on standard blood agar plates in 1–2 wks (J Clin Micro 41: 1710,2003).
Multidrug-Resistant Tuberculosis (MDR TB): Defined as resistant to at least 2 drugs including INH & RIF. Pt clusters with high mortality (AnIM 118:17, 1993; EJCMID 23:174, 2004; MMWR 55:305, 2006; JID 194:1194, 2006; AIM 149:123, 2008).	Resistance to INH & RIF (± SM)	FQ, PZA, ETB, IA, ± alternative agent[7]	18–24	In such cases, extended rx is needed to ↓ the risk of relapse. In cases with extensive disease, the use of an additional agent (alternative agents) may be prudent to ↓ the risk of failure & additional acquired drug resistance. Resectional surgery may be appropriate.	
	Resistance to INH, RIF (± SM), & ETB or PZA	FQ (ETB or PZA if active), IA, & 2 alternative agents[7]	24	Use the first-line agents to which there is susceptibility. Add 2 or more alternative agents in case of extensive disease. Surgery should be considered. Survival ↑ in pts receiving active FQ & surgical intervention (AJRCCM 169:1103, 2004).	
	Resistance to RIF	INH, ETB, FQ, supplemented with PZA for the first 2 mo (an IA may be included for the first 2–3 mos. for pts with extensive disease)	12–18	Q24h & 3 times per wk regimens of INH, PZA, & SM given for 9 mos. were effective in a BMRC trial (ARRD 115:727, 1977). However, extended use of ETB would be as effective as SM in these regimens. An all-oral regimen times 12–18 mos. should be effective. But for more extensive disease &/or to shorten duration (e.g., to 12 mos.), an IA may be added in the initial 2 mos. of rx.	
Extensively Drug-Resistant TB (XDR-TB): Defined as resistant to INH & RIF plus any FQ and at least 1 of the 3 second-line drugs: capreomycin, kanamycin or amikacin (MMWR 56:250, 2007). **See footnotes, page 118**	XDR-TB	See Comments	18–24	Therapy requires administration of 4-6 drugs to which infecting organism is susceptible, including multiple second-line drugs (MMWR 56:250, 2007). Increased mortality seen primarily in HIV+ patients. Cure with outpatient therapy likely in non-HIV+ patients when regimens of 4 or 5 or more drugs to which organism is susceptible are employed (NEJM 359:563, 2008; CID 47:496, 2008). Successful sputum culture conversion corelates to initial susceptibility to FQs and kanamycin (CID 46:42, 2008).	
Reviews of therapy for MDR TB: JAC 54:593, 2004; Med Lett 2:83, 2004. For XDR-TB see MMWR 56:250, 2007; NEJM 359:359, 2008.					

See footnotes, page 118 for footnotes * Dosages are for adults (unless otherwise indicated) and assume normal renal function † DOT = directly observed therapy

See page 3 for abbreviations.

TABLE 12A (5)

CAUSATIVE AGENT/DISEASE; MODIFYING CIRCUMSTANCES	SUGGESTED REGIMENS		COMMENTS
	INITIAL THERAPY	CONTINUATION PHASE OF THERAPY (in vitro susceptibility known)	
B. Extrapulmonary TB	**INH** + **RIF** (or **RFB**) + **PZA** q24h times 2 months. Authors add **pyridoxine** 25–50 mg po q24h to regimens that include INH.	**INH** + **RIF** (or **RFB**)	6 mo regimens probably effective. Most experience with 9–12 mo regimens. Am Acad Ped (1994) recommends 6 mo rx for isolated cervical adenitis, renal and 12 mo for meningitis, miliary, bone/joint. DOT useful here as well as for pulmonary tuberculosis. IDSA recommends 6 mo for lymph node, pleural, pericarditis, disseminated disease, genitourinary & peritoneal TBc; 6–9 mo for bone & joint; 9-12 mo for CNS (including meningeal) TBc. Corticosteroids "strongly rec" only for pericarditis & meningeal TBc [*MMWR 52(RR-11):1, 2003*].
C. Tuberculous meningitis Excellent summary of clinical aspects and therapy (including steroids): *CMR 21:243, 2008.*	**INH** + **RIF** + **ETB** + **PZA**	May omit ETB when susceptibility to **INH** and **RIF** established. See *Table 9, page 81*, for CSF drug penetration. Initial reg of INH + RIF + SM + PZA also effective, even in patients with INH resistant organisms (*JID 192:79, 2005*).	3 drugs often rec for initial rx; we prefer 4. May sub ethionamide for ETB. Infection with MDR TB ↑ mortality & morbidity (*CID 38:851, 2004; JID 192:79, 2005*). Dexamethasone (for 1st mo) has been shown to ↓ complications (*Pediatrics 99:226, 1997*) & ↑ survival in pts >14 yr old (*NEJM 351:1741, 2004*). PCR of CSF markedly ↑ diagnostic sensitivity and provides rapid dx (*Neurol 45:2228, 1995; ArNeurol 53:771, 1996*) but considerable variability in sensitivity depending on method used (*LnID 3:633, 2003*). ↓survival in HIV pts (*JID 192:2134, 2005*).

See page 3 for abbreviations, page 118 for footnotes   * *Dosages are for adults (unless otherwise indicated) and assume normal renal function*   † **DOT** = directly observed therapy

TABLE 12A (6)

FIGURE 1: TREATMENT ALGORITHM FOR TUBERCULOSIS *[Modified from MMWR 52(RR-11):1, 2003]*

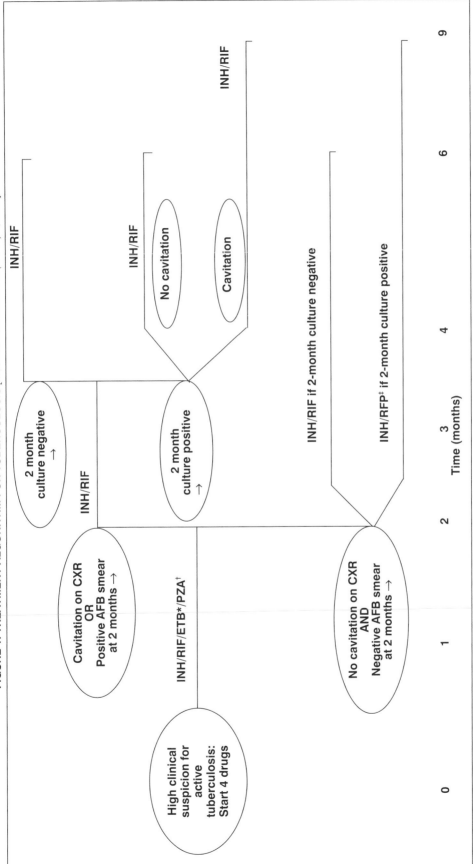

If the pt has HIV infection & the CD4 cell count is <100 per mcL, the continuation phase should consist of q24h or 3 times per wk INH & RIF for 4–7 months.
* ETB may be discontinued in <2 months if drug susceptibility testing indicate no drug resistance. † PZA may be discontinued after 2 months (56 doses).
‡ RFP should not be used in HIV patients with tuberculosis or in patients with extrapulmonary tuberculosis.

See page 3 for abbreviations

TABLE 12A (7)

SUGGESTED REGIMENS

CAUSATIVE AGENT/DISEASE; MODIFYING CIRCUMSTANCES	INITIAL THERAPY	CONTINUATION PHASE OF THERAPY (in vitro susceptibility known)	COMMENTS
III. Mycobacterium tuberculosis (continued)			
D. Tuberculosis during pregnancy	INH + RIF + ETB for 9 mo		PZA not recommended: teratogenicity data inadequate. Because of potential ototoxicity to fetus throughout gestation (16%), SM should not be used unless other drugs contraindicated. Add pyridoxine 25 mg per day for pregnant women on INH. Breast-feeding should not be discouraged in pts on first-line drugs [MMWR 52(RR-11):1, 2003].
E. Treatment failure or relapse: Usually due to poor compliance or resistant organisms (AJM 102:164, 1997)	Directly observed therapy (DOT). Check susceptibilities. (See section III.A, page 114 & above)		Pts whose sputum has not converted after 5–6 mos. = treatment failures. Failures may be due to non-compliance or resistant organisms. Non-compliance common, therefore institute DOT. If isolates show resistance, modify regimen to include at least 2 effective agents, preferably ones which pt has not received. Surgery may be necessary. In HIV+ patients, reinfection is a possible explanation for "failure." NB, patients with MDR-TB usually convert sputum within 12 weeks of successful therapy (AnIM 144:650, 2006).

SUGGESTED REGIMENS

CAUSATIVE AGENT/DISEASE	MODIFYING CIRCUMSTANCES	PRIMARY/ALTERNATIVE	COMMENTS
F. HIV infection or AIDS—pulmonary or extrapulmonary (NOTE: 60–70% of HIV+ pts with TB have extra-pulmonary disease)	INH + RIF (or RFB) + PZA q24h times 2 months. (Authors add **pyridoxine** 25–50 mg po q24h to regimens that include INH)	INH + RIF (or RFB) q24h times 4 months (total 6 mos.). May treat up to 9 mos. in pts with delayed response.	1. Because of possibility of developing resistance to RIF in pts with low CD4 cell counts who receive wkly or biwkly (2x/wk) doses of RFB, it is recom. that such pts receive q24h (or min 3x/wk) doses of RFB for initiation & continuation phase of rx (MMWR 51:214, 2002).

2. Clinical & microbiologic response same as in HIV-neg patient although there is considerable variability in outcomes among currently available studies (CID 32:623, 2001).
3. Post-treatment suppression not necessary for drug-susceptible strains.
4. Rate of INH resistance known to be <4% (for ↑ rates of resistance, see Section III.A).
5. More info: see MMWR 47(RR-20):1, 1998; CID 28:139, 1999; MMWR 52(RR-11):1, 2003
6. May use partially intermittent therapy: 1 dose per day for 2 weeks followed by 2–3 doses per wk for 24wk [MMWR 47(RR-20), 1998].
7. Adjunctive prednisolone of NO benefit in HIV+ patients with CD4 counts >200 (JID 191:856, 2005) or in patients with TBc pleurisy [JID 190:869, 2004].

Initial & cont. therapy:		Alternative regimen:
INH 300 mg + **RFB** (see below for dose) + **PZA** 25 mg per kg + **ETB** 15 mg per kg q24h times 2 mos.; then **INH** + **RFB** times 4 mos. (up to 7 mos.)		**INH** + **SM** + **PZA** + **ETB** times 2 mo; then **INH** + **SM** + **PZA** 2–3 x per wk for 7 mo. May be used with any PI regimen. May be prolonged up to 12 mo in pts with delayed response.

PI Regimen	RFB Dose
Nelfinavir 1250 mg q12h or indinavir 1000 mg q8h or amprenavir 1200 mg q12h	150 mg q24h or 300 mg intermittently
Lopinavir/ritonavir—standard dose	150 mg 2x per wk

Comments: Rifamycins induce cytochrome CYP450 enzymes (RIF > RFP > RFB) & reduce serum levels of concomitantly administered PIs. Conversely, PIs (ritonavir > amprenavir > indinavir = nelfinavir > saquinavir) inhibit CYP450 & cause ↑ serum levels of RFP & RFB. If dose of RFB is not reduced, toxicity ↑. RFB/PI combinations are therapeutically effective (CID 30:779, 1999). RFB has no effect on nelfinavir levels at dose of 1250 mg bid (Can JID 10:21B, 1999). **Although RFB is preferred, RIF can be used for rx of active TB in pts on regimens containing efavirenz or ritonavir. RIF should not be administered to pts on ritonavir + saquinavir because drug-induced hepatitis with marked transaminase elevations has been seen in healthy volunteers receiving this regimen (www.fda.gov).**

Concomitant protease inhibitor (PI) therapy (Modified from MMWR 49:185, 2000; AJRCCM 162:7, 2001)

FOOTNOTES: [1] When DOT is used, drugs may be given 5 days/wk & necessary number of doses adjusted accordingly. Although no studies compare 5 with 7 q24h doses, extensive experience indicates this would be an effective practice. [2] Patients with cavitation on initial chest x-ray & positive cultures at completion of 2 mo of rx should receive a 7 mo (31 wk: either 217 doses [q24h] or 62 doses [2x/wk] continuation phase. [3] 5day/wk admin is always given by DOT. [4] Not recommended for HIV-infected pts with CD4 cell counts <100 cells/mcL. [5] Options 1c & 2b should be used only in HIV-neg. pts who have neg. sputum smears at the time of completion of 2 mo rx & do not have cavitation on initial chest x-ray. For pts started on this regimen & found to have a + culture from 2 mo specimen, rx should be extended extra 3 mo. [6] Options 4a & 4b should be considered only when options 1–3 cannot be given. [7] Alternative agents = ethionamide, cycloserine, p-aminosalicylic acid, clarithromycin, AM-CL, linezolid. [8] Modified from MMWR 52(RR-11):1, 2003. See also IDCP 11:329, 2002. [9] Continuation regimen with INH/ETB less effective than INH/RIF (Lancet 364:1244, 2004).

See page 3 for abbreviations, page 118 for footnotes   * Dosages are for adults (unless otherwise indicated) and assume normal renal function   † DOT = directly observed therapy

TABLE 12A (8)

CAUSATIVE AGENT/DISEASE	MODIFYING CIRCUMSTANCES	SUGGESTED REGIMENS		COMMENTS
		PRIMARY	ALTERNATIVE	
IV. Other Mycobacterial Disease ("Atypical") (See ATS Consensus: AJRCCM 152:51, 1997; IDC No. Amer, March 2002; CMR 15:716, 2002; CID 42:1756, 2006)				
A. M. bovis		INH + RIF + ETB		The M. tuberculosis complex includes M. bovis. All isolates resistant to PZA. 9–12 months of rx used by some authorities. Isolation not required. Increased prevalence of extrapulmonary disease disease in U.S. born Hispanic populations (CID 47:168, 2008; EID 14:909, 2008).
B. Bacillus Calmette-Guerin (BCG) (derived from M. bovis)	Only fever (>38.5°C) for 12–24 hrs	INH 300 mg q24h times 3 months		Intravesical BCG effective in superficial bladder tumors and carcinoma in situ. Adverse effects: fever 2.9%, granulomatosis, pneumonitis, hepatitis 0.7%, sepsis 0.4% (J Urol 147:596, 1992). With sepsis, consider initial adjunctive prednisolone. Resistant to PZA. BCG may cause regional adenitis or pulmonary disease in HIV-infected children (CID 37:1226, 2003).
	Systemic illness or sepsis	INH 300 mg + RIF 600 mg + ETB 1200 mg po q24h times 6 mos.		
C. M. avium-intracellulare complex (MAC, MAI, or Battey bacillus) Clin Chest Med 23:633, 2002; ATS/IDSA Consensus Statement: AJRCCM 175:367, 2007; alternative ref: CID 42:1756, 2006.	**Immunocompetent patients**			See AJRCCM 175:367, 2007 for details of dosing and duration of therapy. Intermittent (tiw) therapy not recommended for patients with cavitary disease, patients who have been previously treated or patients with moderate or severe disease. The primary microbiologic goal of therapy is 12 months of negative sputum cultures on therapy.
	Nodular/Bronchiectatic disease	[Clarithro 1000 mg tiw or azithro 500-600 mg tiw] + ETB 25 mg/kg tiw + RIF 600 mg tiw		"Classic" pulmonary MAC: Men 50–75, smokers, COPD. May be associated with hot tub use (Clin Chest Med 23:675, 2002).
	Cavitary disease	[Clarithro 500-1000 mg/day (lower dose for wt <50 kg) or azithro 250-300 mg/day] +ETB 15 mg/kg/day + RIF 450-600 mg/day ± streptomycin or amikacin		"New" pulmonary MAC: Women 30–70, scoliosis, mitral valve prolapse, (bronchiectasis), pectus excavatum ("Lady Windermere syndrome"). May also be associated with interferon gamma deficiency (AJM 113:756, 2002).
	Advanced (severe) or previously treated disease	[Clarithro 500-1000 mg/day (lower dose for wt <50 kg) or azithro 250-300 mg/day] +ETB 15 mg/kg/day ± streptomycin or amikacin		For cervicofacial lymphadenitis (localized) in immunocompetent children, surgical excision is as effective as chemotherapy (CID 44:1057, 2007). Moxifloxacin and gatifloxacin, active in vitro & in vivo (AAC 51:4071, 2007).
	Immunocompromised pts: Primary prophylaxis—Pt's CD4 count <50-100 per mm³ Discontinue when CD4 count >100 per mm³ in response to HAART (NEJM 342:1085, 2000; CID 34: 662, 2002). Guideline: AnIM 137:435, 2002	Azithro 1200 mg po weekly OR Clarithro 500 mg po bid	RFB 300 mg po q24h OR Azithro 1200 mg po weekly + RIF 300 mg po q24h	RFB reduces MAC infection rate by 55% (no survival benefit); clarithro by 68% (30% survival benefit); azithro by 59% (68% survival benefit) (CID 26:611, 1998). Azithro + RFB more effective than either alone but not as well tolerated (NEJM 335:392, 1996). **Many drug-drug interactions,** see Table 22, pages 195, 198. Drug-resistant MAI disease seen in 29–58% of pts in whom disease develops while taking clarithro prophylaxis & in 11% of those on azithro but has not been observed with RFB prophylaxis (J Inf 38:6, 1999). Clarithro resistance more likely in pts with extremely low CD4 counts at initiation (CID 27:807, 1998). Need to be sure no active M. tbc; RFB used for prophylaxis may promote selection of rifamycin-resistant M. tbc (NEJM 335:384 & 428, 1996).
	Treatment Either presumptive dx or after + culture of blood, bone marrow, or usually, sterile body fluids, eg liver	(Clarithro 500 mg* po bid + ETB 15 mg/kg/day + RFB 300 mg po q24h * Higher doses of clari (1000 mg bid) may be associated with ↑ mortality (CID 29:125, 1999)	Azithro 500 mg po/day + ETB 15 mg/kg/day +/- RFB 300-450 mg po/day	Median time to neg. blood culture: clarithro + ETB 4.4 wks vs azithro + ETB >16 wks. At 16 wks, clearance of bacteremia seen in 37.5% of azithro- & 85.7% of clarithro-treated pts (CID 27:1278, 1998). More recent study suggests similar clearance rates for azithro (46%) vs clarithro (56%) at 24 wks when combined with ETB (CID 31:1245, 2000). Azithro 250 mg po q24h not effective, but azithro 600 mg po q24h as effective as 1200 mg q24h & yields fewer adverse effects (AAC 43: 2869, 1999).
				(continued on next page)

See page 3 for abbreviations.   * Dosages are for adults (unless otherwise indicated) and assume normal renal function   † **DOT** = directly observed therapy

TABLE 12A (9)

CAUSATIVE AGENT/DISEASE	MODIFYING CIRCUMSTANCES	SUGGESTED REGIMENS PRIMARY	SUGGESTED REGIMENS ALTERNATIVE	COMMENTS
IV. Other Mycobacterial Disease ("Atypical") *(continued)*				
C. M. avium-intracellulare complex *(continued)*				*(continued from previous page)* Addition of RFB to clarithro + ETB ↓ emergence of resistance to clari, ↓ relapse rate & improves survival *(CID 37:1234, 2003)*. Data on clofazimine difficult to assess. Earlier study suggested adding CLO of no value *(CID 25:621, 1997)*. More recent study suggests it may be as effective as RFB in 3 drug regimens containing clari & ETB *(CID 29:125, 1999)* although it may not be as effective as RFB at preventing clari resistance *(CID 28:136, 1999)*. Thus, pending more data, we still do not recommend CLO for MAI in HIV+ pts. Drug toxicity: With clarithro, 23% pts had to stop drug 2° to dose-limiting adverse reaction *(AnIM 121: 905, 1994)*. Combination of clarithro, ETB and RFB led to uveitis and pseudojaundice *(NEJM 330:438, 1994)*; result is reduction in max. dose of RFB to 300 mg. Treatment failure rate is high. Reasons: drug toxicity, development of drug resistance, & inadequate serum levels. Serum levels of clarithro ↓ in pts also given RIF or RFB *(JID 171:747, 1995)*. If pt not responding to initial regimen after 2–4 weeks, add one or more drugs. Several anecdotal reports of pts not responding to usual primary regimen who gained weight and became afebrile with dexamethasone 2–4 mg per day po *(AAC 38:2215, 1994; CID 26:682, 1998)*.
	Chronic post-treatment suppression—secondary prophylaxis	**Always necessary.** [**Clarithro** (or azithro) **+ ETB** 15 mg/kg/day (dosage above)	**Clarithro** or **azithro** or **RFB** (dosage above)	Recurrences almost universal without chronic suppression. However, in patients on HAART with robust CD4 cell response, it is possible to discontinue chronic suppression *(JID 178:1446, 1998; NEJM 340:1301, 1999)*.
D. Mycobacterium celatum	Treatment; optimal regimen not defined	May be susceptible to **clarithro**. **FQ** *(Clin Micro Inf 3:582, 1997)*. Suggest rx "like MAI" but often resistant to RIF *(J Inf 38:157, 1999)*. Most reported cases received 3 or 4 drugs, usually clarithro + ETB + CIP ± RFB *(EID 9:399, 2003)*.		Isolated from pulmonary lesions and blood in AIDS patients *(CID 24:144, 1997)*. Easily confused with M. xenopi (and MAC). Susceptibilities similar to MAC, but highly resistant to RIF *(CID 24:140, 1997)*.
E. Mycobacterium chelonae ssp. abscessus — — — — **Mycobacterium chelonae ssp. chelonae**	Treatment; Surgical excision may facilitate clarithro rx in subcutaneous abscess and is important adjunct to rx *(CID 24:1147, 1997)*	**Clarithro** 500 mg po bid times 6 mos. *(AnIM 119:482, 1993; CID 24:1147, 1997; EJCMID 19: 43, 2000)*. Azithro may also be effective. For serious disseminated infections add amikacin + IMP or cefoxitin for 1st 2–6 wks *(Clin Micro Rev 15:716, 2002; AJRCCM 175:367, 2007)*.		M. abscessus susceptible to AMK (70%), clarithro (95%), cefoxitin (70%), CLO, cefmetazole, IMP, azithro, cipro, doxy, mino, tigecycline *(CID 42:1756, 2006)*. Single isolates of M. abscessus often not associated with disease. Clarithro-resistant strains now described *(J Clin Micro 39: 2745, 2001)*. M. chelonae susceptible to AMK (80%), clarithro, azithro, tobramycin (100%), IMP (60%), moxifloxacin (AAC 46:3283, 2002), cipro, mino, doxy, linezolid (94%) *(CID 42:1756, 2006)*. Resistant to cefoxitin, FQ *(CID 24:1147, 1997; AJRCCM 156:S1, 1997)*.
F. Mycobacterium fortuitum	Treatment; optimal regimen not defined. Surgical excision of infected areas.	**AMK + cefoxitin + probenecid** 2–6 wk, then po **TMP- SMX**, or **doxy** 2–6 mo. Usually responds to 6–12 mo of oral rx with 2 drugs to which it is susceptible *(AAC 46: 3283, 2002; Clin Micro Rev 15: 716, 2002)*. Nail salon-acquired infections respond to 4–6 mo of minocycline, doxy, or CIP *(CID 38:38, 2004)*.		**Resistant to all standard anti-TBc drugs.** Sensitive in vitro to doxycycline, minocycline, cefoxitin, IMP, AMK, TMP-SMX, CIP, oflox, azithro, clarithro, linezolid *(Clin Micro Rev 15:716, 2002)*. May be resistant to azithromycin, rifabutin *(JAC 39:567, 1997)*. For M. fortuitum pulmonary disease treat with at least 2 agents active in vitro until sputum cultures negative for 12 months *(AJRCCM 175:367, 2007)*.

See page 3 for abbreviations.   * Dosages are for adults *(unless otherwise indicated)* and assume normal renal function   † **DOT** = directly observed therapy

TABLE 12A (10)

CAUSATIVE AGENT/DISEASE; MODIFYING CIRCUMSTANCES	SUGGESTED REGIMENS		COMMENTS
	PRIMARY	ALTERNATIVE	
IV. Other Mycobacterial Disease ("Atypical") (continued)			
G. Mycobacterium haemophilum	Regimen(s) not defined. In animal model, **clarithro** + **rifabutin** effective (AAC 39:2316, 1995). Combination of **CIP** + **RFB** + **clarithro** reported effective but clinical experience limited (Clin Micro Rev 9:435, 1996). Surgical debridement may be necessary (CID 26:505, 1998).		Clinical: Ulcerating skin lesions, synovitis, osteomyelitis, cervicofacial lymphadenitis in children (CID 41:1569, 2005). Lab: Requires supplemented media to isolate. Sensitive in vitro to: CIP, cycloserine, rifabutin. Over ½ resistant to: INH, RIF, ETB, PZA (AnIM 120:118, 1994). For localized cervicofacial lymphadenitis in immunocompetent children, surgical excision as effective as chemotherapy (CID 44:1057, 2007).
H. Mycobacterium genavense	Regimens used include ≥2 drugs: **ETB, RIF, RFB, CLO, clarithro.** In animal model, **clarithro & RFB** (& to lesser extent amikacin & **ETB**) shown effective in reducing bacterial counts; CIP not effective (JAC 42:483, 1998).		Clinical: CD4 <50. Symptoms of fever, weight loss, diarrhea. Lab: Growth in BACTEC vials slow (mean 42 days). Subcultures grow only on Middlebrook 7H11 agar containing 2 mcg per mL mycobactin J—growth still insufficient for in vitro sensitivity testing (Ln 340:76, 1992; AnIM 117:586, 1992). Survival ↑ from 81 to 263 days in pts rx for at least 1 month with ≥2 drugs (AnIM 155:400, 1995).
I. Mycobacterium gordonae	Regimen(s) not defined, but consider **RIF** + **ETB** + **KM** or **CIP** (J Inf 38:157, 1999) or **linezolid** (AJRCCM 175:367, 2007).		In vitro: sensitive to ETB, RIF, AMK, CIP, clarithro, linezolid (AAC 47:1736, 2003). Resistant to INH (CID 14:1229, 1992). Surgical excision.
J. Mycobacterium kansasii	Q24h po: **INH** (300 mg) + **RIF** (600 mg) + **ETB** (25 mg per kg times 2 mos., then 15 mg per kg). Rx for 18 mos. (until culture-neg. sputum times 12 mos; 15 mos. if HIV+ pt.) (See Comment)	If RIF-resistant, po q24h: [**INH** (900 mg) + **pyridoxine** (50 mg) + **sulfamethox-**ETB (25 mg per kg)] + **azole** (1.0 gm tid). Rx until pt culture-neg. times 12-15 mos. (See Comment). **Clari** + **ETB** + **RIF** also effective in small study (CID 37:1178, 2003).	**All isolates are resistant to PZA.** Rifapentine, azithro, ETB effective alone or in combination in athymic mice (JAC 42:417, 2001). Highly susceptible to linezolid in vitro (AAC 47:1736, 2003) and to clarithro and moxifloxacin (JAC 55:950, 2005). If HIV+ pt taking protease inhibitor, substitute either clarithro (500 mg bid) or RFB (150 mg per day) for RIF (AJRCCM 156:S1, 1997). Because of variable susceptibility to INH, some substitute clarithro 500–750 mg q24h for INH. Resistance to clarithro reported (DMID 31:369, 1998), but most strains susceptible to clarithro as well as moxifloxacin (JAC 55:950, 2005) & levofloxacin (AAC 48:4562, 2004). Prognosis related to level of immunosuppression (CID 37:584, 2003).
K. Mycobacterium marinum	(**Clarithro** 500 mg bid) or (**minocycline** 100–200 mg q24h) or (**doxycycline** 100–200 mg q24h), or (**TMP-SMX** 160/800 mg po bid), or (**RIF** + **ETB**) for 3 mos. (AJRCCM 156:S1, 1997; Eur J Clin Microbiol ID 25:609, 2006). Surgical excision.		Resistant to INH & PZA (AJRCCM 156:S1, 1997). Also susceptible in vitro to linezolid (AAC 47: 1736, 2003). CIP, moxifloxacin also show moderate in vitro activity (AAC 46:1114, 2002).
L. Mycobacterium scrofulaceum	Surgical excision. Chemotherapy seldom indicated. Although regimens not defined, **clarithro** + **CLO** with or **without ETB. INH. RIF. strep** + **cycloserine** have also been used.		In vitro resistant to INH, RIF, ETB, PZA, AMK, CIP (CID 20: 549, 1995). Susceptible to clarithro, strep, erythromycin.
M. Mycobacterium simiae	Regimen(s) not defined. Start 4 drugs as for disseminated MAI.		Most isolates resistant to all 1st-line anti-tbc drugs. Isolates often not clinically significant (CID 26: 625, 1998).
N. Mycobacterium ulcerans (Buruli ulcer)	[**RIF** + **AMK** (7.5 mg per kg IM bid)] or [**ETB** + **TMP-SMX** (160/800 mg po tid)] for 4–6 weeks. Surgical excision most important. WHO recommends **RIF** + **SM** for 8 weeks but overall value of drug therapy not clear (Lancet Infection 6:288, 2006; Lancet 367:1849, 2006; AAC 51:645, 2007). **RIF** + **SM** resulted in 47% cure rate (AAC 51:4029, 2007).		Susceptible in vitro to RIF, strep, CLO, clarithro, CIP, oflox, amikacin, moxi, linezolid (AAC 42:2070, 1998; JAC 45: 231, 2000; AAC 46:3193, 2002; AAC 50:1921, 2006). Monotherapy with RIF selects resistant mutants in mice (AAC 47:1228, 2003). RIF + moxi; RIF + clarithro; moxi + clarithro similar to RIF + SM in mice (AAC 51:3737, 2007). Treatment generally disappointing—see review, Ln 354:1013, 1999. RIF + dapsone only slightly better (82% improved) than placebo (75%) in small study (Intl J Inf Dis 6:60, 2002).
O. Mycobacterium xenopi	Regimen(s) not defined (CID 24:226 & 233, 1997). Some recommend a **macrolide** + (**RIF** or **rifabutin**) (AJRCCM 156:S1, 1997) and many or **RIF** + **INH** ± **ETB** (Resp Med 97:439, 2003) but recent study suggests no need to treat in most pts with HIV (CID 37:1250, 2003).		In vitro: sensitive to clarithro (AAC 36:2841, 1992) and rifabutin (JAC 39:567, 1997) and many standard antimycobacterial drugs. Clarithro-containing regimens more effective than RIF/INH/ETB regimens in mice (AAC 45:3229, 2001). FQs, linezolid also active in vitro.

See page 3 for abbreviations.   * Dosages are for adults (unless otherwise indicated) and assume normal renal function   † **DOT** = directly observed therapy

TABLE 12A (11)

CAUSATIVE AGENT/DISEASE	MODIFYING CIRCUMSTANCES	SUGGESTED REGIMENS		COMMENTS
		PRIMARY	ALTERNATIVE	
Mycobacterium leprae (leprosy) Classification: CID 44:1096, 2007	There are 2 sets of therapeutic recommendations here: one from USA (National Hansen's Disease Programs [NHDP], Baton Rouge, LA) and one from WHO. Both are based on expert recommendations and neither has been subjected to controlled clinical trial (P. Joyce & D. Scollard, Conns Current Therapy 2004; MP Joyce, Immigration Medicine, in press 2006; J Am Acad Dermatol 51:417, 2004).			
Type of Disease		NHDP Regimen	WHO Regimen	COMMENTS
Paucibacillary Forms: (Intermediate, Tuberculoid, Borderline tuberculoid)		**(Dapsone** 100 mg/day (unsupervised) + **RIF** 600 mg po/day) for 12 months	**(Dapsone** 100 mg/day (unsupervised) + **RIF** 600 mg 1x/mo (supervised)) for 6 mo	Side effects overall 0.4%
Single lesion paucibacillary		Treat as paucibacillary leprosy for 12 months.	Single dose **ROM** therapy: **(RIF** 600 mg + **Oflox** 400 mg + **Mino** 100 mg) (Ln 353:655, 1999).	
Multibacillary forms: **Borderline Borderline-lepromatous Lepromatous** See **Comment** for **erythema nodosum leprosum** Rev.: Lancet 363:1209, 2004		**(Dapsone** 100 mg/day + **CLO** 50 mg/day + **RIF** 600 mg/day) for 24 mo **Alternative regimen: (Dapsone** 100 mg/day + **RIF** 600 mg/day + **Minocycline** 100 mg/day) for 24 mo if CLO is refused or unavailable.	**(Dapsone** 100 mg/day + **CLO** 50 mg/day (both unsupervised) + **RIF** 600 mg + **CLO** 300 mg once monthly (supervised)). Continue regimen for 12 months.	Side-effects overall 5.1%. For erythema nodosum leprosum: prednisone 60–80 mg/day or thalidomide 100–400 mg/day (BMJ 44: 775, 1988; AJM 108:487, 2000). Thalidomide available in US at 1-800-4-CELGENE. Altho thalidomide effective, WHO no longer rec because of potential toxicity (JID 193:1743, 2006) however the majority of leprosy experts feel thalidomide remains drug of choice for ENL under strict supervision. **CLO (Clofazimine)** available from NHDP under IND protocol; contact at 1-800-642-2477. **Ethionamide** (250 mg q24h) or **prothionamide** (375 mg q24h) may be subbed for CLO. Oflox 400 mg po q24h: bactericidal and effective clinically with 4 log ↓ in organisms in small trials (AAC 38:662, 1994; AAC 38:61, 1994; Ln 345:4, 1995). Regimens incorporating clarithro, minocycline, RIF, moxifloxacin, and/or oflox also show promise (AAC 44:2919, 2000; AAC 50:1558, 2006). High relapse rate in pts treated with q24h RIF + oflox for 4wk (AAC 41:1953, 1997). Resistance to dapsone, RIF & oflox reported (Ln 349:103, 1997). Dapsone monotherapy has been abandoned due to emergence of resistance, but older patients previously treated with dapsone monotherapy may remain on lifelong maintenance therapy. Dapsone (or acedapsone^NUS) effective for prophylaxis in one study (J Inf 41:137, 2000).

TABLE 12B – DOSAGE AND ADVERSE EFFECTS OF ANTIMYCOBACTERIAL DRUGS

AGENT (TRADE NAME)[1]	USUAL DOSAGE*	ROUTE/1° DRUG RESISTANCE (RES) US[2],§	SIDE-EFFECTS, TOXICITY AND PRECAUTIONS	SURVEILLANCE
FIRST LINE DRUGS				
Ethambutol (Myambutol)	25 mg/kg/day for 2 mo then 15 mg/ kg/day q24h as 1 dose (<10% protein binding) [Bacteriostatic to both extracellular & intracellular organisms]	po RES: 0.3% (0–0.7%)	**Optic neuritis** with decreased visual acuity, central scotomata, and loss of green and red perception; peripheral neuropathy and headache (~1%), rashes (rare), arthralgia (rare), hyperuricemia (rare). Anaphylactoid reaction (rare). Comment: Primarily used to inhibit resistance. Disrupts outer cell membrane in M. avium with ↑ activity to other drugs.	Monthly visual acuity & red/ green with dose >15 mg/kg/ day. ≥10% loss considered significant. Usually reversible if drug discontinued.

[1] Note: Malabsorption of antimycobacterial drugs may occur in patients with AIDS enteropathy. For review of adverse effects, see AJRCCM 167:1472, 2003.

[2] **RES** = % resistance of M. tuberculosis

See page 3 for abbreviations.   * Dosages are for adults (unless otherwise indicated) and assume normal renal function   [†] **DOT** = directly observed therapy

TABLE 12B (2)

AGENT (TRADE NAME)[1]	USUAL DOSAGE*	ROUTE/1° DRUG RESISTANCE (RES) US[2,§]	SIDE-EFFECTS, TOXICITY AND PRECAUTIONS	SURVEILLANCE
FIRST LINE DRUGS *(continued)*				
Isoniazid (INH) (Nydrazid, Laniazid, Teebaconin)	Q24h dose: 5–10 mg/kg/day up to 300 mg/day as 1 dose. 2x/wk dose: 15 mg/kg (900 mg max dose) (< 10% protein binding) [Bactericidal to both extracellular and intracellular organisms] Add pyridoxine in alcoholic, pregnant, or malnourished pts.	po RES: 4.1% (2.6–8.5%) IM (IV route not FDA-approved but has been used, esp. in AIDS)	Overall ~1%. Liver: **Hep** (children 10% mild ↑ SGOT, normalizes with continued rx, age <20 yr rare, 20–34 yr 1.2%, ≥50 yr 2.3%) [also ↑ with q24h alcohol & previous exposure to Hep C (usually asymptomatic—*CID 36:293, 2003*]. May be fatal. With prodromal sx, dark urine do LFTs; discontinue if SGOT >3–5xnormal. **Peripheral neuropathy** (17% on 6 mg/kg per day, less on 300 mg, incidence ↑ in slow acetylators); **pyridoxine 10 mg q24h will ↑ incidence**; other neurologic sequelae: convulsions, optic neuritis, toxic encephalopathy, psychosis, muscle twitching, dizziness, coma (all rare); allergic skin rashes, fever, minor disulfiram-like reaction, flushing after Swiss cheese; blood dyscrasias (rare); + antinuclear (20%). **Drug-drug interactions** common, *see Table 22.*	Pre-rx liver functions. Repeat if symptoms (fatigue, weakness, malaise, anorexia, nausea or vomiting) >3 days (*AJRCCM 152: 1705, 1995*). Some recommend SGOT at 2, 4, 6 mo esp. if age >50 yr. Clinical evaluation every mo.
Pyrazinamide	25 mg per kg per day (maximum 2.5 gm per day) q24h as 1 dose [Bactericidal for intracellular organisms]	po	**Arthralgia; hyperuricemia** (with or without symptoms); hepatitis (not over 2% if recommended dose not exceeded); gastric irritation; photosensitivity (rare).	Pre-rx liver functions. Monthly SGOT, uric acid. Measure serum uric acid if symptomatic gouty attack occurs.
Rifamate®—combination tablet	2 tablets single dose q24h	po (1 hr before meal)	1 tablet contains 150 mg INH, 300 mg RIF	As with individual drugs
Rifampin (Rifadin, Rimactane, Rifocin)	10.0 mg per kg per day up to 600 mg per day q24h as 1 dose (60–90% protein binding) [Bactericidal to all populations of organisms]	po RES: 0.2% (0–0.3%) (IV available, Merrell-Dow)	INH/RIF dc'd in ~3% for toxicity; gastrointestinal irritation, antibiotic-associated colitis, drug fever (1%), pruritus with or without skin rash (1%), anaphylactoid reactions in HIV+ pts, mental confusion, thrombocytopenia (1%), leukopenia (1%), hemolytic anemia, transient **abnormalities in liver function. "Flu syndrome"** (fever, chills, headache, bone pain, shortness of breath) seen if RIF taken irregularly or if q24h dose interrupted after an interval of no rx. **Discolors urine, tears, sweat, contact lens an orange-brownish color.** May cause drug-induced lupus erythematosus (*Ln 349: 1521, 1977*).	Pre-rx liver function. Repeat if symptoms. **Multiple significant drug-drug interactions, see Table 22.**
Rifater®—combination tablet *(See Side-Effects)*	Wt ≥55 kg, 6 tablets single dose q24h	po (1 hr before meal)	1 tablet contains 50 mg INH, 120 mg RIF, 300 mg PZA. Used in 1st 2 months of rx (PZA 25 mg per kg). Purpose is convenience in dosing, ↑ compliance (*AnIM 122: 951, 1995*) but cost 1.58 more. Side-effects = individual drugs.	As with individual drugs, PZA 25 mg per kg
Streptomycin	15 mg per kg IM q24h, 0.75–1.0 gm per day initially for 60–90 days, then 1.0 gm 2–3 times per week (15 mg per kg per day) q24h as 1 dose	IM (or IV) RES: 3.9% (2.7–7.6%)	Overall 8%. **Ototoxicity:** vestibular dysfunction (vertigo): paresthesias; dizziness & nausea (all less in pts receiving 2–3 doses per week); tinnitus and high frequency loss (1%); drug fever. Available from X-Gen Pharmaceuticals, 607-732-4411. Ref. re: IV—*CID 19:1150, 1994.* Toxicity similar with qd vs tid dosing (*CID 38:1538, 2004*).	Monthly audiogram. In older pts, serum creatinine or BUN at start of rx and weekly if pt stable
SECOND LINE DRUGS (more difficult to use and/or less effective than first line drugs)				
Amikacin (Amikin)	7.5–10.0 mg per kg q24h [Bactericidal for extracellular organisms]	IV or IM RES: (est. 0.1%)	*See Table 10, pages 83 & 96* Toxicity similar with qd vs tid dosing (*CID 38:1538, 2004*).	Monthly audiogram. Serum creatinine or BUN weekly if pt stable
Capreomycin sulfate (Capastat sulfate)	1 gm per day (15 mg per kg per day) q24h as 1 dose	IM or IV RES: 0.1% (0–0.9%)	Nephrotoxicity (36%), ototoxicity (auditory 11%), eosinophilia, leukopenia, skin rash, fever, hypokalemia, neuromuscular blockade.	Monthly audiogram, biweekly serum creatinine or BUN
Ciprofloxacin (Cipro)	750 mg bid	po, IV	TB not an FDA-approved indication for CIP. Desired CIP serum levels 4–6 mcg per mL, requires median dose 800 mg (*AJRCCM 151:2006, 1995*). Discontinuation rates 6–7%. CIP well tolerated (*AJRCCM 151:2006, 1995*). FQ-resistant M. Tb identified in New York (*Ln 345:1148, 1995*). *See Table 10, pages 86 & 93 for adverse effects.*	None

See page 3 for abbreviations.   * Dosages are for adults *(unless otherwise indicated)* and assume normal renal function   [†] **DOT** = directly observed therapy
[§] Mean (range) (higher in Hispanics, Asians, and patients <10 years old)

TABLE 12B (3)

AGENT (TRADE NAME)[1]	USUAL DOSAGE*	ROUTE/1° DRUG RESISTANCE (RES) US[2, §]	SIDE-EFFECTS, TOXICITY AND PRECAUTIONS	SURVEILLANCE
SECOND LINE DRUGS *(continued)*				
Clofazimine (Lamprene)	50 mg per day (unsupervised) + 300 mg 1 time per month supervised or 100 mg per day	po (with meals)	Skin: **pigmentation (pink-brownish black)** 75–100%, dryness 20%, pruritus 5%. GI: abdominal pain 50% (rarely severe leading to exploratory laparoscopy), splenic infarction (VR), bowel obstruction (VR), GI bleeding (VR). Eye: conjunctival irritation, retinal crystal deposits.	None
Cycloserine (Seromycin)	750–1000 mg per day (15 mg per kg per day) 2–4 doses per day [Bacteriostatic for both extra-cellular & intracellular organisms]	po RES: 0.1% (0–0.3%)	Convulsions, **psychoses** (5–10% of those receiving 1.0 gm per day); headache: somno-lence; hyperreflexia; increased CSF protein and pressure, **peripheral neuropathy**. 100 mg pyridoxine (or more) q24h should be given concomitantly. Contraindicated in epileptics.	None
Dapsone	100 mg per day	po	Blood: ↓ hemoglobin (1–2 gm) & ↑ retics (2–12%), in most pts. Hemolysis in G6PD deficiency. **Methemoglobinemia**. CNS: peripheral neuropathy (rare). GI: nausea, vomiting. Renal: albuminuria, nephrotic syndrome. Erythema nodosum leprosum in pts rx for leprosy (½ pts 1st year).	None
Ethionamide (Trecator-SC)	500–1000 mg per day (15–20 mg per kg per day) 1–3 doses per day [Bacteriostatic for extracellular organisms only]	po RES: 0.8% (0–1.5%) *(see Comment)*	**Gastrointestinal irritation** (up to 50% on large dose); goiter; peripheral neuropathy (rare); convulsions (rare); changes in affect (rare); difficulty in diabetes control; rashes; hepatitis; purpura; stomatitis; gynecomastia; menstrual irregularity. Give drug with meals or antacids; 50–100 mg pyridoxine per day concomitantly; SGOT monthly. Possibly teratogenic.	
Moxifloxacin (Avelox)	400 mg qd	po, IV	Not FDA-approved indication. Concomitant administration of rifampin reduces serum levels of moxi *(CID 45:1001, 2007)*.	None
Ofloxacin (Floxin)	400 mg bid	po, IV	Not FDA-approved indication. Overall adverse effects 11%, 4% discontinued due to side-effects. GI: nausea 3%, diarrhea 1%. **CNS:** insomnia 3%, headache 1%, dizziness 1%.	
Para-aminosalicylic acid (PAS, Paser) (Na+ or K+ salt)	4–6 gm bid (200 mg per kg per day) [Bacteriostatic for extracellular organisms only]	po RES: 0.8% (0–1.5%) *(see Comment)*	**Gastrointestinal irritation** (10–15%); goitrogenic action (rare); depressed prothrombin activity (rare); G6PD-mediated hemolytic anemia (rare), drug fever, rashes, hepatitis, myalgia, arthralgia. Retards hepatic enzyme induction, may ↓ INH hepatotoxicity. Available from CDC. (404) 639-3670, Jacobus Pharm. Co. (609) 921-7447.	None
Rifabutin (Mycobutin)	300 mg per day (prophylaxis or treatment)	po	Polymyalgia, polyarthralgia, leukopenia, granulocytopenia. Anterior uveitis when given with concomitant clarithromycin; avoid 600 mg dose *(NEJM 330:438, 1994)*. Uveitis reported with 300 mg per day *(AnIM 12:510, 1994)*. Reddish urine, orange skin (pseudojaundice).	None
Rifapentine (Priftin)	600 mg twice weekly for 1st 2 mos., then 600 mg q week	po	Similar to other rifabutins. *(See RIF, RFB)*. Hyperuricemia seen in 21%. Causes red-orange discoloration of body fluids. Note ↑ prevalence of RIF resistance in pts on weekly rx *(Ln 353:1843, 1999)*.	None
Thalidomide (Thalomid)	100–300 mg po q24h (may use up to 400 mg po q24h for severe erythema nodosum leprosum)	po	**Contraindicated in pregnancy. Causes severe life-threatening birth defects. Both male and female patients must use barrier contraceptive methods (Pregnancy Category X). Frequently causes drowsiness or somnolence. May cause peripheral neuropathy.** *(AJM 108:487, 2000)* For review, see *Ln 363:1803, 2004*	Available only through pharma-cists participating in System for Thalidomide Education and Prescribing Safety (S.T.E.P.S.)

See page 3 for abbreviations.   * Dosages are for adults *(unless otherwise indicated)* and assume normal renal function   [†] **DOT** = directly observed therapy
[§] Mean (range) (higher in Hispanics, Asians, and patients <10 years old)

TABLE 13A– TREATMENT OF PARASITIC INFECTIONS*

Many of the drugs suggested are not licensed in the US. The following are helpful resources available through the Center for Disease Control and Prevention (CDC) in Atlanta. Website is www.cdc.gov.
General advice for parasitic diseases other than malaria: (770) 488-7760 or (770) 488-7775.
For CDC Drug Service[1] 8:00 a.m.–4:30 p.m. EST: (404) 639-3670; fax: (404) 639-3717.
For malaria: Prophylaxis advice (770) 488-7788; treatment (770) 488-7788; or after hours (770) 488-7100; website: www.cdc.gov/travel
NOTE: All dosage regimens are for adults with normal renal function unless otherwise stated.
For licensed drugs, suggest checking package inserts to verify dosage and side-effects. Occasionally, post-licensure data may alter dosage as compared to package inserts.
For abbreviations of journal titles, *see page 4.* Reference with peds dosages: *Medical Letter /"Drugs for Parasitic Infections" (Suppl), 2007. General resource: www.gideononline.com*

INFECTING ORGANISM	SUGGESTED REGIMENS		COMMENTS
	PRIMARY	ALTERNATIVE	
PROTOZOA—INTESTINAL (non-pathogenic: E. hartmanni, E. dispar, E. coli, Iodamoeba butschlii, Endolimax nana, Chilomastix mesnili)			
Balantidium coli	Tetracycline 500 mg po qid x 10 days	Metronidazole 750 mg po tid times 5 days	Another alternative: Iodoquinol 650 mg po tid x 20 days.
Blastocystis hominis: Role as pathogen controversial	Nitazoxanide: Adults 500 mg tabs (children 200 mg oral suspension)—both po q12h x 3 days (*AJTMH* 68:384, 2003).	Metronidazole 1.5 gm po as single dose 1x/day x 10 days (placebo-controlled trial in *J Travel Med* 10:128, 2003). Alternatives: iodoquinol 650 mg po tid x 20 days or TMP-SMX-DS, one bid x 7 days	
Cryptosporidium parvum & hominis Treatment is unsatisfactory Ref.: *CID 39:504, 2004*	**Immunocompetent—No HIV:** Nitazoxanide 500 mg po bid x 3 days	**HIV with immunodeficiency:** (1) Effective antiretroviral therapy best therapy. (2) Nitazoxanide is not licensed for immunodeficient pts; no clinical or parasite response compared to placebo	Nitazoxanide: Approved in liquid formulation for rx of children & 500 mg tabs for adults who are immunocompetent. Ref.: *CID 40:1173, 2005.* **C. hominis** assoc. with ↑ in post-infection eye & joint pain, recurrent headache, & dizzy spells (*CID 39:504, 2004*).
Cyclospora cayetanensis	Immunocompetent pts: **TMP-SMX-DS** tab 1 po bid x 7–10 days	AIDS pts: **TMP-SMX-DS** tab 1 po qid x 10 days; then tab 1 po 3x/wk	If sulfa-allergic: **CIP** 500 mg po bid x 7 days & then 1 tab po 3x/wk x 2 wk or **Nitazoxanide** 500 mg po q12h x 7 days (*CID 44:466, 2007*).
Dientamoeba fragilis Treat if patient symptomatic	Iodoquinol 650 mg po tid x 20 days	Tetracycline 500 mg po qid x 10 days OR Metronidazole 500–750 mg po tid x 10 days	Other alternatives: doxy 100 mg po bid x 10 days; paromomycin 25–35 mg/kg/day po in 3 divided doses x 7 days.
Entamoeba histolytica; amebiasis. Reviews: *Ln 361:1025, 2003; NEJM 348:1563, 2003*			
Asymptomatic cyst passer	**Paromomycin** (aminosidine in U.K.) 25–35 mg/kg po in 3 doses x 7 days OR iodoquinol 650 mg po tid x 20 days	**Diloxanide furoate**[NUS] (Furamide) 500 mg po tid x 10 days (Source: Panorama Compound. Pharm., 800-247-9767)	Colitis can mimic ulcerative colitis; ameboma can mimic adenocarcinoma of colon. **Dx:** antigen detection & PCR better than O&P
Patient with diarrhea/dysentery; mild/moderate disease. Oral therapy possible	**Metronidazole** 500–750 mg po tid x 10 days or **tinidazole** 2 gm 1x/day x 3 days, followed by: Either [**paromomycin** 25–35 mg/kg/day po divided in 3 doses x 7 days] or [**iodoquinol** (was diiodohydroxyquin) 650 mg po tid x 20 days] to clear intestinal cysts. See comment.	[**Tinidazole** 1 gm po q12h x 3 days] or [**ornidazole**[NUS] 500 mg po q12h x 5 days) followed by:	**Nitazoxanide** 500 mg po bid x 3 days effective in 2 controlled studies (*JID 184:381, 2001 & Tran R Soc Trop Med & Hyg 101:1025, 2007*).
Severe or extraintestinal infection, e.g., hepatic abscess	(**Metronidazole** 750 mg **IV to PO** tid x 10 days or **tinidazole** 2 gm 1x/day x 5 days) followed by paromomycin 25–35 mg/kg/day po divided in 3 doses	**Metronidazole** 750 mg **IV to PO** tid x 10 days or tinidazole 2 gm 1x/day x 5 days) followed by paromomycin 25–35 mg/kg/day po divided in 3 doses	**Serology positive (antibody present) with extraintestinal disease.** **Refractory pts: (metro 750 mg po + quinacrine**[2] **100 mg po)**—both 3x/day x 3 wk. Ref: *CID 33:22, 2001.* Nitazoxanide ref.: *CID 40:1173, 2005.*
Giardia lamblia; giardiasis	(**Tinidazole** 2 gm po x 1) OR (**nitazoxanide** 500 mg po bid x 3 days)	**Metronidazole** 250 mg po tid x 5 days (high frequency of GI side-effects). See Comment. Rx if preg: **Paromomycin** 500 mg 4x /day x 7 days	
Isospora belli	**TMP-SMX-DS** tab 1 po bid x 10 days; if AIDS pt.: TMP-SMX-DS qid x 10 days & then bid x 3 wk.	(**Pyrimethamine** 75 mg/day po + **folinic acid** 10 mg/day po) x 14 days **CIP** 500 mg po bid x 7 days—87% response (*AnIM 132:885, 2000*).	Chronic suppression in AIDS pts: either 1 TMP-SMX-DS tab 3x/wk OR (pyrimethamine 25 mg/day po + folinic acid 5 mg/day po)

[1] **Drugs available from CDC Drug Service: 404-639-2888 or –3670 or www.cdc.gov/ncidod/srp/drugs/formulary.html: artesunate, Bithionol, diethylcarbamazine (DEC), melarsoprol, nifurtimox, stibogluconate (Pentostam), suramin.**

[2] Quinacrine available from Panorama Compounding Pharmacy, (800) 247-9767; (818) 988-7979.

* *See page 3 for abbreviations. All dosage recommendations are for adults (unless otherwise indicated) and assume normal renal function.*

TABLE 13A (2)

INFECTING ORGANISM	SUGGESTED REGIMENS		COMMENTS
	PRIMARY	ALTERNATIVE	
PROTOZOA—INTESTINAL (continued)			
Microsporidiosis			
Ocular: Encephalitozoon hellum or cuniculi, Vittaforma (Nosema) corneae, Nosema ocularum	For HIV pts: antiretroviral therapy key **Albendazole** 400 mg po bid x 3 wk plus fumagillin eye drops (see Comment).	In HIV+ pts, reports of response of E. hellum to **fumagillin** eyedrops (see Comment). For V. corneae, may need keratoplasty.	To obtain fumagillin: 800-292-6773 or www.leiterx.com. Neutropenia & thrombocytopenia serious adverse events. Dx: Most labs use modified trichrome stain. Need electron micrographs for species identification. FA and PCR methods in development. Peds dose ref.: PIDJ 23:915, 2004
Intestinal (diarrhea): Enterocytozoon bieneusi, Encephalitozoon (Septata) intestinalis	**Albendazole** 400 mg po bid x 3 wk; peds dose: 15 mg/kg per day div. into 2 daily doses x 7 days for **E. intestinalis**	Oral **fumagillin 20 mg po tid** reported effective for **E. bieneusi** (NEJM 346:1963, 2002)—see Comment	
Disseminated: E. hellum, cuniculi or intestinalis; Pleistophora sp., others in Comment	**Albendazole** 400 mg po bid x 3 wk	No established rx for Pleistophora sp.	For Trachipleistophora sp., try itraconazole + albendazole (NEJM 351:42, 2004). Other pathogens: Brachiola vesicularum & algerae (NEJM 351:42, 2004).
PROTOZOA—EXTRAINTESTINAL			
Amebic meningoencephalitis			
Acanthamoeba sp.— no proven rx Rev.: FEMS Immunol Med Micro 50:1, 2007	Success with IV **pentamidine**, topical **chlorhexidine** & 2% **ketoconazole** cream & then po **itra** (NEJM 331:85, 1994). 2 children responded to po rx: **TMP-SMX** + **rifampin** + **keto** (PIDJ 20:623, 2001).		For treatment of keratitis, see Table 1A, page 13
Balamuthia mandrillaris	**Pentamidine** + **clarithro** + **flucon** + **sulfadiazine** + **flucytosine** (MMWR 57:768, 2008).		
Naegleria fowleri. >95% mortality. Ref. MMWR 57:576, 2008. Sappinia diploidea	A cause of chronic granulomatous meningitis **Ampho B** 1.5 mg/kg per day in 2 div. doses x 3 days; then 1 mg/kg/yda x 6 days plus 1.5 mg/day intrathecal a 2 days; then 1 mg/day intrathecal qod x 8 days.		Ampho B + azithro synergistic in vitro & in mouse model (AAC 51:23, 2007).
Babesia microti; babesiosis (CID 32:1117, 2001)	**Azithro** + **pentamidine** + **itra** + **flucytosine** (JAMA 285:2450, 2001) Atovaquone 750 mg bid po x 7–10 days + **azithro** 500 mg po x 1 dose, then 250 mg q24h x 7 days (NEJM 343:1454, 2000).	(**Clindamycin** 600 mg po tid) + (**quinine** 650 mg po tid) x 7–10 days For adults, can give **clinda** IV as 1.2 gm bid.	Can cause overwhelming infection in asplenic patients. In immunocompromised patients, treat for 6 or more weeks (CID 46:370, 2008). Refractory infection responded by adding proguanil (CID 45:1588, 2007).
Ehrlichiosis—See Table 1A, page 53			
Leishmaniasis. Complicated—consultation suggested. Refs: Ln366:1561, 2005 & LnID 6:342, 2006 & LnID 7:581, 2007 & CID 195:1846, 2007			
Cutaneous (C) & Mucocutaneous (MC) Always start with antimony for mucocutaneous disease.			
New World (Mexico/Cen./S. Amer.) **L. viannia** Includes braziliensi (C, MC), guyanensis (C, MC), panamensis C, MC), peruviana (C) & **L. mexicana** Includes mexicana (C), amazonensis (C), venezuelensis (C). **NOTE:** antimony resistance of L. vianna reported (JID 193, 1375, 2006)	**Sodium stibogluconate** (Pentosam) from CDC drug service (404-639-3670) or **meglumine antimoniate (Glucantime)** in France & Latin America. Dose: 20 mg/kg/d IV x 28 days. Dilute in 120 mL of D5W & infuse over 2 hr. Ideally, monitor EKG. Note: only antimony drugs efficacious vs L. braziliensis. In Brazil: **antimony + pentoxifylline** 400 mg po tid x 30 days superior to antimony alone (CID 44:788, 2007).	**Amphotericin B** 1 mg/kg IV qod x 20 doses **or** **Liposomal ampho (Ambisome)** 3 mg/kg per day for 6 days for cutaneous & 3 wks for mucocutaneous. **Or miltefosine**[NUS] effective vs L. paneamensis, marginal vs L. mexicana, failed vs L. braziliensis. Obtain from Zentaris, Germany: Impavido @ Zentaris.de. Dose 2.5 mg/kg po once daily x 28 days. Bolivia results: CID 44:350, 2007.	Concern for species that disseminate to mucosa. Method of choice for speciation is PCR – not widely available: so empirically treat for species with potential to disseminate. Spontaneous resolution varies by species: L. mexicana: 75% in 3 mo; L. braziliensis: 10% in 3 mo; L. major 90% in 2-4 mo; L. tropica: 90% in 6-15 mo. For antimony AEs , see Table 13 B(1).
Old World (Europe, Asia, Africa) L. major, L. tropica, L. aethiopica, L. infantum, L. chagas	**Stibogluconate or meglumine antimoniate** as above. 20 mg/kg/d x 10 days		Other therapies for cutaneous leishmaniasis reviewed in LnID 7:581, 2007; all have limitations.

* See page 3 for abbreviations. All dosage recommendations are for adults (unless otherwise indicated) and assume normal renal function.

TABLE 13A (3)

INFECTING ORGANISM	SUGGESTED REGIMENS		COMMENTS
	PRIMARY	ALTERNATIVE	
PROTOZOA—EXTRAINTESTINAL *(continued)*			
Visceral leishmaniasis – Kala-Azar – New World & Old World *L. donovani:* India, Africa *L. infantum:* Mediterranean *L. chagasi:* New World	**Liposomal ampho B** FDA-approved in immunocompetent hosts: 3 mg/kg once daily days 1-5 & days 14, 21; WHO: 10 mg/kg on 2 consecutive days. All IV.	**Stibogluconate** or **meglumine antimoniate** (resistance in India & Mediterranean): 20 mg/kg/day IV in single dose x 28 days OR **Miltefosine[NUS]** 1.5–2.5 mg/kg/day po x 28 days.	Another alternative: standard **ampho B** 1 mg/kg IV qod daily x 20 days. Ref: liposomal ampho B: *CID 43:917, 2006.*

**Malaria (Plasmodia species)—NOTE: CDC Malaria info—prophylaxis/treatment (770) 488-7788. After hours: 770-488-7100. Refs: *JAMA 297:2251, 2264 & 2285, 2007.*
Websites: www.cdc.gov/malaria; www.who.int/health-topics/malaria.htm.**

Prophylaxis—Drugs plus personal protection: screens, nets, 30–35% DEET skin repellent (avoid 95% products in children), permethrin spray on clothing and mosquito nets			
For areas free of chloroquine (CQ)-resistant P. falciparum: Haiti; Dom. Republic, Cen. America west & north of the Panama Canal, & parts of Middle East	**CQ** 500 mg (300 mg base) po per wk starting 1–2 wk before travel, during travel, & 4 wks post-travel **or atovaquone-proguanil (AP)** 1 adult tab po day (1 day prior to, during, & 7 days post-travel). Note: **CQ** may exacerbate psoriasis.	**CQ Peds dose:** 8.3 mg/kg (5 mg/kg of base) po 1x/wk up to 300 mg (base) max. dose **or AP** by weight (peds tabs): 11–20kg, 1 tab; 21–30 kg, 2 tabs; 31–40 kg, 3 tabs; >40 kg, 1 adult tab per day.	**The areas free of CQ-resistant falciparum malaria continue to shrink:** Central America west of Panama Canal, Haiti, and parts of Middle East. CQ-resistant falciparum malaria reported from Saudi Arabia, Yemen, Oman, & Iran.
For areas with CQ-resistant P. falciparum CDC info on prophylaxis (770) 488-7788 or website: *www.cdc.gov & LnID 6:139, 2006*	**Atovaquone** 250 mg—**proguanil** 100 mg **(Malarone)** comb. tablet, 1 per day with food 1–2 days prior to, during, & 7 days post-travel. Peds dose in footnote[1] **Not in pregnancy**	**Adults: Doxy** or **MQ** as below. **Doxycycline** 100 mg po daily for adults & children >8yr of age[1]. Take 1-2 days before, during & for 4 wks after travel. **OR** **Mefloquine (MQ)**[1] 250 mg (228 mg base) po per wk, 1-2 wks before, during, & for 4 wks after travel. Peds dose in footnote[1]	**Pregnancy: MQ** current best option. Insufficient data with **Malarone. Avoid doxycycline and primaquine.** **Primaquine: Can cause hemolytic anemia if G6PD deficiency present.** **MQ not recommended** if cardiac conduction abnormalities, seizures, or psychiatric disorders, e.g., depression, psychosis. MQ outside U.S.: 275 mg tab, contains 250 mg of base.
	Another option for adults for P. vivax prophylaxis: **primaquine (PQ)** 30 mg base po daily in non-pregnant G6PD-neg. travelers >92% vs P. vivax (*CID 33:1990, 2001*).		

Treatment of Malaria. Diagnosis is by microscopy. Alternative: rapid monoclonal antibody test (Binax NOW): detects 96-100% of P. falciparum and 93% of other plasmodia. Need microscopy to speciate. Can stay positive for over a month after successful treatment.

Clinical Severity/ Plasmodia sp.	Region Acquired	Suggested Treatment Regimens (Drug)		Comments
		Primary—Adults	Alternative & Peds	
Uncomplicated/ P. falciparum (or species not identified)	Cen. Amer., west of Panama Canal; Haiti; Dom. Repub., & most of Mid East—**CQ-sensitive**	**CQ** 1 gm salt (600 mg base) po, then 0.5 gm in 6 hrs, then 0.5 gm daily x 2 days. Total: 2500 mg salt.	**Peds: CQ** 10 mg/kg of base po, then 5 mg/kg of base at 6, 24, & 48 hrs. Total: 25 mg/kg base	**Peds dose should never exceed adult dose.**
Malaria rapid diagnostic test (Binax NOW) approved: *MMWR 56:686, 2007*	CQ-resistant or unknown resistance	[(**QS** 650 mg po tid x 3 days (7 days if SE Asia)] + [(**Doxy** 100 mg po bid) or (**tetra** 250 mg po qid) or **clinda** 20 mg/kg/d divided tid) x 7 days] **OR** **Atovaquone-proguanil** 1 gm–400 mg (4 adult tabs) po 1x/day x 3 days w/ food or mefloquine 750 mg po x 1 dose, then 500 mg po x 1 dose 6-12 hr later.	**Peds: (QS** 10 mg/kg po tid) + (**clinda** 20 mg/kg per day div. tid) —both x 7 days. **MQ Salt:** 15 mg/kg x 1, then 6-12 hrs later, 10 mg/kg ALL po.	Can substitute clinda for doxy/tetra: 20 mg/kg per day po div. tid x 7 days. MQ alternative due to neuropsych. reactions. Avoid if malaria acquired in SE Asia due to resistance. **Peds atovaquone-proguanil dose** (all once daily x 3 d) by weight: 5-8 kg: 2 peds tabs; 9-10 kg: 3 peds tabs; 11-20 kg: 1 adult tab; 21-30 kg: 2 adult tabs; 31-40 kg: 3 adult tabs; >40 kg: 4 adult tabs.
Uncomplicated / P. malariae	All regions	**CQ** as above: adults & peds. In South Pacific, beware of P. knowlesi; looks like P. malariae, but behaves like P. falciparum (*CID 46:165, 2007*).		

[1] **Peds prophylaxis dosages** (Ref.: *CID 34:493, 2002*): **Mefloquine** weekly dose by **weight** in kg: <15 = 5 mg/kg; 15–19 = ¼ adult dose; 20–30 = ½ adult dose; 31–45 = ¾ adult dose; >45 = adult dose. **Atovaquone/proguanil** by **weight** in kg, single daily dose using peds tab (62.5 mg atovaquone & 25 mg proguanil): <11 kg—do not use; 11–20 kg, 1 tab; 21–30 kg, 2 tabs; 31-40 kg, 3 tabs; ≥41 kg, one adult tab. **Doxycycline,** ages >8–12 yrs: 2 mg per kg per day up to 100 mg/day. Continue daily x 4 wks after leaving risk area. Side effects: photosensitivty, nausea, yeast vaginitis
* *See page 3 for abbreviations. All dosage recommendations are for adults (unless otherwise indicated) and assume normal renal function.*

TABLE 13A (4)

INFECTING ORGANISM	SUGGESTED REGIMENS		COMMENTS
Clinical Severity/ Plasmodia sp.	PRIMARY	ALTERNATIVE	Comments
	Region Acquired	Suggested Treatment Regimens (Drug)	
		Primary—Adults	Alternative & Peds	

PROTOZOA—EXTRAINTESTINAL/Malaria/Treatment (continued)

	Region Acquired	Primary—Adults	Alternative & Peds	Comments
Uncomplicated/ P. vivax or P. ovale	All except Papua, New Guinea & Indonesia (CQ-resistant)	**CQ** as above + **PQ** base: 30 mg po once daily x 14 days	**Peds: CQ** as above + **PQ** base 0.5 mg po once daily x 14 days	PQ added to eradicate latent parasites in liver. Screen for G6PD def. before starting PQ; if G6PD positive, dose PQ as 45 mg po once weekly x 8 wk. Avoid PQ in pregnancy.
Uncomplicated/ P. vivax	CQ-resistant: Papua, New Guinea & Indonesia	[**QS** + (**doxy** or **tetra**) + **PQ**] as above	**MQ** + **PQ** as above. **Peds** (<8yrs old): **QS** alone x 7 days or **MQ** alone. If latter fail, add **doxy** or **tetra**	Rarely acute. Lung injury and other serious complications: LnID 8:149, 2008.
Uncomplicated Malaria/Alternatives for Pregnancy Ref: LnID 7:118 & 136, 2007	CQ-sensitive areas	**CQ** as above		Doxy or tetra used if benefits outweigh risks. No controlled studies of AP in pregnancy. Possible association of MQ & ↑ number of stillbirths. If P. vivax or P. ovale, after pregnancy check for G6PD & give PQ 30 mg po daily times 14 days.
	CQ-resistant P. falciparum	**QS** + **clinda** as above	If failing or intolerant, **QS** + **doxy**	
	CQ-resistant P. vivax	**QS** 650 mg po tid x 7 days		
Severe malaria i.e., impaired consciousness, severe anemia, renal failure, pulmonary edema, ARDS, DIC, jaundice, acidosis, seizures, parasitemia >5%. One or more of latter. **Almost always P. falciparum.** Ref: NEJM 358:1829, 2008; Science 320:30, 2008.	All regions Note: Artesunate may be drug of choice. More effective than quinine & safer than quinidine (see Comment)	**Quinidine gluconate** in normal saline: 10 mg/kg (salt) IV over 1hr then 0.02 mg/kg/min by constant infusion OR 24 mg/kg IV over 4 hrs & then 12 mg/kg over 4 hrs q8h. Continue until parasite density <1% & can take po QS. **QS** as above x 7 days (SE Asia) or 3 days elsewhere **PLUS** [**Doxy** 100 mg IV q12h x 7 days) **OR** (**clinda** 100 mg IV q8h IV load & then 5 mg/kg IV q8h x 7 days)	**Peds: Quinidine gluconate** IV—same mg/kg dose as for adults **PLUS** [**Doxy**: if <45 kg, 4 mg per kg IV q12h; if ≥45 kg, dose as for adults) OR **Clinda**, same mg/kg dose as for adults] For **artesunate**, see Comment	During quinidine IV: monitor BP, EKG (prolongation of QTc), & blood glucose (hypoglycemia). Consider exchange transfusion if parasitemia >10%. Switch to oral QS, doxy, & clinda when patient able. Steroids not recommended for cerebral malaria. If quinidine not available, or patient intolerant or high level parasitemia, **IV artesunate** available from CDC Malaria Branch (770-488-7788 or 770-488-7100) (Ref: CID 44:1067 & 1075, 2007). Dose: 2.4 mg/kg IV at 0, 12, 24 & 48 hrs, followed by one week of doxycycline (use clinda in pregnancy). Alternative: atovaquone-proguanil.
Malaria—self-initiated treatment: Only for emergency situation where medical care not available	**Atovaquone-proguanil (AP)** 4 adult tabs (1 gm/400 mg) po daily x 3 days		**Peds:** Using adult **AP** tabs for 3 consecutive days: 11–20 kg, 1 tab; 21–30 kg, 2 tabs; 31–40 kg, 3 tabs; >41 kg, 4 tabs.	Do not use for renal insufficiency pts. Do not use if weight <11kg, pregnant, or breast-feeding.

Pneumocystis carinii pneumonia (PCP), New name is **Pneumocystis jiroveci** (yee-row-vek-ee). Refs:: CID 42:1208, 2006; LnID 7:3, 2007.

	Region Acquired	Primary—Adults	Alternative & Peds	Comments
Not acutely ill, able to take po meds. PaO₂ >70 mmHg Interest in detection of PCP by serum assay for B-Glucan (AnIM 147:70, 2007 & Chest 131:1173, 2007).		(**TMP-SMX-DS**, 2 tabs po q8h x 21 days) OR [(**Dapsone** 100 mg po q24h + **trimethoprim** 5 mg/kg po tid x 21 days] NOTE: Concomitant use of corticosteroids usually reserved for sicker pts with PaO₂ <70 (see below)	[**Clindamycin** 300–450 mg po q6h + **primaquine** 15 mg base po q24h] x21 days OR **Atovaquone** suspension 750 mg po bid with food x 21 days	Mutations in gene of the enzyme target (dihydropteroate synthetase) of sulfamethoxazole identified. Unclear whether mutations result in resist to TMP-SMX or dapsone + TMP (EID 10:1721, 2004). Dapsone ref: CID 27:191, 1998. **After 21 days, chronic suppression in AIDS pts (see below—post-treatment suppression).**
Acutely ill, po rx not possible. PaO₂ <70 mmHg. Still unclear whether antiretroviral therapy (ART) should be started during treatment of PCP (CID 46:625 & 635, 2008).		[**Prednisone** (15–30 min. before TMP-SMX): 40 mg po bid times 5 days, then 40 mg q24h times 5 days, then 20 mg po q24h times 11 days] + [**TMP-SMX** (15 mg of TMP component per kg per day) IV div. q6–8h times 21 days] Can substitute IV prednisolone (reduce dose 25%) for po prednisone	**Prednisone** as in primary rx PLUS [**Clinda** (600 mg IV q8h) + (**primaquine** 30 mg base po q24h)] times 21 days OR **Pentamidine** 4 mg per kg per day IV times 21 days. Caspofungin active in animal models: CID 36:1445, 2003	**After 21 days, chronic suppression in AIDS pts (see post-treatment suppression). PCP** can occur in absence of **HIV infection & steroids (CID 25:215 & 219, 1997).** Wait 4–8 days before declaring treatment failure & switching to clinda + primaquine or pentamidine (JAIDS 48:63, 2008), or adding caspofungin (Transplant 84:685, 2007).

---

* See page 3 for abbreviations. All dosage recommendations are for adults (unless otherwise indicated) and assume normal renal function.

TABLE 13A (5)

INFECTING ORGANISM	SUGGESTED REGIMENS		COMMENTS
	PRIMARY	ALTERNATIVE	
PROTOZOA—EXTRAINTESTINAL/Pneumocystis carinii pneumonia (PCP) *(continued)*			
Primary prophylaxis and post-treatment suppression	(**TMP-SMX-DS or -SS**, 1 tab po q24h or 1 DS 3x/wk) OR (**dapsone** 100 mg po q24h). DC when CD4 >200 x/3mo (*NEJM 344:159, 2001*).	(**Pentamidine** 300 mg in 6 mL sterile water by aerosol q4 wks) OR (**dapsone** 200 mg po + **pyrimethamine** 75 mg po + **folinic acid** 25 mg po —all once a week) or **atovaquone** 1500 mg po q24h with food.	TMP-SMX-DS regimen provides cross-protection vs toxo and other bacterial infections. Dapsone + pyrimethamine protects vs toxo. Atovaquone suspension 1500 mg once daily as effective as daily dapsone (*NEJM 339:1889, 1998*) or inhaled pentamidine (*JID 180:369, 1999*).
Toxoplasma gondii (Reference: *Ln 363:1965, 2004*)			
Immunologically normal patients (*For pediatric doses, see reference*)			
Acute illness w/ lymphadenopathy	No specific rx unless severe/persistent symptoms or evidence of vital organ damage		
Acq. via transfusion (lab accident)	Treat as for active chorioretinitis.		
Active chorioretinitis: meningitis; lowered resistance due to steroids or cytotoxic drugs	[**Pyrimethamine** (pyri) 200 mg po once on 1st day, then 50–75 mg po q24h] + [**sulfadiazine** (*see footnote*) 1–1.5 gm po qid] + [**leucovorin (folinic acid)** 5–20 mg 3x/wk]—**see Comment.** Treat 1–2 wk beyond resolution of signs/symptoms; continue leucovorin 1 wk after stopping pyri.		For congenital toxo, toxo meningitis in adults, & chorioretinitis, **add prednisone** 1 mg/**kg/day in 2 div. doses** until CSF protein conc. falls or vision-threatening inflammation subsides. Adjust folinic acid dose by following CBC results.
Acute in pregnant women. Ref: *CID 47:554, 2008.*	**If <18 wks gestation: Spiramycin**[NUS] 1 gm po q8h until delivery if amniotic fluid PCR is negative. **If >18 wks gestation & documented fetal infection by positive amniotic fluid PCR:** **Pyrimethamine** 50 mg po q12h x 2 days, then 50 mg/day + **sulfadiazine** 75 mg/kg po x 1 dose, then 50 mg/kg q12h (max 4 gm/day) + **folinic acid** 10–20 mg po daily.		Screen patients with IgG/IgM serology at commercial lab. IgG+ /IgM neg = remote past infection; IgG+/IgM+ = seroconversion. Suggest consultation with Palo Alto Medical Foundation Toxoplasma Serology Lab: 650-853-4828 or toxlab@pamf.org
Fetal/congenital	Mgmt complex. Combo rx with pyrimethamine + sulfadiazine + leucovorin—*see Comment*		Details in *Ln 363:1965, 2004*. **Consultation advisable.**
Acquired immunodeficiency syndrome (AIDS)			
Cerebral toxoplasmosis Ref.: *Ln 363:1965, 2004; CID 40(Suppl.3):S131, 2005*	[**Pyrimethamine** (pyri) 200 mg x 1 po, then 75 mg/day po] + **sulfadiazine** 1–1.5 gm po q6h) + (**folinic acid** 10–20 mg/day po) for 4–6 wks after resolution of signs/ symptoms, and then suppressive rx (*see below*) OR **TMP-SMX** 10/50 mg/kg per day po or IV div. q12h x 30 days (*AAC 42:1346, 1998*)	[**Pyri + folinic acid** (as in primary regimen)] + 1 of the following: (1) **Clinda** 600 mg po/IV q6h or (2) **clarithro** 1 gm po bid or (3) **azithro** 1.2–1.5 gm po q24h or (4) **atovaquone** 750 mg po q6h. Treat 4–6 wks after resolution of signs/symptoms, then suppression.	Use alternative regimen for pts with severe sulfa allergy. If multiple ring-enhancing brain lesions (CT or MRI), >85% of pts respond to 7–10 days of empiric rx; if no response, suggest brain biopsy. Pyri penetrates brain even if no inflammation; folinic acid prevents pyrimethamine hematologic toxicity.
Primary prophylaxis AIDS pts—IgG toxo antibody + CD4 count <100 per mcL	(**TMP-SMX-DS**, 1 tab po q24h) or (**TMP-SMX-SS**, 1 tab po q24h)	[(**Dapsone** 50 mg po q24h) + (**pyri** 50 mg po q wk) + (**folinic acid** 25 mg po q24h)] OR **atovaquone** 1500 mg po q24h	Prophylaxis for pneumocystis also effective vs toxo. Refs.: *MMWR 51(RR-8), 6/14/2002; AnIM 137:435, 2002*
Suppression after rx of cerebral toxo	(**Sulfadiazine** 500–1000 mg po 4x/day) + (**pyri** 25–50 mg po q24h) + (**folinic acid** 10–25 mg po q24h). DC if CD4 count >200 x3mo	[(**Clinda** 300–450 mg po q6–8h) + (**pyri** 25–50 mg po q24h) + (**folinic acid** 10–25 mg po q24h)] OR atovaquone 750 mg po q6–12h	(Pyri + sulfa) prevents PCP and toxo; (clinda + pyri) prevents toxo only.
Trichomonas vaginalis	See *Vaginitis, Table 1A, page 24*		
Trypanosomiasis. Ref.: *Ln 362:1469, 2003*			
West African sleeping sickness (T. brucei gambiense)			
Early: Blood/lymphatic—CNS OK	**Pentamidine** 4 mg/kg IM daily x 10 days	**Suramin** 100 mg IV (test dose), then 1 gm IV on days 1, 3, 7, 14, & 21	
Late: Encephalitis	**Melarsoprol** 2.2 mg/kg per day IV x 10 days (melarsoprol/nifurtimox combination superior to melarsoprol a one (*JID 195:311 & 322, 2007*)).	**Eflornithine** 100 mg/kg q6h IV x 14 days (*CID 41:748, 2005*)	Combination of IV eflornithine, 400 mg/kg/day divided q12h x 7 days, plus nifurtimox, 15 mg/kg/day po, divided q8h x 10 days more efficacious than standard dose eflornithine (*CID 45:1435 & 1443, 2007*).
Prophylaxis	**Pentamidine** 3 mg/kg IM q6 mos.	Not for casual visitor	

---

[1] Sulfonamides for toxo. Sulfadiazine now commercially available. Sulfisoxazole much less effective.

* See page 3 for abbreviations. All dosage recommendations are for adults (unless otherwise indicated) and assume normal renal function.

TABLE 13A (6)

INFECTING ORGANISM	SUGGESTED REGIMENS		COMMENTS
	PRIMARY	ALTERNATIVE	
PROTOZOA—EXTRAINTESTINAL/Trypanosomiasis (continued)			
East African sleeping sickness (T. brucei rhodesiense)			
Early: Blood/lymphatic	**Suramin** 100 mg IV (test dose), then 1 gm IV on days 1,3, 7, 14, & 21	None	
Late: Encephalitis	**Melarsoprol**[1] 2–3.6 mg/kg per day IV x 3 days; repeat after 7 days & for 3rd time 7 days after 2nd course	Prednisone may prevent/attenuate encephalopathy	
T. cruzi—**Chagas disease** or acute American trypanosomiasis Ref.: Ln 357:797, 2001 For chronic disease: see Comment.	**Nifurtimox**[1] 8–10 mg/kg per day po div. 4x/day after meals x 120 days Ages 11–16 yrs: 12.5–15 mg/kg per day div. qid po x 90 days Children <11yrs: 15–20 mg/kg per day div. qid po x 90 days	**Benznidazole**[NUS] 5–7 mg/kg per day po div. 2x/day x 30–90 days (AJTMH 63:111, 2000). NOTE: Avoid tetracycline and steroids.	Chronic disease: 1) Immunosuppression for heart transplant can reactivate chronic Chagas disease. 2) Reduced progression with 30 days of benznidazole 5 mg/kg per day: AnIM 144:724, 2006.
NEMATODES—INTESTINAL (Roundworms). Eosinophilia? Think Strongyloides, toxocaria and filariasis: CID 34:407, 2005; 42:1781 & 1655, 2006-- See Table 13C.			
Anisakis simplex (**anisakiasis**) CID 41:1297, 2005; LnID 4:294, 2004	Physical removal: endoscope or surgery IgE antibody test vs A. simplex may help diagnosis.	Anecdotal reports of possible treatment benefit from albendazole (Ln 360:54, 2002; CID 41:1825, 2005)	Anisakiasis acquired by eating raw fish: herring, salmon, mackerel, cod, squid. Similar illness due to Pseudoterranova species acquired from cod, halibut, red snapper.
Ascaris lumbricoides (**ascariasis**) Ln 367:1521, 2006	**Albendazole** 400 mg po x 1 dose or **mebendazole** 100 mg po bid x 3 days or 500 mg po x 1 dose	**Ivermectin** 150–200 mcg/kg po x 1 dose or **Nitazoxanide: Adults**—500 mg po bid x 3 days; **children 4–11**—200 mg oral susp. po q12h	Can present with intestinal obstruction. Review of efficacy of single dose: JAMA 299:1937, 2008.
Capillaria philippinensis (**capillariasis**)	**Mebendazole** 200 mg po bid x 20 days	**Albendazole** 200 mg po bid x 10 days	
Enterobius vermicularis (**pinworm**) Ln 367:1521, 2006	**Albendazole** 400 mg po x 1, repeat in 2 wks OR **mebendazole** 100 mg po x 1, repeat in 2 wks	**Pyrantel pamoate** 11 mg/kg base (to max. dose of 1 gm) po x 1 dose; repeat in 2 wks.	Side-effects in Table 13B, pages 136, 136
Gongylonemiasis	Surgical removal or **albendazole** 400 mg/day po x 3 days		
Hookworm (Necator americanus and Ancylostoma duodenale)	**Albendazole** 400 mg po x 1 dose or **mebendazole** 500 mg po x 1 dose	**Pyrantel pamoate** 11 mg/kg (to max. dose of 1 gm) po daily x 3 days	NOTE: Ivermectin not effective. Eosinophilia may be absent but eggs in stool (NEJM 351:799, 2004).
Strongyloides stercoralis (**strongyloidiasis**)/(See Comment)	**Ivermectin** 200 mcg/kg per day po x 2 days	**Albendazole** 400 mg po bid x 7 days ; less effective	For hyperinfections, repeat at 15 days. For hyperinfection: veterinary ivermectin has been given subcutaneously or rectally
Trichostrongylus orientalis	**Albendazole** 400 mg po x 1 dose	**Pyrantel pamoate** 11 mg/kg (max. 1 gm) po x 1	**Mebendazole** 100 mg po bid x 3 days
Trichuris trichura (**whipworm**) Ln 367:1521, 2006	**Albendazole** 400 mg po 1x/day x 3 days	**Mebendazole** 100 mg po bid x 3 days or 500 mg once	**Ivermectin** 200 mcg/kg daily po x 3 days
NEMATODES—EXTRAINTESTINAL (Roundworms)			
Ancylostoma braziliense & caninum: causes **cutaneous larva migrans** (Dog & cat hookworm)	**Ivermectin** 200 mcg/kg po x 1 dose/day x 1–2 days	**Albendazole** 400 mg po x 1 dose/day po x 3 days	Also called "creeping eruption," dog and cat hookworm. Ivermectin cure rate 77% (1 dose) to 97% (2–3 doses) (CID 31:493, 2000)
Baylisascariasis (Raccoon ascaris)	No drug proven efficacious. Try po **albendazole**, Peds: 25–50 mg/kg per day; Adults: 400 mg bid. Both x 10 days		Some add steroids (CID 39:1484, 2004).
Dracunculus medinensis: **Guinea worm** (CMAJ 170:495, 2004)	Slow extraction of pre-emergent worm	**Metronidazole** 250 mg po tid x 10 days used to ↓ inflammatory response and facilitate removal. Immersion in warm water promotes worm emergence. Mebendazole 400–800 mg/day x 6 days may kill worm.	

[1] Available from CDC Drug Service; see footnote 1 page 125
* See page 3 for abbreviations. All dosage recommendations are for adults (unless otherwise indicated) and assume normal renal function.

TABLE 13A (7)

INFECTING ORGANISM	SUGGESTED REGIMENS — PRIMARY	SUGGESTED REGIMENS — ALTERNATIVE	COMMENTS
NEMATODES—EXTRAINTESTINAL (Roundworms) (continued)			
Filariasis. Wolbachia bacteria needed for filarial development: Rx with doxy 100–200 mg/day x 4–6 wks ↓ number of wolbachia & number of microfilaria but no effect on adult worms (*BMJ 326:207, 2003*)			
Lymphatic (**Elephantiasis**): Wuchereria bancrofti or Brugia malayi or B. timori	**Diethylcarbamazine**[1,2] (DEC): po; Day 1, 50 mg; Day 2, 50 mg tid; Day 3, 100 mg tid; Days 4–14, 2 mg/kg q8h for total of 72 mg over 14 days (see comment)	**Diethylcarbamazine**[1,2] (DEC): Day 1, 50 mg; Interest in combining albendazole with **DEC**; no trials comparing combination vs. DEC alone. **Doxycycline** given as pretreatment followed by **DEC + albendazole** reduced microfilaremia (*CID 46:1358, 2008*).	NOTE: DEC can cause irreversible eye damage if concomitant onchocerciasis. Goal is reducing burden of adult worms.
Cutaneous — Loiasis: **Loa loa**, eyeworm disease	**Diethylcarbamazine** (DEC):[1,2] Day 1, 50 mg; Day 2, 50 mg tid; Day 3, 100 mg tid; Days 4–21, 8–10 mg/kg/day in 3 divided doses	**Albendazole** 200 mg po bid x 21 days	If concomitant oncho & Loa loa, treat oncho first. If over 5,000 microfilaria/mL of blood, DEC can cause encephalopathy. Might start with albendazole x few days ± steroids, then DEC.
Onchocerca volvulus (**onchocerciasis**)—river blindness (*Ln 360:203, 2002*)	**Ivermectin** 150 mcg/kg po for 6–12 months.	If **ivermectin** fails, consider **suramin** (from CDC Drug Service)	Oncho & Loa loa may both be present. Check peripheral smear; if Loa loa microfilaria present, treat oncho first with ivermectin before DEC for Loa loa.
Body cavity — Mansonella perstans (dipetalonemiasis)	Nothing works well. Try DEC as for lymphatic filariasis.	**Albendazole** in high dose x 3 weeks.	Ivermectin has no activity. Ref: *Trans R Soc Trop Med Hyg 100:458, 2006.*
Mansonella streptocerca	**Diethylcarbamazine**[1,2], as above for Wuchereria OR **ivermectin** 150 mcg/kg x 1		Chronic pruritic hypopigmented lesions that may be confused with leprosy. Can be asymptomatic.
Mansonella ozzardi	**Ivermectin** 200 mcg/kg x 1 dose may be effective		Usually asymptomatic. Articular pain, pruritus, lymphadenopathy reported. May have allergic reaction from dying organisms.
Dirofilariasis: **Heartworms** — D. immitis, dog heartworm	No effective drugs; surgical removal only option		Can lodge in pulmonary artery → coin lesion. Eosinophilia rare.
D. tenius (raccoon), D. ursi (bear), D. repens (dogs, cats)	No effective drugs		Worms migrate to conjunctivae, subcutaneous tissue, scrotum, breasts, extremities
Gnathostoma spinigerum: eosinophilic myeloencephalitis	**Albendazole** 400 mg po q24h or bid times 21 days		**Ivermectin** 200 mcg per kg per day times 2 days
Toxocariasis: *Clin Micro Rev 16:265, 2003* — **Visceral larval migrans**	**Albendazole** 400 mg po bid x 5 days	**Mebendazole** 100–200 mg po bid times 5 days	**Rx directed at relief of symptoms as infection self-limited, e.g., steroids & antihistamines; use of anthelminthics controversial.** Severe lung, heart or CNS disease may warrant steroids. Differential dx of larval migrans syndromes: Toxocara canis & catis, Ancylostoma spp., Gnathostoma spp., Spirometra spp.
Ocular larval migrans	First 4 wks of illness: (Oral **prednisone** 30–60 mg po q24h + subtenon **triamcinolone** 40 mg/wk) x 2 wk		No added benefit of antihelminthic drugs. Rx of little effect after 4 wk.
Trichinella spiralis (**trichinosis**)—muscle infection	**Albendazole** 400 mg po bid x 8–14 days. Concomitant **prednisone** 40–60 mg po q24h	**Mebendazole** 200–400 mg po tid x 3 days, then 400–500 mg po tid x 10 days	Use albendazole/mebendazole with caution during pregnancy.

1 Available from CDC Drug Service; see footnote 1 page 125

2 May need antihistamine or corticosteroid for allergic reaction from disintegrating organisms

* See page 3 for abbreviations. All dosage recommendations are for adults (unless otherwise indicated) and assume normal renal function.

TABLE 13A (8)

INFECTING ORGANISM	SUGGESTED REGIMENS		COMMENTS
	PRIMARY	ALTERNATIVE	
TREMATODES (Flukes)			
Clonorchis sinensis (liver fluke)	**Praziquantel** 25 mg/kg po tid x 2 days or **albendazole** 10 mg/kg per day po x 7 days		Same dose in children
Dicrocoelium dendriticum	**Praziquantel** 25 mg/kg po tid x 1 day		Ingestion of raw or undercooked sheep liver (CID 44:145, 2007).
Fasciola buski (intestinal fluke)	**Praziquantel** 25 mg/kg po tid x 1 day		Same dose in children
Fasciola hepatica (sheep liver fluke)	**Triclabendazole**[NUS] (Egaten; Novartis. Contact Victoria Pharmacy, Zurich: +41-211-24-32) 10 mg/kg po x 1 dose (Ref.: Clin Micro Infect 11:859, 2005) or **Nitazoxanide** 500 mg po bid x 7 days.		**Bithionol**[1]. Adults and children: 30–50 mg/kg (max. dose 2 gm/day) every other day times 10–15 doses
Heterophyes heterophyes (intestinal fluke); Metagoninus yokogawai (intestinal fluke); Opisthorchis viverrini (liver fluke)	**Praziquantel** 25 mg/kg po tid x 2 days		Same dose in children. Same regimen for **Metorchis conjunctus (North American liver fluke). Nanophyetus salmincola:** Praziquantel 20 mg/kg po tid x 1 day
Paragonimus westermani (lung fluke)	**Praziquantel** 25 mg/kg po tid x 2 days or **bithionol**[1] 30–50 mg/kg po x 1 every other day x 10 days		Same dose in children
Schistosoma haematobium; GU bilharziasis. (NEJM 346:1212, 2002)	**Praziquantel** 20 mg/kg po bid x 1 day **(2 doses)**		Same dose in children. Alternative: metrifonate 10 mg/kg per dose po q2 wks for 3 doses.
Schistosoma intercalatum	**Praziquantel** 20 mg/kg po bid x 1 day **(2 doses)**		Same dose in children
Schistosoma japonicum; Oriental schisto. (NEJM 346:1212, 2002)	**Praziquantel** 20 mg/kg po **tid** x 1 day **(3 doses)**		Same dose in children. Cures 60–90% pts.
Schistosoma mansoni (intestinal bilharziasis) Possible praziquantel resistance (JID 176:304, 1997) (NEJM 346:1212, 2002)	**Praziquantel** 20 mg/kg po bid x 1 day **(2 doses)**	**Oxamniquine** [NUS] single dose of 15 mg/kg po once; in North and East Africa 20 mg/kg po daily x 3 days Do not use during pregnancy.	Same dose for children. Cures 60–90% pts. Report of success treating myeloradiculopathy with single po dose of praziquantel, 50 mg/kg, + prednisone for 6 mo (CID 39:1618, 2004).
Schistosoma mekongi	**Praziquantel** 20 mg per kg po tid times 1 day **(3 doses)**		Same dose for children
Toxemic schisto; Katayama fever	**Praziquantel** 20 mg per kg po bid or tid x 3-6 days (LnID 7:218, 2007).		Massive infection with either S. japonicum or S. mansoni
CESTODES (Tapeworms)			
Echinococcus granulosus (hydatid disease) (CID 37:1073, 2003; Ln 362:1295, 2003)	Meta-analysis supports percutaneous aspiration-injection-reaspiration (PAIR) + albendazole. Before & after drainage: **albendazole** ≥60 kg, 400 mg po bid or <60 kg, 15 mg/kg per day div. bid, with meals. Then: Puncture (P) & needle aspirate (A) cyst content. Instill (I) hypertonic saline (15–30%) or absolute alcohol, wait 20–30 min, then re-aspirate (R) with final irrigation. **Continue albendazole x 28 days** Cure in 96% as comp to 90% pts with surgical resection.		
Echinococcus multilocularis (alveolar cyst disease) (COID 16:437, 2003)	**Albendazole** efficacy not clearly demonstrated, can try in dosages used for hydatid disease. Wide surgical resection only reliable rx; technique evolving (AJM 18:195, 2005).		
Intestinal tapeworms			
Diphyllobothrium latum (fish), Dipylidium caninum (dog), Taenia saginata (beef), & Taenia solium (pork).	**Praziquantel** 5–10 mg/kg po x 1 dose for children and adults. **Alternative was Niclosamide (Yomesan)** 2 gm po x 1; however, drug no longer available; manufacturer is Bayer, Germany		
Hymenolepis diminuta (rats) and H. nana (humans)	**Praziquantel** 25 mg/kg po x 1 dose for children and adults. **Alternative was Niclosamide (Yomesan)** 500 mg po q24h x 3 days; however, drug no longer available; manufacturer is Bayer, Germany.		
Neurocysticercosis (NCC): Larval form of T. solium Ref.: AJTMH 72:3, 2005	**NOTE: Treat T. solium intestinal tapeworms,** if present, with **praziquantel** 5-10 mg/kg po x 1 dose for children & adults.		

[1] Available from CDC Drug Service; see footnote 1 page 125

* See page 3 for abbreviations. All dosage recommendations are for adults (unless otherwise indicated) and assume normal renal function.

TABLE 13A (9)

INFECTING ORGANISM	SUGGESTED REGIMENS		COMMENTS
	PRIMARY	ALTERNATIVE	

CESTODES (Tapeworms) / Neurocysticercosis (NCC) *(continued)*

Parenchymal NCC

"Viable" cysts by CT/MRI. Meta-analysis: Treatment assoc with cyst resolution, ↓ seizures, and ↓ seizure recurrence. *AnIM 145:43, 2006.*

	PRIMARY	ALTERNATIVE	COMMENTS
	Albendazole ≥60 kg: 400 mg bid with meals or <60 kg: 15 mg/kg per day in 2 div. doses (max. 800 mg/day) + **Dexamethasone** 0.1 mg/kg per day ± Anti-seizure medication]— all x 8-30 days	**(Praziquantel** 100 mg/kg per day in 3 div. doses po x 1 day, then 50 mg/kg/d in 3 doses plus dexamethasone+ **Dexamethasone** 0.1 mg/kg per day ± Anti-seizure medication) — all x 29 days. *See Comment*	Albendazole assoc. with 46% ↓ in seizures *(NEJM 350:249, 2004).* Praziquantel less cysticidal activity. Steroids decrease serum levels of praziquantel. NIH reports methotrexate at ≤20 mg/wk allows a reduction in steroid use *(CID 44:449, 2007).*

"Degenerating" cysts: **Albendazole + dexamethasone as above** — **Treatment improves prognosis of associated seizures.**

Dead calcified cysts: **No treatment indicated**

Subarachnoid NCC (Albendazole + steroids as above) + shunting for hydrocephalus. Without shunt, 50% died within 9yrs *(J Neurosurg 66:686, 1987).*

Intraventricular NCC **Albendazole + dexamethasone + neuroendoscopic removal (if available)**

Sparganosis (Spirometra mansonoides) Larval cysts; source—frogs/snakes — Surgical resection or ethanol injection of subcutaneous masses *(NEJM 330:1887, 1994).*

DISEASE	INFECTING ORGANISM	SUGGESTED REGIMENS		COMMENTS
		PRIMARY	ALTERNATIVE	

ECTOPARASITES. Ref.: *CID 36:1355, 2003; Ln 363:889, 2004.* **NOTE: Due to potential neurotoxicity and risk of aplastic anemia, lindane not recommended.**

Head lice *Med Lett 47:68, 2005*	Pediculus humanus, var. capitis	**Permethrin** 1% generic lotion or cream rinse (Nix): Apply to shampooed dried hair for 10min.; repeat in 1 wk. **OR** **Malathion** 0.5% (Ovide): Apply to dry hair for 8–14 hrs, then shampoo. 2 doses 7 days apart.	**Ivermectin** 200–400 mcg/kg po once; 3 doses at 7 day interval reported effective *(JID 193:474, 2006).*	**Permethrin:** success in 78%. Extra combing of no benefit. Resistance increasing. No advantage to 5% permethrin. **Malathion:** Report that 1–2 20-min. applications 98% effective *(Ped Derm 21:670, 2004).* In alcohol—potentially flammable.
Pubic lice (crabs)	Phthirus pubis	**Pubic hair: Permethrin** OR **malathion** as for head lice	**Eyelids: Petroleum jelly** applied qid x 10 days **OR yellow oxide of mercury** 1% qid x 14 days	
Body lice	Pediculus humanus, var. corporis	No drugs for pt: treat the clothing. Organism lives in & deposits eggs in seams of clothing. Discard clothing; if not possible, treat clothing with 1% malathion powder or 10% DDT powder. Success with ivermectin in home shelter: 12 mg po on days 0, 7, & 14 *(JID 193:474, 2006)*		
Scabies Immunocompetent patients Refs: *LnID 6:769, 2006*	Sarcoptes scabiei	**Primary: Permethrin** 5% cream (ELIMITE). Apply entire skin from chin to toes. Leave on 8–14hr. Repeat in 1 wk. Safe for children >2mo old. **Alternative: Ivermectin** 200 mcg/kg po x 1 ; 2nd dose 14 days later.		Trim fingernails. Reapply to hands after handwashing. Pruritus may persist times 2 wk after mites gone. **Less effective: Crotamiton** 10% cream, apply x 24 hr, rinse off, then reapply x 24 hr.
AIDS patients, CD4 <150 per mm³ (Norwegian scabies—see *Comments*)		For Norweg an scabies: **Permethrin** 5% as above on day 1, then 6% sulfur in petrolatum daily on days 2–7, then repeat times several weeks. **Ivermectin** 200 mcg/kg po x 1 reported effective.		Norwegian scabies in AIDS pts: Extensive, crusted. Can mimic psoriasis. Not pruritic. Highly contagious—isolate!
Myiasis Due to larvae of flies		Usually cutaneous/subcutaneous nodule with central punctum. Treatment: Occlude punctum to prevent gas exchange with petrolatum, fingernail polish, makeup cream or bacon. When larva migrates, manually remove.		

* See page 3 for abbreviations. All dosage recommendations are for adults (unless otherwise indicated) and assume normal renal function.

TABLE 13B – DOSAGE AND SELECTED ADVERSE EFFECTS OF ANTIPARASITIC DRUGS

NOTE: Drugs available from CDC Drug Service indicated by "CDC." Call (404) 639-3670 (or -2888 (Fax)). Doses vary with indication. For convenience, drugs divided by type of parasite; some drugs used for multiple types of parasites, e.g., albendazole.

CLASS, AGENT, GENERIC NAME (TRADE NAME)	USUAL ADULT DOSAGE	ADVERSE REACTIONS/COMMENTS
Antiprotozoan Drugs		
Intestinal Parasites		
Diloxanide furoate^NUS (Furamide)	500 mg po tid x 10 days	Source: Panorama Compounding Pharmacy (800-247-9767). Flatulence, N/V, diarrhea.
Iodoquinol (Yodoxin)	Adults: 650 mg po tid (or 30-40 mg/kg/day div. tid); children: 40 mg/kg per day div. tid.	Rarely causes nausea, abdominal cramps, rash, acne. Contraindicated if iodine intolerance.
Metronidazole/Ornidazole^NUS (Tiberal)	Side-effects similar for all. See metronidazole in Table 10A, page 86, & Table 10C, page 94	
Nitazoxanide (Alinia)	Adults: 500 mg po q12h. Children 4–11: 200 mg susp. po q12h. Take with food.	Abdominal pain 7.8%, diarrhea 2.1%. Rev.: CID 40:1173, 2005; Expert Opin Pharmacother 7:953, 2006. Headaches; rarely yellow sclera (resolves after treatment).
Paromomycin (Humatin) Aminosidine in U.K.	Up to 750 mg qid.	Drug is aminoglycoside similar to neomycin; if absorbed due to concomitant inflammatory bowel disease can result in oto/nephrotoxicity. Doses >3 gm assoc. with nausea, abdominal cramps, diarrhea.
Quinacrine^NUS (Atabrine, Mepacrine)	100 mg tid. No longer available in U.S.; 2 pharmacies will prepare as a service: (1) Connecticut 203-785-6818; (2) California 800-247-9767	Contraindicated for pts with history of psychosis or psoriasis. Yellow staining of skin. Dizziness, headache, vomiting, toxic psychosis (1.5%), hemolytic anemia, leukopenia, thrombocytopenia, urticaria, rash, fever, minor disulfiram-like reactions.
Tinidazole (Tindamax)	500 mg tabs, with food. Regimen varies with indication.	Chemical structure similar to metronidazole but better tolerated. Seizures/peripheral neuropathy reported. **Adverse effects:** Metallic taste 4-6%, nausea 3-5%, anorexia 2-3%.
Antiprotozoan Drugs: Non-Intestinal Protozoa		
Extraintestinal Parasites		
Antimony compounds^NUS Stibogluconate sodium (Pentostam) from CDC or Meglumine antimonate (Glucantime—French tradenames	Dilute in 120 mL of D5W and infuse over 2hr. Ideally, monitor EKG.	Fatigue, myalgia, N/V and diarrhea common. ALT/AST ↑s, ↑amylase and lipase occur. **NOTE: Reversible T wave changes in 30-60%. Risk of QTc prolongation.**
Artesunate Ref: NEJM 358:1829, 2008	Available from CDC Malaria Branch. 2.4 mg/kg IV at 0, 12, 24, & 48 hrs	More effective than quinine & safer than quinidine. Contact CDC at 770-488-7758 or 770-488-7100 after hours. No dosage adjustment for hepatic or renal insufficiency. No known drug interactions.
Atovaquone (Mepron) Ref.: AAC 46:1163, 2002	Suspension: 1 tsp (750 mg) po bid 750 mg/5 mL.	No. pts stopping rx due to side-effects was 9%; rash 22%, GI 20%, headache 16%, insomnia 10%, fever 14%
Atovaquone and proguanil (Malarone) For prophylaxis of P. falciparum; little data on P. vivax	**Prophylaxis:** 1 tab po (250 mg + 100 mg) q24h with food **Treatment:** 4 tabs po (1000 mg + 400 mg) once daily with food x 3 days Adult tab: 250/100 mg; Peds tab 62.5/25 mg. Peds dosage: footnote 1 page 97.	Adverse effects in rx trials: Adults—abd. pain 17%, N/V 12%, headache 10%, dizziness 5%. Rx stopped in 1%. Asymptomatic mild ↑ in ALT/AST. Children—cough, headache, anorexia, vomiting, abd. pain. See drug interactions, Table 22. Safe in G6PD-deficient pts. Can crush tabs for children and give with milk or other liquid nutrients. Renal insufficiency: contraindicated if CrCl <30 mL per min.
Benznidazole^NUS (Rochagan, Roche, Brazil)	7.5 mg/kg per day po	Photosensitivity in 50% of pts. GI: abdominal pain, nausea/vomiting/anorexia. CNS: disorientation, insomnia, twitching/seizures, paresthesias, polyneuritis. **Contraindicated in pregnancy**
Chloroquine phosphate (Aralen)	Dose varies—see Malaria Prophylaxis and rx, pages 127-128.	Minor: anorexia/nausea/vomiting, headache, dizziness, blurred vision, pruritus in dark-skinned pts. Major: protracted rx in rheumatoid arthritis can lead to retinopathy. Can exacerbate psoriasis. Can block response to rabies vaccine. Contraindicated in pts with epilepsy.

See page 3 for abbreviations. All dosage recommendations are for adults (unless otherwise indicated) and assume normal renal function.

TABLE 13B (2)

CLASS, AGENT, GENERIC NAME (TRADE NAME)	USUAL ADULT DOSAGE	ADVERSE REACTIONS/COMMENTS
Antiprotozoan Drugs/Extraintestinal Parasites (*continued*)		
Dapsone Ref.: *CID 27:191, 1998*	100 mg po q24h	Usually tolerated by pts with rash after TMP-SMX. Adverse effects: nausea/vomiting, rash, oral lesions (*CID 18:630, 1994*). Methemoglobinemia (usually asymptomatic); if >10–15%, stop drug. Hemolytic anemia if G6PD deficient. Sulfone syndrome: fever, rash, hemolytic anemia, atypical lymphocytes, and liver injury (*West J Med 156:303, 1992*).
Eflornithine[NUS] (Ornidyl)	Approved in US for trypanosome infections but not market-ed. Aventis product.	Diarrhea in ½ pts, vomiting, abdominal pain, anemia/leukopenia in ½ pts, seizures, alopecia, jaundice, ↓ hearing. Contraindicated in pregnancy.
Fumagillin	Eyedrops + p.o. 20 mg po tid. Leiter's: 800-292-6773.	Adverse events: Neutropenia & thrombocytopenia
Mefloquine (Lariam)	One 250 mg tab/wk for malaria prophylaxis; for rx, 1250 mg x 1 or 750 mg & then 500 mg in 6–8hrs. In U.S.: 250 mg tab = 228 mg base; outside U.S., 275 mg tab = 250 mg base	Side-effects in roughly 3%. Minor: headache, irritability, insomnia, weakness, diarrhea. Toxic psychosis, seizures can occur. Teratogenic—do not use in pregnancy. Do not use with quinine, quinidine, or halofantrine. Rare: Prolonged QT interval and toxic epidermal necrolysis (*Ln 349:101, 1997*). Not used for self-rx due to neuropsychiatric side-effects.
Melarsoprol (*CDC*) (Mel B, Arsobal) (Manufactured in France)	See Trypanosomiasis for adult dose. Peds dose: 0.36 mg/kg IV, then gradual ↑ to 3.6 mg/kg q1–5 days for total of 9–10 doses.	Post-rx encephalopathy (10%) with 50% mortality overall; risk of death 2° to rx 4–8%. Prednisolone 1 mg per kg per day po may ↓ encephalopathy. Other: Heart damage, albuminuria, abdominal pain, vomiting, peripheral neuropathy, Herxheimer-like reaction, pruritus.
Miltefosine[NUS] (Zentaris, Impavido) (Expert Rev Anti Infect Ther 4:177, 2006)	100–150 mg (approx. 2.25 mg/kg per day) po x 28 days Cutaneous leishmaniasis 2.25 mg/kg po q24h x 6 wk	Contact Zentaris (Frankfurt, Ger): info@zentaris.com. **Pregnancy—No:** teratogenic. Side-effects vary: kala-azar pts, vomiting in up to 40%, diarrhea in 17%; "motion sickness", headache & increased creatinine. Daily dose >150 mg can cause severe GI side effects (*Ln 352:1821, 1998*).
Nifurtimox (Lampit) (*CDC*) (Manufactured in Germany by Bayer)	8–10 mg/kg per day po div. 4 x per day	Side-effects in 40–70% of pts. GI: abdominal pain, nausea/vomiting. CNS: polyneuritis (1/3), disorientation, insomnia, twitching, seizures. Skin rash. Hemolysis with G6PD deficiency.
Pentamidine (NebuPent)	300 mg via aerosol q month. Also used IM.	Hypotension, hypocalcemia, hypoglycemia followed by hyperglycemia, pancreatitis. Neutropenia (15%), thrombocytopenia. Nephrotoxicity. Others: nausea/vomiting, ↑ liver tests, rash.
Primaquine phosphate	26.3 mg (=15 mg base). Adult dose is 30 mg of base po daily.	In G6PD def, pts. can cause hemolytic anemia with hemoglobinuria, esp. African, Asian peoples. Methemoglobinemia. Nausea/abdominal pain if pt. fasting. (*CID 39:1336, 2004*). **Pregnancy: No.**
Pyrimethamine (Daraprim, Malocide) Also combined with sulfadoxine as **Fansidar** (25–500 mg)	100 mg po, then 25 mg/day. Cost of folinic acid (leucovorin)	Major problem is hematologic: megaloblastic anemia, ↓ WBC, ↓ platelets. Can give 5 mg folinic acid per day to ↓ bone marrow depression and not interfere with antitoxoplasmosis effect. If high-dose pyrimethamine, ↑ folinic acid to 10–50 mg/day. Pyrimethamine + sulfadiazine can cause mental changes due to carnitine deficiency (*AJM 95:112, 1993*). Other: Rash, vomiting, diarrhea, xerostomia
Quinidine gluconate Cardiotoxicity ref: LnID 7:549, 2007	Loading dose of 10 mg (equiv to 6.2 mg of quinidine base) / kg IV over 1–2hr, then constant infusion of 0.02 mg of quinidine gluconate / kg per minute.	Adverse reactions of quinidine/quinine similar: (1) IV bolus injection can cause fatal hypotension. (2) hyperinsulinemic hypoglycemia, esp. in pregnancy, (3) ↓ rate of infusion if QT interval ↑ >25% of baseline. (4) reduce dose 30–50% after day 3 due to ↓ renal clearance and ↓ vol. of distribution.
Quinine sulfate (300 mg salt = 250 mg base). In U.S. only approved product is Qualaquin.	324 mg tabs. No IV prep. in US. Oral rx of chloro-quine-resistant falciparum malaria: 624 mg po tid x 3 days, then (tetracycline 250 mg po qid or doxy 100 mg bid) x 7 days	Cinchonism; tinnitus, headache, nausea, abdominal pain, blurred vision. Rarely: blood dyscrasias, drug fever, asthma, hypoglycemia. Transient blindness in <1% of 500 pts (*AnIM 136:339, 2002*). **Contraindicated if prolonged QTc, myasthenia gravis, optic neuritis.**

*See page 3 for abbreviations. All dosage recommendations are for adults (unless otherwise indicated) and assume normal renal function.

TABLE 13B (3)

CLASS, AGENT, GENERIC NAME (TRADE NAME)	USUAL ADULT DOSAGE	ADVERSE REACTIONS/COMMENTS
Antiprotozoan Drugs/Extraintestinal Parasites (continued)		
Spiramycin (Rovamycin) (JAC 42:572, 1998)	1 gm po q8h (see Comment).	GI and allergic reactions have occurred. Available at no cost after consultation with Palo Alto Medical Foundation Toxoplasma Serology Lab: 650-853-4828 or from U.S. FDA 301-796-1600.
Sulfadiazine	1–1.5 gm po q6h.	See Table 10C, page 95, for sulfonamide side-effects
Sulfadoxine & pyrimethamine combination (Fansidar)	Contains 500 mg sulfadoxine & 25 mg pyrimethamine	Very long mean half-life of both drugs: Sulfadoxine 169hrs, pyrimethamine 111 hrs allows weekly dosage. Do not use in pregnancy. Fatalities reported due to Stevens-Johnson syndrome and toxic epidermal necrolysis. Renal excretion—use with caution in pts with renal impairment.
DRUGS USED TO TREAT NEMATODES, TREMATODES, AND CESTODES		
Albendazole (Albenza)	Doses vary with indication, 200–400 mg bid po	Teratogenic, Pregnancy Cat. C; give after negative pregnancy test. Abdominal pain, nausea/vomiting, alopecia, ↑ serum transaminase. Rare leukopenia.
Bithionol (CDC)	Adults & children: 30–40 mg/kg (to max. of 2 gm/day) po every other day x 10–15 doses	Photosensitivity, skin reactions, urticaria, GI upset.
Diethylcarbamazine (Hetrazan) (CDC)	Used to treat filariasis. Licensed (Lederle) but not available in US.	Headache, dizziness, nausea, fever. Host may experience inflammatory reaction to death of adult worms: fever, urticaria, asthma, GI upset (Mazzotti reaction). **Pregnancy—No.**
Ivermectin (Stromectol, Mectizan)	Strongyloidiasis dose: 200 mcg/kg x 2 doses po Onchocerciasis: 150 mcg/kg x1 po Scabies: 200 mcg/kg po x 1	Mild side-effects: fever, pruritus, rash. In rx of onchocerciasis, can see tender lymphadenopathy, headache, bone/joint pain. Can cause Mazzotti reaction (see above).
Mebendazole (Vermox)	Doses vary with indication.	Rarely causes abdominal pain, nausea, diarrhea. Contraindicated in pregnancy & children <2 yrs old.
Oxamniquineᴺᵁˢ (Vansil)	For S. mansoni. Some experts suggest 40–60 mg/kg over 2–3 days in all of Africa.	Rarely: dizziness, drowsiness, neuropsychiatric symptoms, GI upset. EKG/EEG changes. Orange/red urine. **Pregnancy—No.**
Praziquantel (Biltricide)	Doses vary with parasite; see Table 13A.	Mild: dizziness/drowsiness, N/V, rash, fever. Only contraindication is ocular cysticercosis. Metab.-induced by anticonvulsants and steroids; can negate effect with cimetidine 400 mg po tid.
Pyrantel pamoate (over-the-counter as Reese's Pinworm Medicine)	Oral suspension. Dose for all ages: 11 mg/kg (to max. of 1 gm) x 1 dose	Rare GI upset, headache, dizziness, rash
Suramin (Germanin) (CDC)	For early trypanosomiasis. Drug powder mixed to 10% solution with 5 mL water and used within 30 min	Does not cross blood-brain barrier; no effect on CNS infection. Side-effects: vomiting, pruritus, urticaria, fever, paresthesias, albuminuria (discontinue drug if casts appear). Do not use if renal/liver disease present. Deaths from vascular collapse reported
Thiabendazole (Mintezol)	Take after meals. Dose varies with parasite; see Table 12A.	Nausea/vomiting, headache, dizziness. Rarely: liver damage, ↓ BP, angioneurotic edema, Stevens-Johnson syndrome. May ↓ mental alertness.

TABLE 13C – PARASITES THAT CAUSE EOSINOPHILIA

Frequent and Intense (>5000 eos/mcL)	Moderate to Marked Early Infections	During Larval Migration: Absent or Mild During Chronic Infections	Other
Strongyloides (absent in compromised hosts); Lymphatic Filariasis; Toxocaria	Ascaris; Hookworm; Clonarchis; Paragonemis	Opisthorchis	Schistosomiasis; Cysticerosis; Trichuris; Angiostrongylus; Non-lymphatic filariasis; Grathasloma; Capillaria; Trichostrongylus

* See page 3 for abbreviations. All dosage recommendations are for adults (unless otherwise indicated) and assume normal renal function.

TABLE 14A – ANTIVIRAL THERAPY (NON-HIV)*

VIRUS/DISEASE	DRUG/DOSAGE	SIDE EFFECTS/COMMENTS
Adenovirus: Cause of RTIs including fatal pneumonia in children & young adults and 60% mortality in transplant pts (*CID 43:331, 2006*). Frequent cause of cystitis in transplant patients. **Findings include:** fever, ↑ liver enzymes, leukopenia, thrombocytopenia, diarrhea, pneumonia, or hemorrhagic cystitis.	In severe cases of pneumonia or post HSCT[1]: **Cidofovir** • 5 mg/kg/wk x 2 wks, then q 2 wks + **probenecid** 1.25 gm/M² given 3hrs before cidofovir and 3 & 9 hrs after each infusion • Or 1 mg/kg IV 3x/wk. For adenovirus hemorrhagic cystitis (*CID 40:199, 2005; Transplantation. 2006; 81:1398*): Intravesical **cidofovir** (5 mg/kg in 100 mL saline instilled into bladder)	Successful in 3/8 immunosuppressed children (*CID 38:45, 2004*) & 8 of 10 children with HSCT (*CID 41: 1812, 2005*). ↓ in virus load predicted response to cidofovir.
Coronavirus—SARS-CoV (Severe Acute Respiratory Distress Syn.) (see *CID 36:1420, 2004*) A new coronavirus, isolated Spring 2003 (*NEJM 348:1953 & 1967, 2003*) emerged from China & spread from Hong Kong to 32 countries. Effective infection control guidelines controlled the epidemic.	**Therapy remains predominantly supportive care.** Therapy tried or under evaluation (see *Comments*): **Ribavirin**—ineffective. Interferon alfa ± steroids—small case series. Pegylated IFN-α effective in monkeys. Value of corticosteroids alone unclear. Inhaled nitric oxide improved oxygenation & improved chest x-ray (*CID 39:1531, 2004*).	Other coronaviruses (HCOV-229E, OC43, NL63, etc.) implicated as cause of croup, asthma exacerbations, & other RTIs in children (*CID 40:1721, 2005; JID 191:492, 2005*). May be associated with Kawasaki disease (*JID 191:489, 2005*).
Enterovirus—Meningitis: most common cause of aseptic meningitis. PCR or CSF valuable for early dx (*Scand J Inf Dis 34:359, 2002*) but ↓ sensitivity >2 days of symptoms. PCR on feces pos. in 12/13 specimens, 5–16 days after clinical onset (*CID 40:982, 2005*).	**No rx currently recommended;** however, **pleconaril** (VP 63843) still under investigation.	No clinical benefit demonstrated in double-blind placebo-controlled study in 21 infants with enteroviral aseptic meningitis (*PIDJ 22:335, 2003*). Large Phase II study underway for enteroviral sepsis syndrome (*www.NIH.gov*).
Hemorrhagic Fever Virus Infections: For excellent reviews, see *Med Lab Observer, May 2005, p. 16, Lancet Infectious Disease Vol 6 No 4.*		
Congo-Crimean Hemorrhagic Fever (HF) (*CID 39:284, 2004*) Tickborne; symptoms include N/V, fever, headache, myalgias, & stupor (1/3). Signs: conjunctival injection, hepatomegaly, petechiae (1/3). Lab: ↓ platelets, ↓ WBC, ↑ ALT, AST, LDH & CPK (100%)	Oral **ribavirin, 30 mg/kg** as initial loading dose & 15 mg/kg q6h x 4 days & then 7.5 mg/kg x 6 days (WHO recommendation) (see *Comment*). Reviewed *Antiviral Therapy 78:181, 2008.*	3/3 healthcare workers in Pakistan had complete recovery (*Ln 346:472, 1995*) & 61/69 (89%) with confirmed CCHF rx with ribavirin survived in Iran (*CID 36:1613, 2003*). Shorter time of hospitalization among ribavirin treated pts (7.7 vs. 10.3 days), but no difference in mortality or transfusion needs in study done in Turkey (*J Infection 52: 207-215, 2006*)
Ebola/Marburg HF (Central Africa) Severe outbreak of Ebola in Angola 308 cases with 277 deaths by 5/3/05 (*NEJM 352:2155, 2005; LnID 5.331, 2005*). Major epidemic of Marburg 1998-2000 in Congo & 2004-5 in Angola (*NEJM355:866, 2006*)	**No effective antiviral rx** (*J Virol 77: 9733, 2003*).	Can infect gorillas & chimps that come in contact with other dead animal carcasses (*Science 303:387, 2004*) Marburg reported in African Fruit Bat, *Rousettus aegyptiacus* (*PLoS ONE, Aug 22, 2007*).
With pulmonary syndrome: Hantavirus pulmonary syndrome, "sin nombre virus"	**No benefit from ribavirin has been demonstrated** (*CID 39:1307, 2004*).	Acute onset of fever, headache, myalgias, non-productive cough, thrombocytopenia and non-cardiogenic pulmonary edema with respiratory insufficiency following exposure to rodents.
With renal syndrome: Lassa, Venezuelan, Korean, HF, Sabia, Argentinian HF, Bolivian HF, Junin, Machupo	Oral **ribavirin, 30 mg/kg** as initial loading dose & 15 mg/kg q6h x 4 days & then 7.5 mg/kg x 6 days (WHO recommendation) (see *Comment*).	Toxicity low, hemolysis reported but recovery when treatment stopped. No significant changes in WBC, platelets, hepatic or renal function. See *CID 36:1254, 2003,* for management of contacts.

[1] HSCT = Hematopoietic stem cell transplant
* See page 3 for abbreviations. NOTE: All dosage recommendations are for adults (unless otherwise indicated) and assume normal renal function.

TABLE 14A (2)

VIRUS/DISEASE	DRUG/DOSAGE	SIDE EFFECTS/COMMENTS
Hemorrhagic Fever Virus Infections *(continued)* **Dengue and dengue hemorrhagic fever (DHF)** www.cdc.gov/ncidod/dvbid/dengue/dengue-hcp.htm Think dengue in traveler to tropics or subtropics (incubation period usually 4-7 days) with fever, bleeding, thrombocytopenia, or hemoconcentration with shock. Dx by viral isolation or serology; serum to CDC (telephone 787-706-2399).	**No data on antiviral rx.** Fluid replacement with careful hemodynamic monitoring critical. Rx of **DHF** with colloids effective: 6% hydroxyethyl starch preferred in 1 study *(NEJM 353:9, 2005). Review in Semin Ped Infect Dis 16: 60-65, 2005.*	Of 77 cases dx at CDC (2001–2004), recent (2-wk) travel to Caribbean island 30%, Asia 17%, Central America 15%, S. America 15% *(MMWR 54:556, June 10, 2005).* 5 pts with severe **DHF** rx with dengue antibody-neg. gamma globulin 500 mg per kg q24h IV for 3-5 days; rapid ↑ in platelet counts *(CID 36:1623, 2003).*
West Nile virus *(see AnIM 104:545, 2004)* A flavivirus transmitted by mosquitoes, blood transfusions, transplanted organs *(NEJM 348: 2196, 2003; CID 38:1257, 2004),* & breast-feeding *(MMWR 51:877, 2002).* Birds (>200 species) are main host with man & horses incidental hosts. The US epidemic continues.	**No proven rx to date.** 2 clinical trials in progress: (1) Interferon alfa-N3 *(CID 40:764, 2005).* See www.nyhq.org/posting/rahal.html. (2) IVIG from Israel with high titer antibody West Nile *(JID 188:5, 2003; Transpl Inf Dis 4:160, 2002).* Contact NIH, 301-496-7453; see www.clinicaltrials.gov/show/NCT00068055. Reviewed in *Lancet Neurology 6: 171-181, 2007.*	Usually nonspecific febrile disease but 1/150 cases develops meningoencephalitis, aseptic meningitis or polio-like paralysis *(AnIM 104:545, 2004; JCI 113: 1102, 2004).* Long-term sequelae (neuromuscular weakness & psychiatric) common *(CID 43:723, 2006).* Dx by ↑ IgM in serum & CSF or CSF PCR (contact State Health Dept./ CDC). Blood supply now tested in U.S. ↑ serum lipase in 11/17 cases *(NEJM 352:420, 2005).*
Yellow fever	**No data on antiviral rx** **Guidelines for use of preventative vaccine (MMWR 51: RR17, 2002)**	Reemergence in Africa & S. Amer. due to urbanization of susceptible population -*(Lancet Inf 5:604, 2005).* Vaccination effective. *(JAMA 276:1157, 1996)*
Chikungunya fever A self limited arborvirus illness spread by Aedes mosquito.	**No antiviral therapy**	Clinical presentation: high fever, severe myalgias & headache, macular papular rash with occ thrombocytopenia. Rarely hemorrhagic complications. Dx by increase in IgM antibody.
Hepatitis Viral Infections **Hepatitis A** *(Ln 351:1643, 1998)*	No therapy recommended. If within 2 wks of exposure, IVIG 0.02 mL per kg IM times 1 protective.	Vaccine recommendations in *Table 20.* 40% of pts with chronic Hep C who developed superinfection with Hep A developed fulminant hepatic failure *(NEJM 338:286, 1998).*

Hepatitis B—Chronic: For pts co-infected with HIV *see Table 12, Sanford Guide to HIV/AIDS Therapy 2009.*
Who to treat? Based on status of e antigen and viral quantification. Adapted from Clin Gastro & Hepatology 4:936-962, 2006. Other useful refs: *Hepatology 45:507, 2007; AnIM 147:58, 2007; Hep B Foundation:* http://www.hepb.org. *New CDC Testing Guidelines published 18 Sept 2008.* www.cdc.gov

	HBV DNA (IU/mL)[1]	ALT	Suggested Management
HBe Ag-Positive	≥20,000	Elevated or normal	Treat if ALT elevated[2] Treat if biopsy abnormal—even if ALT normal[2]
HBe Ag-Negative	≥2,000	Elevated or normal	Treat if ALT elevated[2] Treat if biopsy abnormal—even if ALT normal[2]
Documented cirrhosis (positive or negative HBe Ag)	≥2,000 and compensated cirrhosis	ALT not applicable	Treat with **adefovir** or **entecavir** long term[2]
	<2,000 and compensated cirrhosis	ALT not applicable	Observe or (**adefovir** or **entecavir** long term)[2]
	Decompensated cirrhosis; any HBV DNA level	ALT not applicable	Long term therapy with (**lamivudine** or **entecavir** or **entecavir**) + **adefovir**; waiting list for liver transplantation[2]

[1] IU/mL equivalent to approximately 5.6 copies/mL; if patient treated, monitor every 6 mos if treated with adefovir; every 3 mos. if treated with lamivudine.

[2] Treatment duration varies with viral quantitation, presence/absence of cirrhosis & drug(s) used. *See Clin Gastro & Hepatology 4:936-962, 2006 for details.*

* *See page 3 for abbreviations.* NOTE: All dosage recommendations are for adults (unless otherwise indicated) and assume normal renal function.

TABLE 14A (3)

VIRUS/DISEASE	DRUG/DOSAGE	SIDE EFFECTS/COMMENTS

Hepatitis Viral Infections/Hepatitis B—Chronic (continued)

Comparison of Treatment Options for Chronic Hepatitis B (Patients **not** co-infected with HIV). **Note:** See Table 14B for more dosage details, adverse effects.

	Peg interferon alfa-2A	Telbivudine	Lamivudine	Adefovir	Entecavir	Tenofovir
Dose:	180 mcg sc weekly	600 mg po daily	100 mg po daily	10 mg po daily	0.5 mg po daily	300 mg po daily
Parameter:						
$\log_{10}$ ↓ in serum HBV DNA	4.5	6-6.6 (HBe Ag+)	No data	3.6	6.9	4.7-6.4 (HBeAg+)
HBV DNA below detection, %	25	No data	57	21	67	81% (30% if ADF resistance)
% ALT normalizes	39	75-85	41-72	48	68	76%
% with improved histology	38	65	49-56	53	72	72%
Resistance develops	No	2-3% after 1 yr	70% after 5 yrs	30% after 5 yrs	1% after 4 yrs	No

Hepatitis C (up to 3% of world infected, 4 million in U.S. Co-infection with HIV common—see Sanford Guide to HIV/AIDS Therapy).

Acute

Usually asymptomatic (>75%). Can detect by PCR within 13 days; antibody in 36+ days (CID 40:951, 2005).

Follow plasma HCV viral load by PCR:
It clear within 3-4 mos., no treatment.
It persists: PEG IFN ± ribavirin as below, albeit controversial (NEJM 346:1091, 2002).

15-40% clear infection within 6 mos (JAMA 297:724, 2007).
Sustained viral response with IFN alfa-2b therapy 32% vs. 4% with placebo, P 0.00007 (Cochrane Database Sys & Rev CD000369, 2002).
Alfa-INF alone effective in early infection (CID 42:1673, 2006)

Chronic: NEJM 365:2444, 2006.

Treat if: persistent elevated ALT/AST, + HCV RNA plasma viral load, fibrosis &/or inflam on biopsy.

Genotypes 1, 4, 5 & 6

Pegylated interferon
PEG IFN: Either alfa-2a (Pegasys) 180 mcg subcut. 1x/wk OR
Alfa-2b (PEG-INTRON) 1.5 mcg/kg subcut. 1x/wk
Monitor response by quantification:

HCV RNA	Result
After 4 wks rx:	<1 $\log_{10}$ ↓ IU/mL[1]
After 12 wks rx:	<2 $\log_{10}$ ↓ IU/mL
	>2 $\log_{10}$ ↓ IU/mL or undetectable

+ Ribavirin

Weight	Ribavirin Dose	Action
<75 kg	400 mg am & 600 mg pm	Discontinue therapy
>75 kg	600 mg am & 600 mg pm	Discontinue therapy
		Treat 48 wks

In U.S., 90% due to genotype 1. **Sustained viral response (SVR)** to 48-wk rx of genotype 1: 42-51%; SVR to 24-wk rx of genotype 2 or 3: 76-82%.
Avoid alcohol—accelerates HCV disease.
HIV accelerates HCV disease
See Table 14B for drug adverse effects & cost. Interferon alfa can cause serious depression.
Ribavirin is teratogenic & has dose-related hematologic toxicity.
For drugs in development, see Curr Opin Infect Dis 19:615, 2006.
For genotypes 2 & 3, some use standard IFN; results similar & ↓ cost.
NOTE: High viral load = >800,000 IU/mL. Pts with HCV RNA levels <800,000 IU/mL have 15-35% better response rate.

Genotype 2 or 3 PEG IFN alfa-2a or 2b—dose as for types 1 & 4 above **+ Ribavirin** 400 mg po bid

Quant. HCV RNA	Result	Action
After 4 wks rx:	Undetectable →	Treat 12 wks (NEJM 352:2609, 2005)
	>1 $\log_{10}$ ↓ →	Treat 24 wks (See comment)

For Genotype 2 and 3 12 wks of Rx less effective than 24 wks, except in those with very rapid response (< 1000 c/ml at 1 week) and those < 40 yrs old (if VL undetectable at day 29) Hepatology June 2008.

For prevention of acute and chronic infection, see Table 15D, page 173

---

[1] HCV RNA quantitation. By WHO international standard 8(00,000 IU/mL = 2 million copies/mL. Response to therapy based on $\log_{10}$ fall in IU/mL (JAMA 297:724, 2007).
* See page 3 for abbreviations. NOTE: All dosage recommendations are for adults (unless otherwise indicated) and assume normal renal function.

TABLE 14A (4)

VIRUS/DISEASE	DRUG/DOSAGE	SIDE EFFECTS/COMMENTS
Herpesvirus Infections **Cytomegalovirus (CMV)** Marked ↓ in HIV associated CMV infections & death with Highly Active Antiretroviral Therapy. Initial treatment should optimize HAART.		Risk for developing CMV disease correlates with quantity of CMV DNA in plasma: each log_{10} ↑ associated with 3.1-fold ↑ in disease *(JCI 101:497, 1998; CID 28:758, 1999).* Primary prophylaxis not generally recommended. Preemptive therapy in pts with ↑ CMV DNA titers in plasma & CD4 <100/mm³. Recommended by some: **valganciclovir** 900 mg po q24h *(CID 32: 783, 2001).* Authors rec. primary prophylaxis be dc if response to HAART with ↑ CD4 >100 for 6 mos. *(MMWR 53:98, 2004).*
Colitis, Esophagitis Dx by biopsy of ulcer base/edge *(Clin Gastro Hepatol 2:564, 2004)* with demonstration of CMV inclusions & other pathogen(s).	**Ganciclovir** as with retinitis except induction period extended for 3–6wks. No agreement on use of maintenance; may not be necessary except after relapse. Responses less predictable than for retinitis. **Valganciclovir also likely effective.** Switch to oral valganciclovir when po tolerated & severe enough to interfere with absorption. Antiretroviral therapy is essential in long term suppression.	
Encephalitis, Ventriculitis: Treatment not defined, but should be considered the same as retinitis. Disease may develop while taking ganciclovir as suppressive therapy. *See Herpes 11(Suppl.12):95A, 2004.* Lumbosacral polyradiculopathy: diagnosis by CMV DNA in CSF.	**Ganciclovir**, as with retinitis. Consider combination of ganciclovir & foscarnet, esp. if prior CMV rx used. Switch to **valganciclovir** when possible. Suppression continued until CD4 remains >100/mm³ for 6 mos.	About 50% will respond; survival ↑ (5.4wks to 14.6wks) *(CID 27:345, 1998).* Resistance can be demonstrated genotypically.
Mononeuritis multiplex	Not defined	Due to vasculitis & may not be responsive to antiviral therapy.
Pneumonia— Seen predominantly in transplants (esp. bone marrow), **rare in HIV.** Treat only when histological evidence resent in IDS pts & other pathogens not identified.	**Ganciclovir/valganciclovir**, as with retinitis. In bone marrow transplant pts, combination therapy with CMV immune globulin.	In bone marrow transplant pts, serial measure of pp65 antigen was useful in establishing early diagnosis of CMV interstitial pneumonia with good results if ganciclovir was initiated within 6 days of antigen positivity *(Bone Marrow Transplant 26:413, 2000).* For preventive therapy, see Table 10.
CMV Retinitis Most common cause of blindness in AIDS patients with <50/mm3 CD4 counts. 19/30 pts (63%) with inactive CMV retinitis who responded to HAART (↑ of ≥60 CD4 cells/mL) developed immune recovery vitreitis (vision ↓ & floaters with posterior segment inflammation — vitreitis, papillitis & macular changes) an average of 43 wks after rx started *(JID 179: 697, 1999).* Corticosteroid rx ↓ inflammatory reaction of immune recovery vitreitis without reactivation of CMV retinitis, either periocular corticosteroids or short course of systemic steroid.	**For immediate sight-threatening lesions:** **Ganciclovir** intraocular implant & **valganciclovir** 900 mg po q24h. **For peripheral lesions:** **Valganciclovir** 900 mg po q12h x 14–21d, then 900 mg po q24h for maintenance therapy	Differential diagnosis: HIV retinopathy, herpes simplex retinitis, varicella-zoster retinitis (rare, hard to diagnose) *(NEJM 346:1119, 2002).* Cannot use ganciclovir ocular implant alone as approx. 50% risk of CMV retinitis other eye at 6 mos. & 31% risk visceral disease. Risk ↓ with systemic rx but when contralateral retinitis does occur, ganciclovir-resistant mutation often present *(JID 189:611, 2004).* **Concurrent systemic rx recommended!**
	Ganciclovir 5 mg/kg IV q12h x 14–21d, then **valganciclovir** 900 mg po q24h **OR** **Foscarnet** 60 mg/kg IV q8h or 90 mg/kg IV q12h x 14–21d, then 90–120 mg/kg IV q24h **OR** **Cidofovir** 5 mg/kg IV x 2wks, then 5 mg/kg every other wk: each dose should be administered with IV saline hydration & oral probenecid **OR** Repeated intravitreal injections with **fomivirsen** (for relapses only, not as initial therapy)	Because of unique mode of action, **fomivirsen** may have a role as isolates become resistant to other therapies. Retinal detachments 50–60% within 1yr of dx of retinitis. *(Ophthal 111:2232, 2004.)* Equal efficacy of IV GCV & FOS. GCV avoids nephrotoxicity of FOS; FOS avoids bone marrow suppression of GCV. Although bone marrow toxicity may be similar to ganciclovir. **Oral valganciclovir should replace both.**
Pts who discontinue suppression therapy should undergo regular eye examination for early detection of relapses!	**Post treatment suppression** (Prophylactic) if CD4 count <100/mm³: **Valganciclovir** 900 mg po q24h.	Discontinue if CD4 >100/mm³ × 6 mos on HAART0.
CMV in Transplant patients: *See Table 15E.* Use of **valganciclovir** to prevent infections in CMV seronegative recipients who receive organs from a seropositive donor & in seropositive receivers has been highly effective *(Ln 365:2105, 2005).* Others suggest preemptive rx when pt develops CMV antigenemia or positive PCR post-transplant *(Transplant 79:85, 2005).*		

* *See page 3 for abbreviations.* NOTE: All dosage recommendations are for adults (unless otherwise indicated) and assume normal renal function.

TABLE 14A (5)

VIRUS/DISEASE	DRUG/DOSAGE	SIDE EFFECTS/COMMENTS
Herpesvirus Infections *(continued)*		
Epstein Barr Virus (EBV)—Mononucleosis *(Ln ID 3:131, 2003)*	**No treatment.** Corticosteroids for tonsillar obstruction, CNS complications, or threat of splenic rupture.	*(See JAC 56:277, 2005 for current status of drugs in development.)*
HHV-6—Implicated as cause of roseola (exanthem subitum) & other febrile diseases of childhood *(NEJM 352:768, 2005)*. Fever & rash documented in transplant pts *(JID 179:311, 1999)*. Reactivation in 47% of 110 U.S. hematopoietic stem cell transplant pts assoc. with delayed monocytes & platelet engraftment *(CID 40:932, 2005)*. Recognized in assoc. with meningoencephalitis in immunocompetent adults. Diagnosis made by pos. PCR in CSF. ↓ viral copies in response to **ganciclovir** rx *(CID 40:890 & 894, 2005)*. Foscarnet therapy improved thrombotic microangiopathy *(Am J Hematol 76:156, 2004)*.		
HHV-7—ubiquitous virus (>90% of the population is infected by age 3 yrs). No relationship to human disease. Infects CD4 lymphocytes via CD4 receptor; transmitted via saliva.		
HHV-8—The agent of Kaposi's sarcoma, Castleman's disease, & body cavity lymphoma	**No antiviral treatment.** Effective anti-HIV therapy may help.	Localized lesions: radiotherapy, laser surgery or intralesional chemotherapy. Systemic: chemotherapy. Castleman's disease responded to ganciclovir *(Blood 103:1632, 2004)* & valganciclovir *(JID 2006)*.
Herpes simplex virus (HSV Types 1 & 2)		
Bell's palsy H. simplex most implicated etiology. Other etiologic considerations: VZV, HHV-6, Lyme disease.	As soon as possible after onset of palsy: 1) **Prednisone** 1 mg/kg po divided bid x 5 days then taper to 5 mg bid over the next 5 days (total of 10 days prednisone) + 2) **Valacyclovir** 500 mg bid x 5 days	Prospective randomized double blind placebo controlled trial compared prednisone vs acyclovir vs (prednisolone + acyclovir) vs placebo. Best result with prednisolone: 85% recovery with placebo, 96% recovery with prednisolone, 93% with combination of steroid & prednisolone *(NEJM 357:1598 & 1653, 2007)*. Similar study design using valaciclovir showed best outcome with combination of steroid & valacyclovir *(Otol Neurol 28:408, 2007)*
Encephalitis (Excellent reviews: *CID 35: 254, 2002)*. UK experience *(EID 9:234, 2003; Eur J Neurol 12:331, 2005; Antiviral Res : 141-148, 2006)*	**Acyclovir** IV 10 mg/kg IV (infuse over 1 hr) q8h x 14–21 days. Up to 20 mg/kg q8h in children <12 yrs	HSV-1 is most common cause of sporadic encephalitis. Survival & recovery from neurological sequelae are related to mental status at time of initiation of rx. **Early dx and rx imperative.** Mortality rate reduced from >70% to 19% with acyclovir rx. PCR analysis of CSF for HSV-1 DNA is 100% specific & 75–98% sensitive. 8/33 (25%) CSF samples drawn before day 3 were neg. by PCR; neg. PCR assoc. with ↓ protein & <10 WBC per mm^3 in CSF *(CID 36:1335, 2003)*. All were + after 3 days. Relapse after successful rx reported in 7/27 (27%) children. Relapse was associated with a lower total dose of initial acyclovir rx (285 ± 82 mg per kg in relapse group vs. 462 ± 149 mg per kg, p <0.03) *(CID 30:185, 2000; Neuropediatrics 35:371, 2004)*.
Genital Herpes: Sexually Transmitted Treatment Guidelines 2006: www.cdc.gov/std/treatment/2006/genital-ulcers.htm, MMWR Recomm Rep. 2006 Aug 4:55 (RR-11):1-94.		
Primary (initial episode)	**Acyclovir** (Zovirax or generic) 400 mg po tid x 7–10 days OR	↓ by 2 days time to resolution of signs & symptoms, ↓ by 4 days time to healing of lesions, ↓ by 7 days duration of viral shedding. Does not prevent recurrences. For severe cases only: 5 mg per kg IV q8h times 5–7 days.
	Valacyclovir (Valtrex) 1000 mg po bid x 7-10 days OR	An ester of acyclovir, which is well absorbed, bioavailability 3–5 times greater than acyclovir.
	Famciclovir (Famvir) 250 mg po tid x 7–10 days	Metabolized to penciclovir, which is active component. Side effects and activity similar to acyclovir. **Famciclovir** 250 mg po tid **equal to acyclovir** 200 mg 5 times per day.
Episodic recurrences	**Acyclovir** 800 mg po tid **x 2 days** or 400 mg po tid **x 5 days** or **Famciclovir** 1000 mg bid **x 1 day** or 125 mg po bid x 5 days or **Valacyclovir** 500 mg po bid **x 3 days** or 1 gm po once daily **x 5 days** For HIV patients, *see Comment*	For episodic recurrences in HIV patients: **acyclovir** 400 mg po tid x 5-10 days or **famciclovir** 500 mg po bid x 5-10 days or **valacyclovir** 1 gm po bid x 5-10 days

* *See page 3 for abbreviations.* NOTE: All dosage recommendations are for adults (unless otherwise indicated) and assume normal renal function.

TABLE 14A (6)

VIRUS/DISEASE	DRUG/DOSAGE *(continued)*	SIDE EFFECTS/COMMENTS

Herpesvirus Infections/Herpes Simplex Virus (HSV Types 1 & 2)/Genital Herpes

VIRUS/DISEASE	DRUG/DOSAGE	SIDE EFFECTS/COMMENTS
Chronic daily suppression	**Suppressive therapy reduces the frequency of genital herpes recurrences by 70–80% among pts who have frequent recurrences (i.e., >6 recurrences per yr) & many report no symptomatic outbreaks.** **Acyclovir** 400 mg po bid, **or famciclovir** 250 mg po bid, **or valacyclovir** 1 gm po q24h; pts with <9 recurrences per yr could use 500 mg po q24h and then use valaciclovir 1 gm po q24h if breakthrough at 500 mg. For HIV patients, see *Comment*	For chronic suppression in HIV patients: **acyclovir** 400-800 mg po bid or tid or **famciclovir** 500 mg po bid or **valacyclovir** 500 mg po bid
Genital, immunocompetent Gingivostomatitis, primary (children)	**Acyclovir** 15 mg/kg po 5x/day x 7 days	Efficacy in randomized double-blind placebo-controlled trial *(BMJ 314:1800, 1997)*.
Kerato-conjunctivitis and recurrent epithelial keratitis	**Trifluridine** (Viroptic). 1 drop 1% solution q2h (max. 9 drops per day) for max. of 21 days *(see Table 1A, page 13)*	In controlled trials, response % > idoxuridine. Suppressive rx with acyclovir (400 mg bid) reduced recurrences of ocular HSV from 32% to 19% *(NEJM 339:300, 1998)*.
Mollaret's recurrent "aseptic" meningitis (usually HSV-2) *(Ln 363:1772, 2004)*	No controlled trials of antiviral rx & resolves spontaneously. If therapy is to be given, IV acyclovir (15–30 mg/kg/day) should be used.	Pos. PCR for HSV in CSF confirms dx *(EJCMID 23:560, 2004)*. Daily suppression rx might ↓ frequency of recurrence but no clinical trials.

Mucocutaneous *(for genital see previous page)*
Oral labial, "fever blisters":

VIRUS/DISEASE	DRUG/DOSAGE	SIDE EFFECTS/COMMENTS
Normal host See *Ann Pharmacotherapy 38:705, 2004; JAC 53:703, 2004*	Start rx with prodrome symptoms (tingling/burning) before lesions show. <table><tr><td>**Drug**</td><td>**Dose**</td><td>**Sx Decrease**</td></tr><tr><td>**Oral:** Valacyclovir</td><td>2 gm po q12h x 1 day</td><td>↓ 1 day</td></tr><tr><td>Famciclovir[1]</td><td>500 mg po bid x 7 days</td><td>↓ 2 days</td></tr><tr><td>Acyclovir[NFDA]</td><td>400 mg po 5 x per day (q4h while awake) x 5 daysc)</td><td>↓ ½ day</td></tr></table> **Topical:** Penciclovir 1% cream — q2h during day x 4 days — ↓ 1 day Acyclovir 5% cream[2] — 6x/day (q3h) x 7 days — ↓ ½ day [1] FDA approved only for HIV pts; [2] Approved for immunocompromised pts. See *Table 1A, page 25*	Penciclovir *(J Derm Treat 13:67, 2002; JAMA 277:1374, 1997; AAC 46: 2848, 2002)*. Docosanol *(J Am Acad Derm 45:222, 2001)*. Oral acyclovir 5% cream *(AAC 46:2238, 2002)*. Oral famciclovir *(JID 179:303, 1999)*. Topical fluocinonide (0.05% Lidex gel) q8h times 5 days in combination with famciclovir ↓ lesion size and pain when compared to famciclovir alone *(JID 181:1906, 2000)*.

(dashed line — Herpes Whitlow)

VIRUS/DISEASE	DRUG/DOSAGE	SIDE EFFECTS/COMMENTS
Oral labial or genital: immunocompromised (includes pts with AIDS) and critically ill pts in ICU setting/large necrotic ulcers in perineum or face. *(See Comment)*	**Acyclovir** 5 mg per kg IV (infused over 1 hr) q8h times 7 days (250 mg per M[2]) or 400 mg po 5 times per day times 14–21 days *(see Comment if suspect acyclovir-resistant)* **OR Famciclovir**: In HIV infected, 500 mg po bid for 7 days for recurrent episodes of genital herpes **OR Valacyclovir[NFDA-I]**: In HIV-infected, 500 mg po bid for 5–10 days for recurrent episodes of genital herpes or 500 mg po bid for chronic suppressive rx.	**Acyclovir-resistant HSV**: IV foscarnet *(For dose see Table 14A)*. Suppressive therapy with famciclovir (500 mg po bid), valacyclovir (500 mg po bid) or acyclovir (400-800 mg po bid) reduces viral shedding and clinical recurrences.
Pregnancy and genital H. simplex	Acyclovir safe even in first trimester. No proof that acyclovir at delivery reduces risk/severity of neonatal Herpes. In contrast, C-section in women with active lesions reduces risk of transmission. Ref. *Obstet Gyn 106:845, 2006.*	

* *See page 3 for abbreviations. NOTE: All dosage recommendations are for adults (unless otherwise indicated) and assume normal renal function.*

TABLE 14A (7)

VIRUS/DISEASE	DRUG/DOSAGE	SIDE EFFECTS/COMMENTS
Herpesvirus Infections (continued)		
Herpes simiae (Herpes B virus): **Monkey bite** CID 35:1191, 2002	**Postexposure prophylaxis:** Valacyclovir 1 gm po q8h times 14 days or acyclovir 800 mg po 5 times per day times 14 days. **Treatment of disease:** (1) CNS symptoms absent: Acyclovir 12.5–15 mg per kg IV q8h or ganciclovir 5 mg per kg IV q12h. (2) CNS symptoms present: Ganciclovir 5 mg per kg IV q12h	Fatal human cases of myelitis and hemorrhagic encephalitis have been reported following bites, scratches, or eye inoculation of saliva from monkeys. Initial sx include fever, headache, myalgias and diffuse adenopathy, incubation period of 2–14 days (EID 9:246, 2003). In vitro ACV and ganciclovir less active than other nucleosides (pencyclovir or 5-ethyldeoxyuridine may be more active; clinical data needed)(AAC 51:2028, 2007).
Varicella-Zoster Virus (VZV) **Varicella:** Vaccination has markedly ↓ incidence of varicella & morbidity (NEJM 352:450, 2005; NEJM 353:2377, 2005 & NEJM 356:1338, 2007).		
Normal host (chickenpox) Child (2–12 years)	**In general, treatment not recommended.** Might use oral **acyclovir** for healthy persons at ↑ risk for moderate to severe varicella, ie, >12yrs of age; chronic cutaneous or pulmonary diseases; chronic salicylate rx (↑ risk of Reye syndrome), **acyclovir** dose: 20 mg/kg po qid x 5 days (start within 24 hrs of rash).	Acyclovir slowed development and ↓ number of new lesions and ↓ duration of disease in children: 9 to 7.6 days (PIDJ 21:739, 2002). Oral dose of acyclovir in children should not exceed 80 mg per kg per day or 3200 mg per day.
Adolescents, young adults	**Acyclovir** 800 mg po 5x/day x 5–7 days (start within 24 hrs of rash) or **valacyclovir**[NFDA-1] 1000 mg po 3x/day x 5 days. **Famciclovir**[NFDA-1] 500 mg po 3x/day probably effective but data lacking.	↓ duration of fever, time to healing, and symptoms (AnIM 130:922, 1999).
Pneumonia or chickenpox in 3rd trimester of pregnancy	**Acyclovir** 800 mg po 5 times per day or 10 mg per kg IV q8h times 5 days. Risks and benefits to fetus and mother still unknown. Many experts recommend rx, especially in 3rd trimester. Some would add VZIG (varicella-zoster immune globulin).	Varicella pneumonia associated with 41% mortality in pregnancy Acyclovir ↓ incidence and severity (JID 185:422, 2002). If varicella-susceptible mother exposed and respiratory symptoms develop within 10 days after exposure, start acyclovir
Immunocompromised host	**Acyclovir** 10–12 mg per kg (500 mg per M²) IV (infused over 1 hr) q8h times 7 days	Disseminated 1° varicella infection reported during infliximab rx of rheumatoid arthritis (J Rheum 31:2517, 2004). Continuous infusion of high-dose acyclovir (2 mg per kg per hr) successful in 1 pt with severe hemorrhagic varicella (NEJM 336:732, 1997). Mortality high (43%) in AIDS pts (Int J Inf Dis 6:6, 2002).
Prevention—Post-exposure prophylaxis Varicella deaths still occur in unvacci-nated persons (MMWR 56 (RR-4) 1–40, 2007)	**CDC Recommendations for Prevention:** Since <5% of cases of varicella but >50% of varicella-related deaths occur in adults >20 yrs of age, the CDC recommends a more aggressive approach in this age group: **1st, varicella-zoster immune globulin** (VZIG) (125units/10 kg (22 lbs) body weight IM up to a max. of 625 units; minimum dose is 125 units) is recommended for post-exposure prophylaxis in susceptible persons at greater risk for complications (immunocompromised such as HIV, malignancies, pregnancy, and steroid therapy) as soon as possible after exposure (<96 hrs). If varicella develops, initiate treatment quickly (<24 hrs of rash) with **acyclovir** as below. Some would rx presumptively with acyclovir in high-risk pts. **2nd,** susceptible adults should be vaccinated. Check antibody in adults with negative or uncertain history of varicella (10–30% will be Ab-neg.) and vaccinate those who are Ab-neg. **3rd,** susceptible children should receive vaccination. Recommended routinely before age 12–18 mos. but OK at any age.	

* See page 3 for abbreviations. NOTE: All dosage recommendations are for adults (unless otherwise indicated) and assume normal renal function.

TABLE 14A (8)

VIRUS/DISEASE	DRUG/DOSAGE	SIDE EFFECTS/COMMENTS
Herpesvirus Infections/Herpes Varicella-Zoster Virus (VZV) *(continued)*		
Herpes zoster (shingles) *(See NEJM 342:635, 2000 & 347:340, 2002)*	**[NOTE: Trials showing benefit of therapy: only in pts treated within 3 days of onset of rash]**	
Normal host Effective therapy most evident in pts >50 yrs.	**Valacyclovir** 1000 mg po tid times 7 days (adjust dose for renal failure) *(See Table 17)* **OR**	Valacyclovir ↓ post-herpetic neuralgia more rapidly than acyclovir in pts >50 yrs of age: median duration of zoster-associated pain was 38 days with valacyclovir and 51 days on acyclovir *(AAC 39:1546, 1995)*. Toxicity of both drugs similar *(Arch Fam Med 9:863, 2000)*.
(For treatment of post-herpetic neuralgia, see CID 36: 877, 2003) 25-fold ↓ in zoster after immunization *(MMWR 48:R-6, 1999)*	**Famciclovir** 500 mg tid x 7 days. Adjust for renal failure *(see Table 17)*	Time to healing more rapid. Reduced post-herpetic neuralgia (PHN) vs placebo in pts >50 yrs of age: duration of PHN with famciclovir 63 days, placebo 163 days. Famciclovir similar to acyclovir in reduction of acute pain and PHN *(J Micro Immunol Inf 37:75, 2004)*.
New vaccine ↓ herpes zoster & post-herpetic neuralgia *(NEJM 352: 2271, 2005; JAMA 292:157, 2006)*. Reviewed in *J Am Acad Derm 58:361, 2008*.	**OR** **Acyclovir** 800 mg po 5 times per day times 7–10 days	A meta-analysis of 4 placebo-controlled trials (691 pts) demonstrated that acyclovir accelerated by approx. 2-fold pain resolution by all measures employed and reduced post-herpetic neuralgia at 3 & 6 mos *(CID 22:341, 1996)*; med. time to resolution of pain 41 days vs 101 days in those >50 yrs.
	Add **Prednisone** in pts over 50 yrs old to decrease discomfort during acute phase of zoster. Does not decrease incidence of post-herpetic neuralgia. Dose: 30 mg po bid days 1–7, 15 mg bid days 8–14 and 7.5 mg bid days 15–21.	Prednisone added to acyclovir improved quality of life measurements (↓ acute pain, sleep, and return to normal activity) *(AnIM 125:376, 1996)*. In post-herpetic neuralgia, controlled trials demonstrated effectiveness of gabapentin, the lidocaine patch (5%) & opioid analgesic in controlling pain *(Drugs 64:937, 2004; J Clin Virol 29:248, 2004)*. Nortriptyline & amitriptyline are equally effective but nortriptyline is better tolerated *(CID 36:877, 2003)*. Role of antiviral drugs in rx of PHN unproven *(Neurol 64:21, 2005)* but 8 of 15 pt improved with IV acyclovir 10 mg/kg q 8 hrs x 14 days followed by oral valacyclovir 1 gm 3x a day for 1 month *(Arch Neur 63:940, 2006)*.
Immunocompromised host Not severe	**Acyclovir** 800 mg po 5 times per day times 7 days. (Options: **Famciclovir** 750 mg po q24h or 500 mg bid or 250 mg 3 times per day times 7 days **OR valacyclovir** 1000 mg po tid times 7 days, though both are not FDA-approved for this indication)	If progression, switch to IV
Severe: >1 dermatome, trigeminal nerve or disseminated	**Acyclovir** 10–12 mg per kg IV (infusion over 1 hr) q8h times 7–14 days. In older pts, ↓ to 7.5 mg per kg. If nephrotoxicity and pt improving, ↓ to 5 mg per kg q8h.	A common manifestation of immune reconstitution following HAART in HIV-infected children *(J All Clin Immun 113:742, 2004)*. Rx must be begun within 72 hrs. Acyclovir-resistant VZV occurs in HIV+ pts previously treated with acyclovir. Foscarnet (40 mg per kg IV q8h for 14–26 days) successful in 4/5 pts but 2 relapsed in 7 and 14 days *(AnIM 115:19, 1991)*.

* See page 3 for abbreviations. NOTE: All dosage recommendations are for adults (unless otherwise indicated) and assume normal renal function.

TABLE 14A (9)

VIRUS/DISEASE	DRUG/DOSAGE	SIDE EFFECTS/COMMENTS
Influenza (A & B) (*MMWR 56:1, 2007*) **Suspect or proven acute disease** Rapid diagnostic tests available but sensitivity limited. Antiviral therapy cost-effective without viral testing in febrile pt with typical symptoms during influenza season. New IDSA Guidelines due in Spring 2009.	**If fever & cough; known community influenza activity; and 1st 48 hrs of illness, consider:** **For influenza A & B; also avian (H5N1):** **Oseltamivir** 75 mg po bid times 5 days (also approved for rx of children age 1–12 yrs, dose 2 mg per kg up to a total of 75 mg bid times 5 days) or **Zanamivir** 2 inhalations (2 times 5 mg) bid times 5 days.	Pts with COPD or asthma, **potential risk of bronchospasm with zanamivir.** All ↓ duration of symptoms by approx. 50% (1–2 days) if given within 30–36 hrs after onset of symptoms. Benefit influenced by duration of sx before rx; initiation of oseltamivir within 1st 12 hrs after fever onset ↓ total median illness duration by 74.6 hrs (*JAC 51:123, 2003*). ↓ risk of pneumonia (*Curr Med Res Opin 21:761, 2005*). **Watch for Emergence of Resistance:** oseltamivir-resistant virus detected after 4 days of rx (*Ln 364: 733 & 759, 2004*). In another study of 298 rx cases of adults & children, no oseltamivir-resistant viruses found (*JID 189:440, 2004*).
Pathogenic avian influenza (H5N1) emerged in poultry (mainly chickens & ducks) in East & South-east Asia. From Dec 1, 2003 to August 30, 2006, 246 laboratory confirmed cases reported in 10 countries with 144 deaths (see *www.cdc.gov/flu/avian*). Human-to-human transmission reported; most have had direct contact with poultry. Mortality highest in young age 10-19 (73%) vs. 50% overall and associated with high viral load and cytokine-storm (*Nature Medicine Sept, 2006*). Human isolates resistant to amantadine/rimantadine. Oseltamivir therapy recommended if avian H5N1 suspected. ↑ dose & duration of oseltamivir necessary for maximum effect in mouse model (*JID 192:665, 2005; Nature 435:419, 2005*).	Note: CDC Advisory 12/19/2008. New treatment recommendations due to near 100% resistance of influenza A/H1N1 isolates to oseltamivir. The A/H1N1 isolates are (so far) sensitive to zanamivir, amantadine, and rimantadine. For full treatment recommendations: www.cdc.gov/flu/professionals/antivirals/recommendations.htm	Report of increasing resistance in up to 18% of children with H5N1 treated with oseltamivir and less responsive H5N1 virus in several patients (*J Virology 79(10):1577-86*). Less resistance to zanamivir so far. ↑ concern about post-influenza complications including community-associated MRSA pneumonia (*CID 40:1693, 2005*). Review in *Crit Care Med 39:2660, Sept 2008*.
Prevention	**Prevention of influenza A & B:** give vaccine and if ≥13 yrs age, consider **oseltamivir** 75 mg po q24h for duration of peak influenza in community or for outbreak control in high-risk populations (*CID 39:459, 2004*). (Consider for similar populations as immunization recommendations.)	Immunization contraindicated if hypersensitivity to hen's eggs. Zanamavir also approved for prophylaxis: 2 inhalations (10 mg) once daily x 10 days (household exposure) or 28 days (community exposure).
Measles While measles in the US is at the lowest rates ever (55/100,000) much higher rates reported in developing countries (*CID 42:322, 2006*).		
Children	No therapy or **vitamin A** 200,000 units po daily times 2 days	Vitamin A may ↓ severity of measles.
Adults	No rx or **ribavirin** IV: 20–35 mg per day times 7 days	↓ severity of illness in adults (*CID 20:454, 1994*).
Metapneumovirus (HMPV) A paramyxovirus isolated from pts of all ages, with mild bronchiolitis/bronchospasm to pneumonia (*PIDJ 23:S215, 2004*). Can cause lethal pneumonia in HSCT pts (*Ann Intern Med 144:344, 2006*).	**No proven antiviral therapy** (intravenous ribavirin used anecdotally with variable results)	Human metapneumovirus isolated from 6-21% of children with RTIs (*JID 190, 20 & 27, 2004; NEJM 350:443, 2004 & PIDJ 23:436, 2004*). Dual infection with RSV assoc. with severe bronchiolitis (*JID 191:382, 2005*).
Monkey pox (orthopox virus) (see *LnID 4:17, 2004*) Outbreak from contact will kill prairie dogs. Source likely imported Gambian giant rats (*MMWR 42:642, 2003*).	**No proven antiviral therapy.** Cidofovir is active in vitro & in mouse model (*AAC 46:1329, 2002; Antiviral Res 57:13, 2003*) (*Potential new drugs Virol J 4:8, 2007*)	Incubation period of 12 days, then fever, headache, cough, adenopathy, & a vesicular papular rash that pustulates, umbilicates, & crusts on the head, trunk, & extremities. Transmission in healthcare setting rare (*CID 40:789, 2005; CID 41:1742, 2005, CID 41:1765, 2005*).
Norovirus (Norwalk-like virus, or NLV) Vast majority of outbreaks of non-bacterial gastroenteritis.	**No antiviral therapy.** Replete volume. Transmission by contaminated food, fecal-oral contact with contaminated surfaces, or fomites.	Sudden onset of nausea, vomiting, and/or watery diarrhea lasting 12–60 hours. Ethanol-based hand rubs effective (*J Hosp Inf 60:144, 2005*).

* *See page 3 for abbreviations.* NOTE: All dosage recommendations are for adults (unless otherwise indicated) and assume normal renal function.

146

TABLE 14A (10)

VIRUS/DISEASE	DRUG/DOSAGE	SIDE EFFECTS/COMMENTS
Papillomaviruses: Warts. For human papillomavirus vaccine, see *TABLE 20B*, page 187		
External Genital Warts	***Patient applied:*** **Podofilox** (0.5% solution or gel): apply 2x/day x 3 days, 4th day no therapy, repeat cycle 4x; OR **Imiquimod** 5% cream: apply once daily hs 3x/wk for up to 16 wks. **Provider administered:** Cryotherapy with liquid nitrogen; repeat q1-2 wks; OR **Podophyllin resin** 10-25% in tincture of benzoin. Repeat weekly as needed; OR **Trichloroacetic acid** (TCA): repeat weekly as needed; OR surgical removal.	**Podofilox:** Inexpensive and safe (pregnancy safety not established). Mild irritation after treatment. **Imiquimod:** Mild to moderate redness & irritation. Safety in pregnancy not established. **Cryotherapy:** blistering and skin necrosis common. **Podophyllin resin:** Must air dry before treated area contacts clothing. Can irritate adjacent skin. **TCA:** caustic. Can cause severe pain on adjacent normal skin. Neutralize with soap or sodium bicarbonate.
Warts on cervix	Need evaluation for evolving neoplasia	Gynecological consult advised
Vaginal warts	Cryotherapy with liquid nitrogen or **TCA**	
Urethral warts	Cryotherapy with liquid nitrogen or **Podophyllin resin** 10-25% in tincture of benzoin	
Anal warts	Cryotherapy with liquid nitrogen or **TCA** or surgical removal	Advise anoscopy to look for rectal warts.
Skin papillomas	Topical α-lactalbumin. **Oleic acid** (from human milk) applied 1x/day for 3 wks	↓ lesion size & recurrence vs placebo (p <0.001) (*NEJM 350:2663, 2004*). Further studies warranted.
Parvo B19 Virus (Erythrovirus B19). *Review: NEJM 350:586, 2004. Wide range of manifestation.* **Treatment options for common symptomatic infections:**		
Erythema infectiosum	Symptomatic treatment only	Diagnostic tools: IgM and Igb antibody titers. Perhaps better: blood parvovirus PCR.
Arthritis/arthalgia	Nonsteroidal anti-inflammatory drugs (NSAID)	Dose of IVIG not standardized; suggest 400 mg/kg IV of commercial IVIG for 5 or 10 days or 1000 mg/kg IV for 3 days.
Transient aplastic crisis	Transfusions and oxygen	Most dramatic anemias in pts with pre-existing hemolytic anemia.
Fetal hydrope	Intrauterine blood tranfusion	Bone marrow shown erythrocyte maturation arrest with giant pronormoblasts.
Chronic infection with anemia	**IVIG** and transfusion	
Chronic infection without anemia	perhaps **IVIG**	
Papovavirus/Polyomavirus		
Progressive multifocal leukoencephalopathy (PML) Serious demyelinating disease due to JC virus in immunocompromised pts.	No specific therapy for JC virus. Two general approaches: 1. In HIV pts: HAART 2. Stop or decrease immunosuppressive therapy.	Failure of treatment with interferon alfa-2b, cytarabine and topotocan. Immunosuppressive natalizumab temporarily removed from market due to reported associations with PML. Mixed reports on cidofovir. Most likely effective in pts with HAART experience.
BK virus induced nephropathy in immunocompromised pts: e.g., hemorrhagic cystitis, urethral stenosis, interstitial nephritis	Decrease immunosuppression if possible. Suggested antiviral therapy based on anecdotal data. If progressive renal dysfunction: 1. **Fluoroquinolone** first; 2. **IVIG** 500 mg/kg IV; 3. **Leflunomide** 100 mg po daily x 3 days, then 10-20 mg po daily; 4. **Cidofovir** only if refractory to all of the above (*see Table 14B for dose*).	Use PCR to monitor viral "load" in urine and/or plasma.

* *See page 3 for abbreviations.* NOTE: All dosage recommendations are for adults (unless otherwise indicated) and assume normal renal function.

TABLE 14A (11)

VIRUS/DISEASE	DRUG/DOSAGE	SIDE EFFECTS/COMMENTS
Rabies (see Table 20D, page 191; see MMWR 54:RR-3:1, 2005, CDC Guidelines for Prevention and Control 2006, MMWR/55/RR-5,2006) Rabid dogs account for 50,000 cases per yr worldwide. Most cases in the U.S. are cryptic, i.e., no documented evidence of bite or contact with a rabid animal (CID 35:738, 2003). 70% assoc. with 2 rare bat species (EID 9:151, 2003). An organ donor with early rabies infected 4 recipients (2 kidneys, liver & artery) who all died of rabies avg. 13 days after transplant (NEJM 352:1103, 2005).	**Mortality 100% with only survivors those who receive rabies vaccine before the onset of illness/symptoms** (CID 36:61, 2003). A 15-year-old female who developed rabies 1 month post-bat bite survived after drug induction of coma (+ other rx) for 7 days; did not receive immunoprophylaxis (NEJM 352:2508, 2005).	Corticosteroids ↑ mortality rate and ↓ incubation time in mice. Therapies that have failed after symptoms develop include rabies vaccine, rabies immuno-globulin, rabies virus neutralizing antibody, ribavirin, alfa interferon, & ketamine.
Respiratory Syncytial Virus (RSV) Major cause of morbidity in neonates/infants.	Hydration, supplemental oxygen. Routine use of ribavirin not recommended. Ribavirin therapy associated with small increases in O₂ saturation. No consistent decrease in need for mech. ventilation or ICU stays. High cost, aerosol administration & potential toxicity (Red Book of Pediatrics, 2006).	In adults, RSV accounted for 10.6% of hospitalizations for pneumonia, 11.4% for COPD, 7.2% for asthma & 5.4% for CHF in pts >65 yrs of age (NEJM 352:1749, 2005). RSV caused 11% of clinically important respiratory illnesses in military recruits (CID 41:311, 2005).
Prevention of RSV in: (1) Children <24 mos. old with chronic lung disease of prematurity (formerly broncho-pulmonary dysplasia) requiring supple-mental O₂ or (2) Premature infants (<32 wks gestation) and <6 mos. old at start of RSV season or (3) Children with selected congenital heart diseases	**Palivizumab** (Synagis) 15 mg per kg IM q month Nov.-April. Ref: Red Book of Pediatrics, 2006.	Expense argues against its use, but in 2004 approx. 100,000 infants received drug annually in U.S. (PIDJ 23:1051, 2004). Significant reduction in RSV hospitalization among children with congenital heart disease (Expert Opin Biol Ther.7:1471-80, 2007)
Rhinovirus (Colds) See Ln 361:51, 2003 Found in 1/2 of children with community-acquired pneumonia; role in pathogenesis unclear (CID 39:681, 2004). Antiviral Kleenex may reduce spread (Med Lett 47:3, 2005).	No antiviral rx indicated (Ped Ann 34:53, 2005). Symptomatic rx: • ipratropium bromide nasal (2 sprays per nostril tid) • clemastine 1.34 mg 1–2 tab po bid–tid (OTC)	Sx relief: ipratropium nasal spray ↓ rhinorrhea and sneezing vs placebo (AnIM 125:89, 1996). Clemastine (an antihistamine) ↓ sneezing, rhinorrhea but associated with dry nose, mouth & throat in 6–19% (CID 22:656, 1996). Oral **pleconaril** given within 24 hrs of onset reduced duration (1 day) & severity of "cold symptoms" in DBPCT (p < .001) (CID 36:1523, 2003). Echinacea didn't work (CID 38:1367, 2004 & 40:807, 2005)—put it to rest!
Rotavirus: Leading recognized cause of diarrhea-related illness among infants and children world-wide and kills ½ million children annually.	No antiviral rx available; oral hydration life-saving. In one study, **Nitazoxanide 7.5 mg/kg 2x/d x 3 days** reduced duration of illness from 75 to 31 hrs in Egyptian children. Impact on rotavirus or other parameters not measured. (Lancet 368:100 & 124, 2006) Too early to recommend routine use (Lancet 368:100, 2006)	Two live-attenuated vaccines highly effective (85 and 98%) and safe in preventing rotavirus diarrhea and hospitalization (NEJM 354: 1 & 23, 2006)
SARS-CoV: See page 137		
Smallpox (NEJM 346:1300, 2002) **Contact vaccinia** (JAMA 288:1901, 2002)	Smallpox vaccine (if within 4 days of exposure) + cidofovir (dosage uncertain; contact CDC: 770-488-7100) From vaccination: Progressive vaccinia—vaccinia immune globulin may be of benefit. To obtain immune globulin, contact CDC: 770-488-7100 (CID 39:759, 776 & 819, 2004)	
West Nile virus: See page 138		

* See page 3 for abbreviations. NOTE: All dosage recommendations are for adults (unless otherwise indicated) and assume normal renal function.

TABLE 14B – ANTIVIRAL DRUGS (OTHER THAN RETROVIRAL)

DRUG NAME(S) GENERIC (TRADE)	DOSAGE/ROUTE IN ADULTS*	COMMENTS/ADVERSE EFFECTS
CMV (See *SANFORD GUIDE TO HIV/AIDS THERAPY*)		
Cidofovir (Vistide)	5 mg per kg IV once weekly for 2 weeks, then once every other week. **Properly timed IV prehydration with normal saline & Probenecid must be used with each cidofovir infusion:** 2 gm po 3 hrs before each dose and further 1 gm doses 2 & 8 hrs after completion of the cidofovir infusion. Renal function (serum creatinine and urine protein) must be monitored prior to each dose (*see pkg insert for details*). Contraindicated if creatinine >1.5 mg/dL, CrCl ≤55 mL/min or urine protein ≥100 mg/dL.	**Adverse effects: Nephrotoxicity;** dose-dependent proximal tubular injury (Fanconi-like syndrome): proteinuria, glycosuria, bicarbonaturia, phosphaturia, polyuria (nephrogenic diabetic insipidus, *Ln 350:413, 1997*), acidosis, ↑ creatinine. Concomitant saline prehydration, probenecid, extended dosing intervals allowed use but still highly nephrotoxic. Other toxicities: nausea 69%, fever 58%, alopecia 27%, myalgia 16%, probenecid hypersensitivity 16%, neutropenia 29%. Iritis and uveitis reported; also ↓ intraocular pressure. **Black Box warning.** Renal impairment can occur after ≤2 doses. Contraindicated in pts receiving concomitant nephrotoxic agents. Monitor for ↓ WBC. In animals, carcinogenic, teratogenic; causes ↓ sperm and ↓ fertility. FDA indication only CMV retinitis in HIV pts. **Comment:** Recommended dosage, frequency or infusion rate must not be exceeded. Dose must be reduced or discontinued if changes in renal function occur during rx. For ↑ of 0.3–0.4 mg per dL in serum creatinine, cidofovir dose must be ↓ from 5 to 3 mg per kg; discontinue cidofovir if ↑ of 0.5 mg per dL above baseline or 3+ proteinuria develops (for 2+ proteinuria, observe pts carefully and consider discontinuation).
Ganciclovir (Cytovene)	IV: 5 mg per kg q12h times 14 days (induction) 5 mg per kg IV q24h or 6 mg per kg 5 times per wk (maintenance) Dosage adjust. with renal dysfunction (*see Table 17*)	**Adverse effects: Black Box warnings:** cytopenias, carcinogenicity/teratogenicity & aspermia in animals. Absolute neutrophil count dropped below 500 per mm³ in 15%, thrombocytopenia 21%, anemia 6%. Fever 48%. GI 50%: nausea, vomiting, diarrhea, abdominal pain 19%, rash 10%. Retinal detachment 11% (relationship to ganciclovir?). Confusion, headache, psychiatric disturbances and seizures. Neutropenia may respond to granulocyte colony stimulating factor (G-CSF or GM-CSF). Severe myelosuppression may be ↑ with coadministration of zidovudine or azathioprine. 32% dc/interrupted rx, principally for neutropenia. Avoid extravasation.
	Oral: 1.0 gm tid with food (fatty meal) (250 mg & 500 mg cap)	Hematologic less frequent than with IV. Granulocytopenia 18%, anemia 12%, thrombocytopenia 6%. GI, skin same as with IV. Retinal detachment 8%.
Ganciclovir (Vitrasert)	Intraocular implant	**Adverse effects:** Late retinal detachment (7/30 eyes). Does not prevent CMV retinitis in good eye or visceral dissemination. **Comment:** Replacement every 6 months recommended
Valganciclovir (Valcyte)	900 mg (two 450 mg tabs) po bid times 21 days for induction, followed by 900 mg po q24h. Take with food. Dosage adjustment for renal dysfunction (*See Table 17A*).	A prodrug of ganciclovir with better bioavailability than oral ganciclovir: 60% with food. **Adverse effects:** Similar to ganciclovir.
Herpesvirus (non-CMV) **Acyclovir** (Zovirax or generic)	Doses: see *Table 14A* 400 mg or 800 mg tab 200 mg cap Suspension 200 mg per 5 mL Ointment or cream 5% IV injection Dosage adjustment for renal dysfunction (*See Table 17A*).	**po:** Generally well-tolerated with occ. diarrhea, vertigo, arthralgia. Less frequent rash, fatigue, insomnia, fever, menstrual abnormalities, acne, sore throat, muscle cramps, lymphadenopathy. **IV:** Phlebitis, caustic with vesicular lesions with IV infiltration, CNS (1%): lethargy, tremors, confusion, hallucinations, delirium, seizures, coma—all reversible. Renal (5%): ↑ creatinine, hematuria. With high doses may crystallize in renal tubules → obstructive uropathy (rapid infusion, dehydration, renal insufficiency and ↑ dose ↑ risk). Adequate pre-hydration may prevent such nephrotoxicity. Hepatic: ↑ ALT, AST. Uncommon: neutropenia, rash, diaphoresis, hypotension, headache, nausea.

* *See page 3 for abbreviations. NOTE: All dosage recommendations are for adults (unless otherwise indicated) and assume normal renal function.*

TABLE 14B (2)

DRUG NAME(S) GENERIC (TRADE)	DOSAGE/ROUTE IN ADULTS*	COMMENTS/ADVERSE EFFECTS
Herpesvirus (non-CMV) (continued)		
Famciclovir (Famvir)	125 mg, 250 mg, 500 mg tabs. Dosage depends on indication: (see label and Table 14A).	Metabolized to penciclovir. **Adverse effects:** similar to acyclovir, included headache, nausea, diarrhea, and dizziness but incidence does not differ from placebo. May be taken without regard to meals. Dose should be reduced if CrCl <60 mL per min (see package insert & Table 14A, page 141 & Table 17, page 184). May be taken with or without food.
Penciclovir (Denavir)	Topical 1% cream	Apply to area of recurrence of herpes labialis with start of sx, then q2h while awake times 4 days. Well tolerated.
Trifluridine (Viroptic)	Topical 1% solution:1 drop q2h (max. 9 drops/day) until corneal re-epithelialization, then dose is ↓ for 7 more days (one drop q4h for at least 5 drops/day) not to exceed 21 days total rx.	Mild burning (5%), palpebral edema (3%), punctate keratopathy, stromal edema. For HSV keratoconjunctivitis or recurrent epithelial keratitis.
Valacyclovir (Valtrex)	500 mg, 1 gm tabs. Dosage depends on indication and renal function (see label, Table 14A & Table 17A)	An ester pro-drug of acyclovir that is well-absorbed, bioavailability 3–5 times greater than acyclovir. **Adverse effects** similar to acyclovir (see JID 186:540, 2002). Thrombotic thrombocytopenic purpura/hemolytic uremic syndrome reported in pts with advanced HIV disease and transplant recipients participating in clinical trials at doses of 8 gm per day.
Hepatitis		
Adefovir dipivoxil (Hepsera)	10 mg po q24h (with normal CrCl); see Table 17A if renal impairment. 10 mg tab	Adefovir dipivoxil is a prodrug of adefovir. It is an acyclic nucleotide analog with activity against hepatitis B (HBV) at 0.2–2.5 mM (IC$_{50}$). See Table 9 for Cmax & T½. Active against YMDD mutant lamivudine-resistant strains and in vitro vs. entecavir-resistant strains. Primarily renal excretion—adjust dose. No food interactions. Remarkably few side effects. At 10 mg per day potential for delayed nephrotoxicity. Monitor renal function, esp. with pts with pre-existing or other risks for renal impairment. Lactic acidosis reported with nucleoside analogs, esp. in women. Pregnancy Category C. Hepatitis may exacerbate when treatment discontinued; Up to 25% of pts developed ALT ↑ 10 times normal within 12 wks; usually responds to re-treatment or self-limited, but hepatic decompensation has occurred.
Entecavir (Baraclude)	0.5 mg q24h. If refractory to lamivudine: 1 mg per day. Tabs: 0.5 mg & 1 mg. Oral solution: 0.05 mg/mL.	A nucleoside analog active against HBV including lamivudine-resistant mutants. Minimal adverse effects reported: headache, fatigue, dizziness, & nausea reported in 22% of pts. Potential for lactic acidosis and exacerbation of hepB at discontinuation. Do not use as single anti-retroviral agent in HIV co-infected pts; M134 mutation can emerge (NEJM 356:2614, 2007). Adjust dosage in renal impairment (see Table 17, page 184).
Interferon alfa is available as alfa-2a (Roferon-A), alfa-2b (Intron-A)	For hepC, usual Roferon-A and Intron-A doses are 3 million international units thrice weekly subQ	Depending on agent, available in pre-filled syringes, vials of solution, or powder. **Black Box warnings:** include possibility of serious neuropsychiatric effects, autoimmune disorders, ischemic events, infection.
PEG interferon alfa-2b (PEG-Intron)	0.5–1.5 mcg/kg subQ q wk	**Adverse effects:** Flu-like syndrome is common, esp. during 1st wk of rx: fever 98%, fatigue 89%, myalgia 73%, headache 71%. GI: anorexia 46%, diarrhea 29%. CNS: dizziness 21%. Hemorrhagic or ischemic stroke. Rash 18%, may progress to Stevens Johnson or exfoliative dermatitis. Profound fatigue & psychiatric symptoms in up to ½ of pts (J Clin Psych 64:708, 2003) (depression, anxiety, emotional lability
Pegylated-40k interferon alfa-2a (Pegasys)	180 mcg subQ q wk	& agitation); consider prophylactic antidepressant in pts with history. Alopecia. ↑ TSH, autoimmune thyroid disorders with ↓- or ↑- thyroidism. Hematol: ↓ WBC 49%, ↓ Hgb 27%, ↓ platelets 35%. Acute reversible hearing loss &/or tinnitus in up to 1/3 (Ln 343:1134, 1994). Optic neuropathy (retinal hemorrhage, cotton wool spots, ↓ in color vision) reported (AIDS 18:1805, 2004). Doses may require adjustment (or dc) based on individual response or adverse events, and can vary by product, indication (eg, HCV or HBV) and mode of use (mono- or combination-rx). (Refer to labels of individual products and to ribavirin if used in combination for details of use.)

* See page 3 for abbreviations. NOTE: All dosage recommendations are for adults (unless otherwise indicated) and assume normal renal function.

TABLE 14B (3)

DRUG NAME(S) GENERIC (TRADE)	DOSAGE/ROUTE IN ADULTS*	COMMENTS/ADVERSE EFFECTS
Hepatitis (continued)		
Lamivudine (3TC) (Epivir-HBV)	Hepatitis B dose: 100 mg po q24h. Dosage adjustment with renal dysfunction (see label). Tabs 100 mg and oral solution 5 mg/mL.	**Black Box warnings:** caution, dose is lower than HIV dose, so must exclude co-infection with HIV before using this formulation; lactic acidosis/hepatic steatosis; severe exacerbation of liver disease can occur on dc. YMDD-mutants resistant to lamivudine may emerge on treatment. **Adverse effects:** See Table 14D.
Ribavirin (Rebetol, Copegus)	For use with an interferon for hepatitis C. Available as 200 mg caps and 40 mg/mL oral solution (Rebetol) or 200 mg tabs (Copegus) (See Comments regarding dosage).	**Black Box warnings:** ribavirin monotherapy of HCV is ineffective; hemolytic anemia may precipitate cardiac events; teratogenic/ embryocidal **(Preg Category X)**. Drug may persist for 6 mo, avoid pregnancy for at least 6 mo after end of rx of women or their partners. Only approved for pts with Ccr > 50 mL/min. Also should not be used in pts with severe heart disease or some hemoglobinopathies. ARDS reported (Chest 124:406, 2003). **Adverse effects:** hemolytic anemia (may require dose reduction or dc), dental/periodontal disorders, and all adverse effects of concomitant interferon used (see above). See Table 14A for specific regimens, but dosing depends on: interferon used, weight, HCV genotype, and is modified (or dc) based on side effects (especially degree of hemolysis, with different criteria in those with/without cardiac disease). For example, initial Rebetol dose with Intron A (interferon alfa-2b) is wt-based: 400 mg am & 600 mg pm for ≤ 75 kg, and 600 mg am & 600 mg pm for wt > 75 kg, but with Pegintron approved dose is 400 mg am & 400 mg pm with meals. Doses and duration of Copegus with peg-interferon alfa-2a are less in pts with genotype 2 or 3 (800 mg per day divided into 2 doses, for 24 wks) than with genotypes 1 or 4 (1000 mg per day divided into 2 doses for wt < 75 kg and 1200 mg per day divided into 2 doses for ≥ 75 kg for 48 wks). (See individual labels for details, including initial dosing and criteria for dose modification in those with/without cardiac disease.)
Telbivudine (Tyzeka)	One 600 mg tab orally q24h, without regard to food. Dosage adjustment with renal dysfunction, Ccr < 50 mL/min (see label).	An oral nucleoside analog approved for Rx of Hep B. It has ↑ rates of response and superior viral suppression than lamivudine (NEJM 357:2576, 2007). **Black Box warnings** regarding lactic acidosis/hepatic steatosis with nucleosides and potential for severe exacerbation of HepB on dc. Generally well-tolerated with ↓ mitochondrial toxicity vs other nucleosides and no dose limiting toxicity observed (Ann Pharmacother 40:472, 2006; Medical Letter 49:11, 2007). Myalgias and myopathy reported. Genotypic resistance rate was 4.4% by one yr, ↑ to 21.5% by 2 yrs of rx of eAg+ pts. Selects for YMDD mutation like lamivudine. Combination with lamivudine was inferior to monotherapy (Hepatology 45:507, 2007).
Tenofovir (TDF)(Viread)	300 mg tabs. Dose and dose-reduction with renal impairment same as for HIV.	In 2008, FDA approved for treatment of chronic hepB in adults. **Black box warnings**—lactic acidosis, hepatic steatosis; exacerbation hepB when rx stopped, monitor closely. (See Table 14D for additional comments.)
Influenza A Amantadine (Symmetrel) or Rimantadine (Flumadine)	At present, these adamantanes are not recommended for routine use in treatment or prophylaxis of influenza because of high resistance rates*. **Amantadine** 100 mg caps, tabs; 50 mg/mL oral solution & syrup. Treatment or prophylaxis: 100 mg bid: or 100 mg daily if age ≥65 y; dose reductions with Ccr starting at ≤50 mL/min. **Rimantadine** 100 mg tabs, 50 mg/5 mL syrup. Treatment or prophylaxis: 100 mg bid, or 100 mg daily in elderly nursing home pts, or severe hepatic disease, or Ccr ≤10 mL/min. For children, rimantadine only approved for prophylaxis.	**Side-effects/toxicity:** CNS (nervousness, anxiety, difficulty concentrating, and lightheadedness). Symptoms occurred in 6% on rimantadine vs 14% on amantadine. They usually ↓ after 1st week and disappear when drug dc. GI (nausea, anorexia). Some serious side-effects—delirium, hallucinations, and seizures—are associated with high plasma drug levels resulting from renal insufficiency, esp. in older pts, those with prior seizure disorders, or psychiatric disorders. Activity restricted to influenza A viruses. * Rimantadine combined with oseltamivir can be used as alternative to zanamivir in specific circumstances (see www2a.cdc.gov/HAN/ArchiveSys/ViewMsgV.asp?AlertNum=00279).

* See page 3 for abbreviations. NOTE: All dosage recommendations are for adults (unless otherwise indicated) and assume normal renal function.

TABLE 14B (4)

DRUG NAME(S) GENERIC (TRADE)	DOSAGE/ROUTE IN ADULTS*	COMMENTS/ADVERSE EFFECTS
Influenza A and B—For both drugs, initiate within 48 hrs of symptom onset		
Zanamivir (Relenza) For pts ≥ 7 yrs of age (treatment) or ≥ 5 yrs (prophylaxis)	Powder is inhaled by specially designed inhalation device. Each blister contains 5 mg zanamivir. **Treatment:** oral inhalation of 2 blisters (10 mg) bid for 5 days. **Prophylaxis:** oral inhalation of 2 blisters (10 mg) once daily for 10 days (household outbreak) to 28 days (community outbreak).	Active by inhalation against neuraminidase of both influenza A and B and inhibits release of virus from epithelial cells of respiratory tract. Approx. 4–17% of inhaled dose absorbed into plasma. Excreted by kidney but with low absorption, dose reduction not necessary in renal impairment. Minimal side-effects: <3% cough, sinusitis, diarrhea, nausea and vomiting. **Reports of respiratory adverse events in pts with or without h/o airways disease, should be avoided in pts with underlying respiratory disease.** Allergic reactions and neuropsychiatric events have been reported.
Oseltamivir (Tamiflu) For pts ≥ 1 yr	For adults: **Treatment:** 75 mg po bid for 5 days; **Prophylaxis:** 75 mg po once daily for 10 days to 6 wk. *(See label for pediatric weight-based dosing.)* Adjust doses for Ccr ≤30 mL/min. 30 mg, 45 mg, 75 mg caps; powder for oral suspension.	Well absorbed (80% bioavailable) from GI tract as ethyl ester of active compound GS 4071. T½ 6–10 hrs; excreted unchanged by kidney. Adverse effects in 15% include diarrhea 1.6%, nausea 0.5%, vomiting, headache *(J Am Ger Soc 50:608, 2002)*. Nausea ↓ with food. Rarely, severe skin reactions. Delirium & abnormal behavior reported.
Respiratory Syncytial Virus (RSV)		
Palivizumab (Synagis) Used for prevention of RSV infection in high-risk children	15 mg per kg IM q month throughout RSV season Single dose 100 mg vial	A monoclonal antibody directed against the F glycoprotein on surface of virus; side-effects are uncommon, occ. ↑ ALT. Anaphylaxis <1/10⁵ pts; acute hypersensitivity reaction <1/1000. Preferred over polyclonal immune globulin in high risk infants & children.
Warts *(See CID 28:S37, 1999)*	Regimens are from drug labels specific for external genital and/or perianal condylomata acuminata only *(see specific labels for indications, regimens, age limits).*	
Interferon alfa-2b (IntronA)	Injection of 1 million international units into base of lesion, thrice weekly on alternate days for up to 3 wks. Maximum 5 lesions per course.	Interferons may cause "flu-like" illness and other systemic effects. 88% had at least one adverse effect.
Interferon alfa-N3 (Alferon N)	Injection of 0.05 mL into base of each wart, up to 0.5 mL total per session, twice weekly for up to 8 weeks.	Flu-like syndrome and hypersensitivity reactions. Contraindicated with allergy to mouse IgG, egg proteins, or neomycin.
Imiquimod (Aldara)	5% cream. Thin layer applied at bedtime, washing off after 6-10 hr, thrice weekly to maximum of 16 wks.	Erythema, itching & burning, erosions. Flu-like syndrome, increased susceptibility to sunburn (avoid UV).
Podofilox (Condylox)	0.5% gel or solution twice daily for 3 days, no therapy for 4 days; can use up to 4 such cycles.	Local reactions—pain, burning, inflammation in 50%. Can ulcerate. Limit surface area treated as per label.
Sinecatechins (Veregen)	15% ointment. Apply 0.5 cm strand to each wart three times per day until healing but not more than 16 weeks.	Application site reactions, which may result in ulcerations, phimosis, meatal stenosis, superinfection.

* See page 3 for abbreviations. *NOTE: All dosage recommendations are for adults (unless otherwise indicated) and assume normal renal function.*

TABLE 14C – AT A GLANCE SUMMARY OF SUGGESTED ANTIVIRAL AGENTS AGAINST TREATABLE PATHOGENIC VIRUSES

ANTIVIRAL AGENT

Antiviral Agent	Adenovirus	BK virus	Cytomegalovirus	Hepatitis B	Hepatitis C	Herpes simplex virus	Influenza A / Influenza B	JC Virus	Respiratory Syncytial Virus	Varicella-zoster virus
Zanamivir	-	-	-	-	-	-	+++ / +++	-	-	-
Valganciclovir	±	-	+++	-	-	+	-	-	-	+
Valacyclovir	-	-	±	-	-	+++	-	-	-	+++
Rimantadine	-	-	-	-	-	-	+** / ±	-	-	-
Ribavirin	-	-	-	±	+++*	-	-	-	+	-
Oseltamivir	-	-	-	-	-	-	+++ / ++	-	-	-
αInterferon Or PEG INF	-	-	-	+++	+++*	-	-	- -	-	-
Ganciclovir	±	-	+++	-	-	++	-	-	-	+
Foscarnet	-	-	+++	-	-	++	-	-	-	++
Famciclovir	-	-	±	-	-	+++	-	-	-	++
Cidofovir	+	+	+++	-	-	+	-	+	-	+
Adefovir / Entecavir / Lamivudine / Tenofovir	-	-	-	+++	-	-	-	-	-	-
Amantadine	-	-	-	-	-	-	+** / ±	-	-	-
Acyclovir	-	-	±	-	-	+++	-	-	-	+++

* 1st line rx = an IFN + Ribavirin   ** not CDC recommended due to high prevalence of resistance

- = no activity; ± = possible activity; + = active; + = active, 3rd line therapy (least active clinically)
++ = Active, 2nd line therapy (less active clinically); +++ = Active, 1st line therapy (usually active clinically)

TABLE 14D – ANTIRETROVIRAL THERAPY IN TREATMENT-NAÏVE ADULTS

(See the 2009 SANFORD GUIDE TO HIV/AIDS THERAPY, Table 6, for additional information regarding treatment and complications of antiretroviral agents)

The U.S. Dept of Health & Human Services (DHHS) updated guidelines for treatment of adults and adolescents with HIV-1 infection in November 2008. These, and guidelines for pediatric patients and pregnant women, can be found at www.aidsinfo.nih.gov. Since the previous edition, the first of 2 new classes of antiretrovirals (CCR5 co-receptor antagonist and integrase inhibitor) were approved in the US. Whenever starting antiretroviral therapy, **resistance testing** should be performed to help guide choice of agents Note that **immune reconstitution syndromes** may result from initiation of antiretroviral therapy, and may require medical intervention. For additional explanation and other acceptable alternatives relating to these tables, see www.aidsinfo.nih.gov.

The following concepts guide therapy:
- **The goal of rx is to inhibit maximally viral replication, allowing re-establishment & persistence of an effective immune response that will prevent or delay HIV-related morbidity.**
- **The lower the viral RNA can be driven, the lower the rate of accumulation of drug resistance mutations & the longer the therapeutic effect will last.**
- **To achieve maximal & durable suppression of viral RNA, combinations of potent antiretroviral agents are required, as is a high degree of adherence to the chosen regimens.**
- **Treatment regimens must be tailored to the individual as well as to the virus. Antiretroviral drug toxicities can compromise adherence in the short term & can cause significant negative health effects over time. Carefully check for specific risks to the individual, for interactions between the antiretrovirals selected & between those & concurrent drugs, & adjust doses as necessary for body weight, and for renal or hepatic dysfunction, & for possible pharmacokinetic interactions.**

A. **When to start therapy?** *(see www.aidsinfo.nih.gov for additional indications: pregnancy, nephropathy, HBV co-infection requiring rx)*

HIV Symptoms	CD4 cells/µl	Start Treatment	Comment
Yes	Any	Yes	
No	<200	Yes	*New DHHS recommendation.
No	≥200 – <350	Yes*	*Maybe if CD4 decreasing rapidly &/or viral load >100,000 copies/mL. Whether there is long-term
No	≥350	No*	immunological benefit of starting ART at CD4>350 remains a topic of investigation. IAS-USA Guidelines suggest considering ARV Rx in all patients regardless of CD4 count *(JAMA 300:555, 2008).*

B. **Acute HIV Infection.** The benefits of ARV treatment in acute HIV infection are uncertain, but may include improved immunological response to the virus and decreased potential for transmission. However, treatment also exposes the patient to risks of drug adverse events, and the optimal duration of rx is unknown. Therefore, treatment is considered optional and is best undertaken in a research setting. Optimal regimens in this setting have not yet been defined. An observational study of acute or early HIV-1 infection showed comparable results from either PI-based or NNRTI-based regimens *(CID 42:1024, 2006),* although some feel that the higher barrier to resistance of PIs might be advantageous *(JAMA 300: 255, 2008).*

C. **Approach to constructing ARV regimens for treatment naïve adults.** (From Guidelines for the Use of Antiretroviral Agents in HIV-1-Infected Adults and Adolescents at www.aidsinfo.nih.gov. See that document for explanations, qualifications and further alternatives.)

Design a regimen consisting of
[either an NNRTI *OR* a Protease Inhibitor] *PLUS* [a dual-NRTI component]

- See section D of this table for specific regimens and tables which follow for drug characteristics, usual doses, adverse effects and additional details
- Selection of components will be influenced by many factors, such as
  - Co-morbidities (e.g., lipid effects of PIs, liver or renal disease, etc)
  - Pregnancy (e.g., avoid efavirenz—pregnancy class D)
  - HIV status (e.g., avoid nevirapine in women with CD4 >250)
  - Results of viral resistance testing
  - Potential drug interactions or adverse drug effects
  - Convenience of dosing

Co-formulations increase convenience, but sometimes prescribing the two constituents individually is preferred, as when dose-adjustments are needed for renal disease.

TABLE 14D (2)

Preferred components by class (alphabetical order)

NNRTI	Protease Inhibitor	Dual-NRTI
Efavirenz	Atazanavir + ritonavir or	Tenofovir/ Emtricitabine (co-formulated)
	Lopinavir/ritonavir (co-formulated, twice-daily regimen)	

Alternative components by class

NNRTI	Protease Inhibitor	Dual-NRTI
Nevirapine	Atazanavir or	Abacavir/Lamivudine (co-formulated) or
	Fosamprenavir or	Didanosine + (emtricitabine or lamivudine) or
	Fosamprenavir + ritonavir (once-daily regimen) or	Zidovudine + lamivudine (co-formulated)
	Lopinavir/ritonavir	
	(co-formulated, once-daily regimen) or	
	Fosamprenavir + ritonavir (twice-daily regimen)	

D. **Suggested Initial Therapy Regimens for Untreated Chronic HIV-1 Infection** Doses & use assume normal renal & hepatic function unless otherwise stated. *(For pregnancy, see below; also, Table 8B of The Sanford Guide to HIV/AIDS Therapy 2009 for additional explanation & alternatives, see www.aidsinfo.nih.gov)*

1. **Preferred Regimens**

	Regimen	Pill strength (mg)	Usual Daily Regimen (oral)	No. pills/ day	Comment (See also individual agents & Table 14E)
a.	(Tenofovir + Emtricitabine) + Efavirenz	(300 + 200) + 600	(Combination—Truvada 1 tab q24h) + 1 tab q24h at bedtime, empty stomach	2	Analysis at 48 wks of ongoing trial reported superior virus suppression, higher CD4 & fewer AEs of tenofovir/ emtricitabine/ efavirenz as compared to ZDV/3TC/efavirenz (NEJM 354:251, 2006). Tenofovir: reports of renal toxicity (CID 42:283, 2006). Avoid efavirenz in pregnancy or in women who might become pregnant (**Pregnancy Category D**). Food may ↑ serum efavirenz concentration, which can lead to ↑ adverse events. See section F.2 re how to stop efavirenz.
	OR				
b.	(Tenofovir + Emtricitabine + Efavirenz)	(300 + 200 + 600)	Combination—Atripla 1 tab q24h at bedtime, empty stomach	1	
	OR				
c.	(Tenofovir + Emtricitabine) + Atazanavir + Ritonavir (low dose)	(300 + 200) + 300 + 100	(Combination – Truvada 1 tab q24h) + 1 cap q24h + 1 cap q24h both with food	3	
	OR				
d.	(Tenofovir + Emtricitabine) + Darunavir + Ritonavir (low dose)	(300 + 200) + 800 + 100	(Combination – Truvada 1 tab q24h) + 2 (400 mg) caps q24h + 1 cap q24h both with food	4	

TABLE 14D (3)

	Regimen	Pill strength (mg)	Usual Daily Regimen (oral)	No. pills/ day	Comment (See also *individual agents & Table 14E*)
2.	**Alternative Regimens**				
a.	(Zidovudine + Lamivudine) + Efavirenz	(300 + 150) + 600	(Combination—Combivir 1 tab bid) + 1 tab q24h at bedtime, empty stomach	3	Good efficacy; low pill burden; low AE profile. Avoid efavirenz in pregnancy or in women who might become pregnant **(Pregnancy Category D)**. Food may ↑ serum efavirenz concentration, which can lead to ↑ adverse events. See section F.2 re how to stop efavirenz.
b.	(Zidovudine + Lamivudine) + Lopinavir/ Ritonavir	(300 + 150) + 200/50	(Combination—Combivir 1 tab bid) + (Combination—Kaletra 2 tabs bid) without regard to food	6	Good virologic efficacy & durable effect. Tolerable AEs. *Preferred regimen is* to use lopinavir/ritonavir twice daily. As an alternative regimen, lopinavir/ritonavir can be given as 4 tabs once daily in rx-naïve pts.
c.	(Zidovudine + Lamivudine) + Atazanavir + Ritonavir	(300 + 150) + 300 + 100	(Combination—Combivir 1 tab bid) + 1 cap q24h + 1 cap q24h both with food	4	Lower potential for lipid derangement by (unboosted) atazanavir than w/other PIs. May ↑ EKG PR interval & bilirubin. Acid-lowering agents can markedly ↓ absorption; avoid with PPIs & give 2 hr before or 10 hr after H2-blockers. As an alternative regimen, atazanavir can be used without ritonavir, at a dose of 400 mg q24h with food, in combination therapy for Rx-naïve patients.
d.	(Zidovudine + Lamivudine) + Fosamprenavir + Ritonavir	(300 + 150) + 700 + 100	(Combination—Combivir 1 tab bid) + 1 tab bid fed or fasting + 1 cap bid fed or fasting	6	Can take without regard to meals. Skin rash, GI symptoms. Fosamprenavir contains sulfa moiety. Alternative fosamprenavir regimens available for rx-naïve pts, including fosamprenavir without ritonavir & once-daily fosamprenavir/ritonavir regimens (*see label for use & doses*).
e.	Didanosine EC + Lamivudine + Efavirenz	400 + 300 + 600	1 cap q24h at bedtime, fasting + 1 tab q24h + 1 tab q24h at bedtime, empty stomach **Didanosine dosage shown for ≥60 kg**	3	Low pill burden. Efficacy & durability under study. Potential didanosine AEs (pancreatitis, peripheral neuritis). Avoid efavirenz in pregnancy or in women who might become pregnant **(Pregnancy Category D)**. Food may ↑ serum efavirenz concentration, which can lead to ↑ adverse events. Can substitute emtricitabine 200 mg po q24h for lamivudine 300 mg po q24h.
f.	(Abacavir + Lamivudine) + Efavirenz	(600 + 300) + 600	(Combination—Epzicom 1 tab q24h) without regard to food + 1 tab q24h at bedtime, empty stomach	2	Low pill burden. **Risk of abacavir hypersensitivity reaction (see Comment Table 14E)**. Comparison of abacavir/lamivudine with tenofovir/emtricitabine as backbone in rx-naïve pts under study. Avoid efavirenz in pregnancy or in women who might become pregnant **(Pregnancy Category D)**. Food may ↑ serum efavirenz concentration, which can lead to ↑ adverse events.

156

TABLE 14D (4)

Regimen	Pill strength (mg)	Usual Daily Regimen (oral)	No. pills/ day	Comment (See also individual agents)

3. Triple nucleoside regimen: Due to inferior virologic activity, use only when preferred or alternative regimen not possible. Seek expert advice about alternatives.

a. (Zidovudine + Lamivudine + Abacavir)	(300 + 150 + 300)	(Combination-Trizivir 1 tab bid)	2	Reduced activity as compared with preferred or alternative regimens. Potentially serious abacavir AEs (see comments for individual agents.)

4. During pregnancy. Expert consultation mandatory. Timing of rx initiation & drug choice must be individualized. Viral resistance testing should be performed. Long-term effects of agents unknown. Certain drugs hazardous or contraindicated. (See Table 8A of the Sanford Guide to HIV/AIDS Therapy). For additional information & alternative options, see www.aidsinfo.nih.gov. For regimens to prevent perinatal transmission, see Table 8A of the Sanford Guide to HIV/AIDS Therapy. See JID 193:1191, 2006 re pre-term delivery with PIs.

a. (Zidovudine + Lamivudine) + Nevirapine	(300 + 150) + 200	(Combination-Combivir 1 tab bid) + 1 tab bid fed or fasting [after 14-day lead-in period of 1 tab q24h]	4	See especially nevirapine **Black Box warnings**—among others ↑ risk of **potentially fatal hepatotoxicity** in women with CD4 >250. Avoid in this group unless benefits clearly > risks; monitor intensively if drug must be used. **Nevirapine contraindicated in Childs Pugh B & C liver disease.**
b. (Zidovudine + Lamivudine) + Lopinavir/ritonavir	(300 + 150) + 200/50	(Comination—Combivir 1 tab bid) + 2 tabs bid without regard to food	6	Optimal dose in 3rd trimester unknown. May need to monitor levels as ↑ dose may be required. Once-daily dosing of lopinavir/ritonavir not recommended.

5. Alternative Regimen (DHHS 2008: www.aidsinfo.nih.gov)

a. (Zidovudine + Lamivudine) + Saquinavir + Ritonavir	(300 + 150) + 500 + 100	(Combination-Combivir 1 tab bid) + 2 tabs bid + 1 cap bid	8	Use saquinavir tabs only in combination with ritonavir. Certain drugs metabolized by CYP3A are contra-indicated with saquinavir/ritonavir. (Original DHHS recommendations were based on saquinavir soft gel caps, which are no longer available, plus ritonavir).

TABLE 14D (5)

E. **Selected Characteristics of Antiretroviral Drugs**

1. **Selected Characteristics of Nucleoside or Nucleotide Reverse Transcriptase Inhibitors (NRTIs)**
   All agents have Black Box warning: Risk of lactic acidosis/hepatic steatosis. Also, labels note risk of fat redistribution/accumulation with ARV therapy. For combinations, see warnings for component agents.

Generic/Trade Name	Pharmaceutical Prep.	Usual Adult Dosage & Food Effect	% Absorbed, po	Serum T½, hrs	Intracellular T½, hrs	Elimination	Major Adverse Events/Comments *(See Table 14E)*
Abacavir (ABC; Ziagen)	300 mg tabs or 20 mg/ml oral solution	300 mg po bid or 600 mg po q24h. Food OK	83	1.5	20	Liver metab., renal excretion of metabolites, 82%	**Hypersensitivity reaction:** fever, rash, N/V, malaise, diarrhea, abdominal pain, respiratory symptoms. (Severe reactions may be ↑ with 600 mg dose.) **Do not rechallenge!** Report to 800-270-0425. **Test HLA-B*5701 before use. See Comment Table 14E.** Study raises concerns re ABC/3TC regimens in pts with VL ≥100,000 (www3.niaid.nih.gov/news/newsreleases/2008/actg5202bulletin.htm). Recent report suggests possible ↑ risk of cardiac event in pts with other cardiac risk factors (*Ln 371:1417, 2008*).
Abacavir/lamivudine/ zidovudine (Trizivir)	Film-coated tabs: ABC 300 mg + 3TC 150 mg + ZDV 300 mg	1 tab po bid (not recommended for wt <40 kg or CrCl <50 mL/min or im-paired hepatic function)		*(See individual components)*			*(See Comments for individual components)* Note: **Black Box warnings** for ABC hyper-sensitivity reaction & others. Should only be used for regimens intended to include these 3 agents. Black Box warning— limited data for VL >100,000 copies/mL. Not recommended as initial therapy because of inferior virologic efficacy.
Didanosine (ddI; Videx or Videx EC)	125, 200, 250, 400 enteric-coated caps; 100, 167, 250 mg powder for oral solution;	≥60 kg. Usually 400 mg enteric-coated po q24h 0.5 hr before or 2 hrs after meal. Do not crush. <60 kg: 250 mg EC po q24h. Food ↓ levels. See Comment	30–40	1.6	25–40	Renal excretion, 50%	**Pancreatitis,** peripheral neuropathy, lactic acidosis & hepatic steatosis (rare but life-threatening, esp. combined with stavudine in pregnancy). Retinal, optic nerve changes. **The combination ddI + TDF is generally avoided, but if used,** reduce dose of ddI-EC from 400 mg to 250 mg EC q24h (or from 250 mg EC to 200 mg EC for adults <60 kg). **Monitor for ↑ toxicity & possible ↓ in efficacy of this combination; may result in ↓ CD4.** Possible increased risk of cardiovascular disease (*Ln 371:1417, 2008*).

TABLE 14D (6)

Generic/Trade Name	Pharmaceutical Prep.	Usual Adult Dosage & Food Effect	% Absorbed, po	Serum T½, hrs	Intracellular T½, hrs	Elimination	Major Adverse Events/Comments (See Table 14E)
Emtricitabine (FTC, Emtriva)	200 mg caps; 10 mg per mL oral solution.	200 mg po q24h. Food OK.	93 (caps), 75 (oral sol'n)	Approx. 10	39	Renal excretion 86%, minor biotransformation, 14% excretion in feces	Well tolerated; headache, nausea, vomiting & diarrhea occasionally, skin rash rarely. Skin hyperpigmentation. Differs only slightly in structure from lamivudine (5-fluoro substitution). **Exacerbation of Hep B reported in pts after stopping FTC.** Monitor at least several months after stopping FTC in Hep B pts; some may need anti-HBV therapy.
Emtricitabine/tenofovir disoproxil fumarate (Truvada)	Film-coated tabs: FTC 200 mg + TDF 300 mg	1 tab po q24h for CrCl ≥50 ml/min. Food OK	93/25	10/17	—	Primarily renal/renal	*See Comments for individual agents* **Black Box warning—Exacerbation of HepB after stopping FTC;** but preferred therapy for those with Hep B.
Emtricitabine/tenofovir/efavirenz (Atripla)	Film-coated tabs: FTC 200 mg + TDF 300 mg + efavirenz 600 mg	1 tab po q24h on an empty stomach, preferably at bedtime. Do not use if CrCl <50 ml/min	*(See individual components)*				Not recommended for pts <18yrs. *(See warnings for individual components).* **Exacerbation of Hep B** reported in pts discontinuing component drugs; some may need anti-HBV therapy (preferred anti-Hep B therapy). **Pregnancy category D-** may cause fetal harm. Avoid in pregnancy or in women who may become pregnant.
Lamivudine (3TC; Epivir)	150, 300 mg tabs; 10 mg/ml oral solution	150 mg po bid or 300 mg po q24h. Food OK	86	5-7	18	Renal excretion, minimal metabolism	**Use HIV dose, not Hep B dose.** Usually well-tolerated. **Risk of exacerbation of Hep B after stopping 3TC.** Monitor at least several months after stopping 3TC in Hep B pts; some may need anti-HBV therapy.
Lamivudine/abacavir (Epzicom)	Film-coated tabs: 3TC 300 mg + abacavir 600 mg	1 tab po q24h. Food OK Not recommended for CrCl <50 ml/min or impaired hepatic function	86/86	5-7/1.5	16/20	Primarily renal/metabolism	*See Comments for individual agents.* **Note abacavir hypersensitivity Black Box warnings** (severe reactions may be somewhat more frequent with 600 mg dose) and 3TC Hep B warnings. Test HLA-B*5701 before use.
Lamivudine/zidovudine (Combivir)	Film-coated tabs: 3TC 150 mg + ZDV 300 mg	1 tab po bid. Not recommended for CrCl <50 ml/min or impaired hepatic function Food OK	86/64	5-7/0.5-3	—	Primarily renal/metabolism with renal excretion of glucuronide	*See Comments for individual agents* See **Black Box warning**—exacerbation of Hep B in pts stopping 3TC

TABLE 14D (7)

Generic/Trade Name	Pharmaceutical Prep.	Usual Adult Dosage & Food Effect	% Absorbed, po	Serum T½, hrs	Intracellular T½, hrs	Elimination	Major Adverse Events/Comments *(See Table 14E)*
Stavudine (d4T; Zerit)	15, 20, 30, 40 mg capsules; 1 mg per mL oral solution	≥60 kg: 40 mg po bid <60 kg: 30 mg po bid Food OK	86	1.2–1.6	3.5	Renal excretion, 40%	Not recommended by DHHS as initial therapy because of adverse reactions. **Highest incidence of lipoatrophy, hyperlipidemia, & lactic acidosis of all NRTIs.** Pancreatitis. Peripheral neuropathy. *(See didanosine comments.)*
Tenofovir disoproxil fumarate (TDF; Viread)—a nucleotide	300 mg tabs	CrCl ≥50 ml/min: 300 mg po q24h. Food OK; high-fat meal ↑ absorption	39 (with food) 25 (fasted)	17	>60	Renal excretion	Headache, N/V. **Cases of renal dysfunction reported:** avoid concomitant nephrotoxic agents. One study found ↑ renal disfunction at 48-wk in pts receiving TDF with a PI (mostly lopinavir/ritonavir) than with a NNRTI *(JID 197:102, 2008)*. Must adjust dose of ddI (↓) if used concomitantly but best to avoid this combination *(see ddI Comments)*. Atazanavir & lopinavir/ritonavir ↑ tenofovir concentrations: monitor for adverse effects. **Black Box warning—exacerbations of Hep B reported after stopping tenofovir.** Monitor several months after stopping TDF in Hep B pts; some may need anti-HBV Rx.
Zidovudine (ZDV, AZT; Retrovir)	100 mg caps, 300 mg tabs; 10 mg per mL IV solution; 10 mg/mL oral syrup	300 mg po q12h. Food OK	64	1.1	11	Metabolized to glucuronide & excreted in urine	Bone marrow suppression, GI intolerance, headache, insomnia, malaise, myopathy.

2. **Selected Characteristics of Non-Nucleoside Reverse Transcriptase Inhibitors (NNRTIs)**

Generic/Trade Name	Pharmaceutical Prep.	Usual Adult Dosage & Food Effect	% Absorbed, po	Serum T½, hrs	Elimination	Major Adverse Events/Comments
Delavirdine (Rescriptor)	100, 200 mg tabs	400 mg po three times daily. Food OK	85	5.8	Cytochrome P450 (3A inhibitor). 51% excreted in urine (<5% unchanged), 44% in feces	Rash severe enough to stop drug in 4.3%. ↑ AST/ALT, headaches. **Use of this agent is not recommended.**

TABLE 14D (8)

Generic/Trade Name	Pharmaceutical Prep.	Usual Adult Dosage & Food Effect	% Absorbed, po	Serum T½, hrs	Elimination	Major Adverse Events/Comments
Efavirenz (Sustiva) **(Pregnancy Category D)**	50, 100, 200 mg capsules; 600 mg tablet	600 mg po q24h at bedtime, without food. Food may ↑ serum conc., which can lead to ↑ in risk of adverse events.	42	40–55 See *Comment*	Cytochrome P450 2B6 (3A mixed inducer/inhibitor). 14–34% of dose excreted in urine as glucuronidated metabolites, 16–61% in feces	Rash severe enough to dc use of drug in 1.7%. High frequency of diverse CNS AEs: somnolence, dreams, confusion, agitation. Serious psychiatric symptoms. Certain CYP2B6 polymorphisms may predict exceptionally high plasma levels with standard doses (*CID 45:1230, 2007*). False-pos. cannabinoid screen. **Pregnancy Category D—may cause fetal harm—avoid in pregnant women or those who might become pregnant.** (Note: No single method of contraception is 100% reliable). Very long tissue T½. **If rx to be discontinued, stop efavirenz 1–2 wks before stopping companion drugs.** Otherwise, risk of developing efavirenz resistance, as after 1–2 days only efavirenz in blood &/or tissue. Some authorities bridge this gap by adding a PI to the NRTI backbone if feasible after efavirenz is discontinued. (*CID 42:401, 2006*)
Etravirine (Intelence)	100 mg tabs	200 mg twice daily after a meal	Unknown (↓ systemic exposure if taken fasting)	41	Metabolized by CYP 3A4 (inducer) & 2C9, 2C19 (inhibitor). Excreted into feces (> 90%), mostly unchanged drug.	For pts with HIV-1 resistant to NNRTIs & others. Active in vitro against most such isolates. Rash common, but rarely can be severe. Potential for multiple drug interactions. Generally, multiple mutations are required for high-level resistance (*JAC 2008: advanced access, June 19*). Because of interactions, do not use with boosted atazanavir, boosted tipranavir, unboosted PIs, or other NNRTIs.
Nevirapine (Viramune)	200 mg tabs; 50 mg per 5 mL oral suspension	200 mg po q24h x14 days & then 200 mg po bid (*see Comments & Black Box warning*) Food OK	>90	25–30	Cytochrome P450 (3A4, 2B6) inducer; 80% of dose excreted in urine as glucuronidated metabolites, 10% in feces	**Black Box warning—fatal hepatotoxicity.** Women with CD4 >250 esp. vulnerable, inc. pregnant women. Avoid in this group unless benefits clearly > risks (*www.fda.gov/ cder drug/advisory/nevirapine.htm*). If used, intensive monitoring required. Men with CD4 >400 also at ↑ risk. Rash severe enough to stop drug in 7%, **severe or life-threatening skin reactions** in 2%. Do not restart if any suspicion of such reactions. 2wk dose escalation period may ↓ skin reactions. As with efavirenz, because of long T½, consider continuing companion agents for several days if nevirapine is discontinued. **Nevirapine is contraindicated in pts with Childs Pugh B & C liver disease.**

TABLE 14D (9)

3. **Selected Characteristics of Protease Inhibitors (PIs).**

All PIs: Glucose metabolism: new diabetes mellitus or deterioration of glucose control; fat redistribution; possible hemophilia bleeding; hypertriglyceridemia or hypercholesterolemia. Exercise caution re: potential drug interactions & contraindications. QTc prolongation has been reported in a few pts taking PIs; some PIs can block HERG channels in vitro (*Lancet 365:682, 2005*)

Generic/Trade Name	Pharmaceutical Prep.	Usual Adult Dosage & Food Effect	% Absorbed, po	Serum T½, hrs	Elimination	Major Adverse Events/Comments (See Table 14E)
Atazanavir (Reyataz)	100, 150, 200, 300 mg capsules	400 mg po q24h with food. Ritonavir-boosted dose (atazanavir 300 mg po q24h + ritonavir 100 mg po q24h), with food, is recommended for ARV rx-experienced pts. The boosted dose is also used when combined with either efavirenz 600 mg po q24h or TDF 300 mg po q24h. If used with buffered ddI, take with food 2 hrs pre or 1 hr post ddI.	Good oral bioavailability; food enhances bioavailability & ↓ pharmacokinetic variability. Absorption ↓ by antacids, H₂-blockers, proton pump inhibitors. Avoid unboosted drug with PPIs/H₂-blockers. Boosted drug can be used with or > 10 hr after H2-blockers or > 12 hr after a PPI, as long as limited doses of the acid agents are used (*see 2008 drug label changes*).	Approx. 7	Cytochrome P450 (3A4, 1A2 & 2C9 inhibitor) & UGT1A1 inhibitor), 13% excreted in urine (7% unchanged), 79% excreted in feces (20% unchanged)	Lower potential for ↑ lipids. Asymptomatic unconjugated hyperbilirubinemia common; jaundice especially likely in Gilbert's syndrome (*JID 192:1381, 2005*). Headache, rash, GI symptoms. Prolongation of PR interval (1st degree AV block) reported. Caution in pre-existing conduction system disease. Efavirenz & tenofovir ↓ atazanavir exposure: use atazanavir/ritonavir regimen; also, atazanavir ↑ tenofovir concentrations—watch for adverse events. In rx-experienced pts taking TDF and needing H2 blockers, atazanavir 400 mg with ritonavir 100 mg can be given; do not use PPIs. Rare reports of renal stones
Darunavir (Prezista)	300 mg, 400 mg (new), 600 mg tablets	[600 mg darunavir + 100 mg ritonavir] po bid, with food [800 mg darunavir + 100 mg ritonavir] po q24h with food (naive patients).	82% absorbed (taken with ritonavir). Food ↑ absorption.	Approx 15 hr (with ritonavir)	Metabolized by CYP3A and is a CYP3A inhibitor	Contains sulfa moiety. Rash, nausea, headaches seen. Coadmin of certain drugs cleared by CYP3A is contraindicated (*see label*). Use with caution in pts with hepatic dysfunction. (Recent FDA warning about occasional hepatic dysfunction early in the course of treatment). Monitor carefully, esp. first several months and with pre-existing liver disease. May cause hormonal contraception failure.

TABLE 14D (10)

Generic/Trade Name	Pharmaceutical Prep.	Usual Adult Dosage & Food Effect	% Absorbed, po	Serum T½, hrs	Elimination	Major Adverse Events/Comments (See Table 14E)
Fosamprenavir (Lexiva)	700 mg tablet, 50 mg/ml oral suspension	1400 mg (two 700 mg tabs) po bid **OR** with ritonavir: [1400 mg fosamprenavir (2 tabs) + ritonavir 200 mg] po q24h **OR** [1400 mg fosamprenavir (2 tabs) + ritonavir 100 mg] po q24h **OR** [700 mg fosamprenavir (1 tab) + ritonavir 100 mg] po bid	Bioavailability not established. Food OK	7.7 Amprenavir	Hydrolyzed to amprenavir, then acts as cytochrome P450 (3A4 substrate, inhibitor, inducer)	Amprenavir prodrug. Contains sulfa moiety. Potential for serious drug interactions (see label). Rash, including Stevens-Johnson syndrome. Once daily regimens: (1) not recommended for PI-experienced pts, (2) additional ritonavir needed if given with efavirenz (see label). Boosted twice daily regimen is recommended for PI-experienced pts.
Indinavir (Crixivan)	100, 200, 400 mg capsules Store in original container with desiccant	Two 400 mg caps (800 mg) po q8h, without food or with light meal. Can take with ritonavir (e.g., 800 mg indinavir + 100 mg ritonavir po q12h), no food restrictions]	65	1.2–2	Cytochrome P450 (3A4 inhibitor)	**Maintain hydration. Nephrolithiasis,** nausea, inconsequential ↑ of indirect bilirubin (jaundice in Gilbert syndrome), ↑ AST/ALT, headache, asthenia, blurred vision, metallic taste, hemolysis. ↑ urine WBC (>100/hpf) has been assoc. with nephritis/medullary calcification, cortical atrophy.
Lopinavir + ritonavir (Kaletra)	(200 mg lopinavir + 50 mg ritonavir), and (100 mg lopinavir + 25 mg ritonavir) tablets. Tabs do not need refrigeration. Oral solution: (80 mg lopinavir + 20 mg ritonavir) per mL. Refrigerate, but can be kept at room temperature (≤77°F) x2 mos.	(400 mg lopinavir + 100 mg ritonavir)—2 tabs po bid. Higher dose may be needed in non-rx-naïve pts when used with efavirenz, nevirapine, or unboosted fosamprenavir. [Dose adjustment in concomitant drugs may be necessary; see Table 22B & Table 22C]	No food effect with tablets.	5–6	Cytochrome P450 (3A4 inhibitor)	Nausea/vomiting/diarrhea (worse when administered with zidovudine), ↑ AST/ALT, pancreatitis. Oral solution 42% alcohol. Lopinavir + ritonavir can be taken as a single daily dose of 4 tabs (total 800 mg lopinavir + 200 mg ritonavir), except in treatment-experienced pts or those taking concomitant efavirenz, nevirapine, amprenavir, or nelfinavir.
Nelfinavir (Viracept)	625, 250 mg tabs; 50 mg/gm oral powder	Two 625 mg tabs (1250 mg) po bid, with food	20–80 Food ↑ exposure & ↓ variability	3.5–5	Cytochrome P450 (3A4 inhibitor)	Diarrhea. Coadministration of drugs with life-threatening toxicities & which are cleared by CYP34A is contraindicated. Not recommended in initial regimens because of inferior efficacy.

TABLE 14D (11)

Generic/Trade Name	Pharmaceutical Prep.	Usual Adult Dosage & Food Effect	% Absorbed, po	Serum T½, hrs	Elimination	Major Adverse Events/Comments (See Table 14E)
Ritonavir (Norvir)	100 mg capsules; 600 mg per 7.5 mL solution. Refrigerate caps but not solution. Room temperature for 1 mo. is OK.	Full dose not recommended (see comments). **With rare exceptions, used exclusively to enhance pharmacokinetics of other PIs, using lower ritonavir doses.**	Food ↑ absorption	3-5	Cytochrome P450. Potent 3A4 & 2D6 inhibitor	Nausea/vomiting/diarrhea, extremity & circumoral paresthesias, hepatitis, pancreatitis, taste perversion, ↑ CPK & uric acid. **Black Box warning—** potentially fatal drug interactions. Many drug interactions—see Table 22A – Table 22C
Saquinavir (Invirase—hard gel caps or tabs) + ritonavir	Saquinavir 200 mg caps, 500 mg film-coated tabs; ritonavir 100 mg caps	[2 tabs saquinavir (1000 mg) + 1 cap ritonavir (100 mg)] po bid with food	Erratic, 4 (saquinavir alone)	1-2	Cytochrome P450 (3A4 inhibitor)	Nausea, diarrhea, headache, ↑ AST/ ALT. Avoid rifampin with saquinavir + ritonavir: ↑ hepatitis risk. **Black Box warning—** Invirase to be used only with ritonavir.
Tipranavir (Aptivus)	250 mg caps. Refrigerate unopened bottles. Use opened bottles within 2 mo. 100 mg/mL solution	[500 mg (two 250 mg caps) + ritonavir 200 mg] po bid with food. Solution: Adults: 5 mL oral solution with 200 mg ritonavir twice daily Pediatrics: (age 2-18 yrs). Calculate dose based on body weight or BSA.	May be taken with or without food, ↓ with Al⁺⁺⁺ & mg⁺⁺ antacids.	5.5-6	Cytochrome 3A4 but with ritonavir, most of drug is eliminated in feces.	Contains sulfa moiety. **Black Box warning—reports of fatal/nonfatal intracranial hemorrhage, hepatitis, fatal hepatic failure.** Use cautiously in liver disease, esp. hepB, hepC; contraindicated in Child-Pugh class B-C. Monitor LFTs. Coadministration of certain drugs contraindicated (see label). **For treatment-experienced pts or for multiple-PI resistant virus.**

4. **Selected Characteristics of Fusion Inhibitors**

Selected Characteristics of Fusion Inhibitors

Generic/Trade Name	Pharmaceutical Prep.	Usual Adult Dosage	% Absorbed	Serum T½, hrs	Elimination	Major Adverse Events/Comments (See Table 14E)
Enfuvirtide (T20, Fuzeon)	Single-use vials of 90 mg/mL when reconstituted. Vials should be stored at room temperature. Reconstituted vials can be refrigerated for 24 hrs only.	90 mg (1 ml) subcut. bid. Rotate injection sites, avoiding those currently inflamed.	84	3.8	Catabolism to its constituent amino acids with subsequent recycling of the amino acids in the body pool. Elimination pathway(s) have not been performed in humans. Does not alter the metabolism of CYP3A4, CYP2D6, CYP1A2, CYP2C19 or CYP2E1 substrates.	Local reaction site reactions 98%, 4% discontinue; erythema/induration ~80–90%, nodules/cysts ~80% **Hypersensitivity reactions reported** (fever, rash, chills, N/V, ↓ BP, &/or ↑ AST/ALT)—do not restart if occur. Including background regimens, peripheral neuropathy 8.9%, insomnia 11.3%, ↓ appetite 6.3%, myalgia 5%, lymphadenopathy 2.3%, eosinophilia ~10%. ↑ incidence of bacterial pneumonias: Alone offers little benefit to a failing regimen (NEJM 348:2249, 2003).

TABLE 14D (12)

5. Selected Characteristics of CCR-5 Co-receptor Antagonists

Generic/ Trade name	Pharmaceutical Prep. (Avg. Wholesale Price)	Usual Adult Dosage (po) & Food Effect	% Absorbed po	Serum T½, hrs	Elimination	Major Adverse Effects/Comments
Maraviroc (Selzentry)	150 mg, 300 mg film-coated tabs	Without regard to food: 150 mg bid if concomitant meds include CYP3A inhibitors including PIs (except tipranavir/ritonavir) and delavirdine (with/without CYP3A inducers) 300 mg bid without significantly interacting meds including NRTIs, tipranavir/ritonavir, nevirapine 600 mg bid if concomitant meds include CYP3A inducers, including efavirenz, (without strong CYP3A inhibitors)	Est. 33% with 300 mg dosage	14-18	CYP3A and P-glycoprotein substrate. Metabolites (via CYP3A) excreted feces > urine.	**Black Box Warning- Hepatotoxicity,** may be preceded by rash, ↑ eos or IgE. NB: no hepatoxicity was noted in MVC trials. Data lacking in hepatic/renal insufficiency; ↑ concern with either could ↑ risk of ↓ BP. Currently for treatment-experienced patients with multi-resistant strains. Document CCR-5-tropic virus before use, as treatment failures assoc. with appearance of CXCR-4 or mixed-tropic virus.

6. Selected Characteristics of Integrase Inhibitors

Generic/ Trade name	Pharmaceutical Prep. (Avg. Wholesale Price)	Usual Adult Dosage (po) & Food Effect	% Absorbed po	Serum T½, hrs	Elimination	Major Adverse Effects/Comments
Raltegravir (Isentress)	400 mg film-coated tabs	400 mg po bid, without regard to food	Unknown	~ 9	Glucuronidation via UGT1A1, with excretion into feces and urine. (Therefore does NOT require ritonavir boosting)	For treatment experienced pts with multiply-resistant virus. Generally well-tolerated. Nausea, diarrhea, headache, fever similar to placebo. CK ↑ & rhabdomyolysis reported, with unclear relationship to drug.

TABLE 14E– ANTIRETROVIRAL DRUGS AND ADVERSE EFFECTS
(www.aidsinfo.nih.gov)
See also www.aidsinfo.nih.gov; for combinations, see individual components

DRUG NAME(S): GENERIC (TRADE)	MOST COMMON ADVERSE EFFECTS	MOST SIGNIFICANT ADVERSE EFFECTS
Nucleoside Reverse Transcriptase Inhibitors (NRTI) (Black Box warning for all nucleoside/nucleotide RTIs: lactic acidosis/hepatic steatosis, potentially fatal. Also carry Warnings that fat redistribution has been observed)		
Abacavir (Ziagen)	Headache 7-13%, nausea 7-19%, diarrhea 7%, malaise 7-12%	**Black Box warning-Hypersensitivity reaction (HR)** in 8% with malaise, fever, GI upset, rash, lethargy & respiratory symptoms most commonly reported; myalgia, arthralgia, edema, parethesia less common. **Rechallenge contraindicated; may be life-threatening.** Severe HR may be more common with once-daily dosing. **HLA-B*5701 allele** predicts ↑ risk of HR in Caucasian pop.; excluding pts with B*5701 markedly ↓'d HR incidence (*NEJM 358:568, 2008; CID 46:1111-1118, 2008*). DHHS guidelines recommend testing for B*5701 and use of abacavir-containing regimens only if HLA-B*5701 negative; Vigilance essential in all groups. Possible increased risk of MI under study (*www.fda.gov/CDER*).
Didanosine (ddI) (Videx)	Diarrhea 28%, nausea 6%, rash 9%, headache 7%, fever 12%, hyperuricemia 2%	**Pancreatitis 1-9%. Black Box warning—Cases of fatal & nonfatal pancreatitis** have occurred in pts receiving ddI, especially when used in combination with d4T or d4T + hydroxyurea. Fatal lactic acidosis in pregnancy with ddI + d4T. Peripheral neuropathy in 20%, 12% required dose reduction. Rarely, retinal changes. Possible increased risk of MI under study (*www.fda.gov/CDER*).
Emtricitabine (FTC) (Emtriva)	Well tolerated. Headache, diarrhea, nausea, rash, skin hyperpigmentation	Potential for lactic acidosis (as with other NRTIs). Also **in Black Box—severe exacerbation of hepatitis B on stopping drug reported—monitor clinical/labs for several months after stopping in pts with hepB.** Anti-HBV rx may be warranted if FTC stopped.
Lamivudine (3TC) (Epivir)	Well tolerated. Headache 35%, nausea 33%, diarrhea 18%, abdominal pain 9%, insomnia 11% (all in combination with ZDV). Pancreatitis more common in pediatrics (15%).	**Black Box warning.** Make sure to use HIV dosage, not Hep B dosage. **Exacerbation of hepatitis B on stopping drug. Patients with hepB who stop lamivudine require close clinical/lab monitoring for several months.** Anti-HBV rx may be warranted if 3TC stopped.
Stavudine (d4T) (Zerit)	Diarrhea, nausea, vomiting, headache	**Peripheral neuropathy** 15-20%. Pancreatitis 1%. Appears to produce lactic acidosis more commonly than other NRTIs. **Black Box warning—Fatal & nonfatal pancreatitis with d4T + ddI + hydroxy-urea. Fatal lactic acidosis/steatosis in pregnant women receiving d4T + ddI.** Motor weakness in the setting of lactic acidosis mimicking the clinical presentation of Guillain-Barre syndrome (including respiratory failure) (rare).
Zidovudine (ZDV, AZT) (Retrovir)	Nausea 50%, anorexia 20% vomiting 17%, **headache 62%.** Also reported: asthenia, insomnia, myalgias, nail pigmentation. Macrocytosis expected with all dosage regimens.	**Black Box warning—hematologic toxicity, myopathy. Anemia** (<8 gm, 1%), granulocytopenia (<750, 1.8%). Anemia may respond to epoetin alfa if endogenous serum erythropoietin levels are ≤500 milliUnits/mL.
Nucleotide Reverse Transcriptase Inhibitor (NtRTI) (Black Box warning for all nucleoside/nucleotide RTIs: lactic acidosis/hepatic steatosis, potentially fatal. Also carry Warnings that fat redistribution has been observed)		
Tenofovir disoproxil fumarate (TDF) (Viread)	Diarrhea 11%, nausea 8%, vomiting 5%, flatulence 4% (generally well tolerated)	**Black Box Warning—Severe exacerbations of hepatitis B reported in pts who stop tenofovir.** Monitor carefully if drug is stopped; anti-HBV rx may be warranted if TDF stopped. Possible ↑ bone demineralization. Reports of Fanconi syndrome & **renal injury induced by tenofovir** (*CID 37:e174, 2003; J AIDS 35:269, 2004; CID 42:283,2006*). Modest decline in Ccr with TDF may be greater than with other NRTIs (*CID 40:1194, 2005*). Monitor creatinine clearance, especially carefully in those with pre-existing renal dysfunction. **Dose reduce to every 48 hrs if CrCl<50 cc/min.** Decline in renal function may be more rapid in pts receiving TDF with a PI vs. TDF with an NNRTI (*JID 197:102, 2008*).

TABLE 14E (2)

DRUG NAME(S): GENERIC (TRADE)	MOST COMMON ADVERSE EFFECTS	MOST SIGNIFICANT ADVERSE EFFECTS
Non-Nucleoside Reverse Transcriptase Inhibitors (NNRTI)		
Delavirdine (Rescriptor)	Nausea, diarrhea, vomiting, headache	**Skin rash** has occurred in 18%; can continue or restart drug in most cases. Stevens-Johnson syndrome & erythema multiforme have been reported rarely. ↑ in liver enzymes in <5% of patients.
Efavirenz (Sustiva)	**CNS side-effects 52%;** symptoms include dizziness, insomnia, somnolence, impaired concentration, psychiatric sx, & abnormal dreams; symptoms are worse after 1st or 2nd dose & improve over 2–4 weeks; discontinuation rate 2.6%. Rash 26% (vs. 17% in compartors); often improves with oral antihistamines; discontinuation rate 1.7%. Can cause false-positive urine test results for cannabinoid with CEDIA DAU multi-level THC assay.	Serious neuropsychiatric symptoms reported, including severe depression (2.4%) & suicidal ideation (0.7%). Elevation in liver enzymes. **Teratogenicity reported in primates; pregnancy category D—may cause fetal harm, avoid in pregnant women or those who might become pregnant** (see Table 8A of The Sanford Guide to HIV/AIDS Therapy 2009). NOTE: No single method of contraception is 100% reliable. Contraindicated with certain drugs metabolized by CYP3A4. Slow metabolism in those homozygous for the CYP-2B6 G516T allele resulting in exaggerated toxicity and intolerance. This allele much more common in blacks and women (CID 42:408, 2006).
Etravirine (Intelence)	Rash 9%, generally mild to moderate and spontaneously resolving; 2% dc clinical trials for rash. More common in women. Nausea 5%.	Hypersensitivity or severe rash (erythema multiforme or Stevens-Johnson) < 0.1%. Potential for CYP-mediated drug interactions.
Nevirapine (Viramune)	**Rash 37%:** usually occurs during 1st 6 wks of therapy. Follow recommendations for 14-day lead-in period to ↓ risk of rash (see Table 14D). Women experience 7-fold ↑ in risk of rash (CID 32:124, 2001). 50% resolve within 2 wks of dc drug & 80% by 1 month. 6.7% discontinuation rate.	**Black Box warning—Severe life-threatening skin reactions reported:** Stevens-Johnson syndrome, toxic epidermal necrolysis, & hypersensitivity reaction or drug rash with eosinophilia & systemic symptoms (DRESS) (ArIM 161:2501, 2001). For severe rashes, dc drug immediately & do not restart. In a clinical trial, the use of prednisone ↑ the risk of rash. **Black Box warning—Life-threatening hepatotoxicity reported,** 2/3 during the first 12 wks of rx. Overall 1% develop hepatitis. Pts with pre-existing ↑ in ALT or AST &/or history of chronic Hep B or C ↑ susceptible (Hepatol 35:182, 2002). Women with CD4 >250, including pregnant women, at ↑ risk. Avoid in this group unless no other option. Men with CD4 >400 also at ↑ risk. Monitor pts intensively (clinical & LFTs), esp. during the first 12 wks of rx. If clinical hepatotoxicity, severe skin or hypersensitivity reactions occur, dc drug & never rechallenge.
Protease inhibitors (PI)		
Abnormalities in glucose metabolism, dyslipidemias, fat redistribution syndromes are potential problems. Pts taking PI may be at increased risk for developing osteopenia/osteoporosis. Spontaneous bleeding episodes have been reported in HIV+ pts with hemophilia being treated with PI. Rheumatoid complications have been reported with use of PIs (An Rheum Dis 61:82, 2002). Potential of some PIs for QTc prolongation has been suggested (Lancet 365:682, 2005). **Caution for all PIs**—Coadministration with certain drugs dependent on CYP3A for elimination & for which ↑ levels can cause serious toxicity may be contraindicated.		
Atazanavir (Reyataz)	Asymptomatic unconjugated hyperbilirubinemia in up to 60% of pts, jaundice in 7–9% (especially with Gilbert syndrome (JID 192: 1381, 2005)). Moderate to severe events: Diarrhea 1–3%, nausea 6–14%, abdominal pain 4%, headache 6%, rash 5–7%.	Prolongation of PR interval (1st degree AV block) reported; rarely 2° AV block. QTc increase and torsades reported (CID 44:e67, 2007). Acute interstitial nephritis (Am J Kid Dis 44:E81, 2004) and urolithiasis (atazanavir stones) reported (AIDS 20:2131, 2006; NEJM 355:2158, 2006).
Darunavir (Prezista)	With background regimens, headache 15%, nausea 18%, diarrhea 20%, ↑ amylase 17%. Rash in 17% of treated; 0.3% discontinuation.	Hepatitis in 0.5%, some with fatal outcome. Use caution in pts with HBV or HCV co-infections or other hepatic dysfunction. Monitor for clinical symptoms and LFTs. Stevens-Johnson syndrome, erythema multiforme. Potential for major drug interactions. May cause failure of hormonal contraceptives.
Fosamprenavir (Lexiva)	Skin rash ~ 20% (moderate or worse in 3–8%), nausea, headache, diarrhea.	Rarely Stevens-Johnson syndrome, hemolytic anemia. Pro-drug of amprenavir. Contains sulfa moiety.

TABLE 14E (3)

DRUG NAME(S): GENERIC (TRADE)	MOST COMMON ADVERSE EFFECTS	MOST SIGNIFICANT ADVERSE EFFECTS
Protease inhibitors *(continued)*		
Indinavir (Crixivan)	↑ in indirect bilirubin 10–15% (≥2.5 mg/dl), with overt jaundice especially likely in those with Gilbert syndrome *(JID 192:1381, 2005)*. Nausea 12%, vomiting 4%, diarrhea 5%. Paronychia of big toe reported *(CID 32:140, 2001)*.	**Kidney stones.** Due to indinavir crystals in collecting system. Nephrolithiasis in 12% of adults, higher in pediatrics. Minimize risk with good hydration (at least 48 oz. water/day) *(AAC 42:332, 1998)*. Tubulointerstitial nephritis/renal cortical atrophy reported in association with asymptomatic ↑ urine WBC. Severe hepatitis reported in 3 cases *(Ln 349:924, 1997)*. Hemolytic anemia reported.
Lopinavir/Ritonavir (Kaletra)	GI: **diarrhea** 14–24%, nausea 2–16%. More diarrhea with q24h dosing.	Lipid abnormalities in up to 20–40%. Hepatitis, with hepatic decompensation; caution especially in those with pre-existing liver disease. Pancreatitis. Inflammatory edema of legs *(AIDS 16:673, 2002)*.
Nelfinavir (Viracept)	Mild to moderate **diarrhea** 20%. Oat bran tabs, calcium, or oral anti-diarrheal agents (e.g., loperamide, diphenoxylate/ atropine sulfate) can be used to manage diarrhea.	Potential for drug interactions.
Ritonavir (Norvir) (With rare exceptions, only use is to enhance levels of other anti-retrovirals, because of ↑ toxicity/ interactions with full-dose ritonavir)	GI: bitter aftertaste ↓ by taking with chocolate milk, Ensure, or Advera; nausea 23%; ↓ by initial dose esc (titration) regimen; vomiting 13%; diarrhea 15%. Circumoral paresthesias 5–6%. ↑ dose >100 mg bid assoc. with ↑ GI side-effects & ↑ in lipid abnormalities.	Hepatic failure *(AnIM 129:670, 1998)*. Black Box warning relates to many important drug-drug interactions—inhibits P450 CYP3A & CYP2D6 system—may be life-threatening *(see Table 22A)*. Rarely Stevens-Johnson syndrome, anaphylaxis.
Saquinavir (Invirase: hard cap, tablet)	**Diarrhea,** abdominal discomfort, nausea, headache	**Black Box Warning—Use Invirase only with ritonavir.** Avoid garlic capsules (may reduce SQV levels) and use cautiously with proton-pump inhibitors (increased SQV levels significant; may lead to increased GI sx, triglycerides, DVT).
Tipranavir (Aptivus)	Nausea & vomiting, diarrhea, abdominal pain. Rash in 8-10%, more common in women, & 33% in women taking ethinyl estradiol. Discontinue drug if skin rash develops. Major lipid effects.	**Black Box Warning—associated with hepatitis & fatal hepatic failure.** Risk of hepatotoxicity increased in hepB & hepC co-infection. **Associated with fatal/nonfatal intracranial hemorrhage (can inhibit platelet aggregation).** Caution in those with bleeding risks. Potential for major drug interactions. Contains sulfa moiety.
Fusion Inhibitor		
Enfuvirtide (T20, Fuzeon)	Local injection site reactions (98% at least 1 local ISR, 4% dc because of ISR) (pain & discomfort, induration, erythema, nodules & cysts, pruritus, & ecchymosis). Diarrhea 32%, nausea 23%, fatigue 20%.	↑ Rate of bacterial pneumonia (6.7 pneumonia events/100 pt yrs), **hypersensitivity reactions ≤1%** (rash, fever, nausea & vomiting, chills, rigors, hypotension, & ↑ serum liver transaminases); can occur with reexposure.
CCR5 Co-receptor Antagonists		
Maraviroc (Selzentry)	With ARV background: cough 13%, fever 12%, rash 10%, abdominal pain 8%. Also, dizziness, myalgia, arthralgias. ↑ Risk of URI, HSV infection.	**Black box warning-Hepatotoxicity.** May be preceded by allergic features. No hepatoxicity was noted in clinical trials. Use with caution in pt with HepB or C. Cardiac ischemia/infarction in 1.3%. May cause ↓ BP, syncope. Significant interactions with CYP3A inducers/inhibitors. Long-term risk of malignancy unknown.
Integrase Inhibitors		
Raltegravir (Isentress)	Diarrhea, headache, nausea. LFT ↑ may be more common in pts co-infected with HBV or HCV.	Hypersensitivity can occur. ↑ CK with myopathy or rhabdomyolysis reported, with unclear relationship to drug.

TABLE 15A – ANTIMICROBIAL PROPHYLAXIS FOR SELECTED BACTERIAL INFECTIONS*

CLASS OF ETIOLOGIC AGENT/DISEASE/CONDITION	PROPHYLAXIS AGENT/DOSE/ROUTE/DURATION	COMMENTS
Group B streptococcal disease (GBS), neonatal: Approaches to management [CDC Guidelines, *MMWR* 51(RR-11):1, 2002]:		
Pregnant women—intrapartum antimicrobial prophylaxis procedures: 1. Screen all pregnant women with vaginal & rectal swab for GBS at 35-37 wks gestation (unless other indications for prophylaxis exist: GBS bacteriuria during this pregnancy or previously delivered infant with invasive GBS disease; even then cultures may be useful for susceptibility testing). Use transport medium; GBS survive at room temp. up to 96 hrs. **Rx during labor if swab culture positive.** 2. Rx during labor if previously delivered infant with invasive GBS infection, or if any GBS bacteriuria during this pregnancy (*MMWR* 53:506, 2004). 3. Rx if GBS status unknown but if any of the following are present: (a) delivery at <37 wks gestation [see *MMWR* 51(RR-11):1, 2002 algorithm for threatened preterm delivery]; or (b) duration of ruptured membranes ≥18 hrs; or (c) intrapartum temp. ≥100.4°F (≥38.0°C).	**Prophylactic regimens during labor:** **Pen G** 5 million units IV (load) then 2.5 million units IV q4h. Alternative rx: **Ampicillin** 2 gm IV (load) then give 1 gm IV q4h. **Pen-allergic: Pts not at high risk for anaphylaxis: Cefazolin** 2 gm IV initial dose, then 1 gm IV q8h. **Pts at high risk for anaphylaxis:** GBS susceptible to clinda & erythro: **Clindamycin** 900 mg IV q8h or **erythromycin** 500 mg IV q6h. Vancomycin for pts at high risk for anaphylaxis when alternative to clindamycin or erythromycin needed (e.g., GBS-resistant or unknown susceptibility). Continue treatment until delivery.	
Neonate of mother given prophylaxis	Careful observation of signs & symptoms. 95% of infants will show clinical signs of infection during the 1st 24 hrs whether mother received intrapartum antibiotics or not (*Pediatrics* 106:244, 2000). For gestational age <35 wks or intrapartum antibiotics <4 hrs, lab evaluation (CBC, diff, blood culture) & ≥48 hr observation recommended. See algorithm: *MMWR* 51(RR-11):1, 2002.	
Preterm, premature rupture of the membranes in Group B strep-negative women	[IV **ampicillin** 2 gm q6h + IV **erythromycin** 250 mg q6h) for 48 hrs followed by **amoxicillin** 250 mg q8h + po **erythromycin** base 333 mg q8h times 5 days.	Antibiotic rx reduced infant respiratory distress syndrome (50.6% to 40.8%, p = 0.03), necro-tizing enterocolitis (5.8% to 2.3%, p = 0.03) and prolonged pregnancy (2.9 to 6.1 days, p < 0.001) vs placebo. In 1 large study (4809 pts), po erythromycin rx improved neonatal outcomes vs placebo (11.2% vs 14.4% poor outcomes, p=0.02 for single births) but not co-AM-CL or both drugs in combination (both assoc. with ↑ necrotizing enterocolitis) (*Ln* 357:979, 2001). (See ACOG discussion, *Ob Gyn* 102:875, 2003; *Practice Bulletin in ObGyn* 109:1007, 2007; *Rev Obstet Gynecol* 1:11, 2008).
	Decreases infant morbidity. (*JAMA* 278:989, 1997) (*Note:* May require additional antibiotics for therapy of specific existing infections)	
Post-splenectomy bacteremia. Likely agents: Pneumococci (90%), meningococci , H. influenzae type b (also at ↑ risk of fatal malaria, severe babesiosis , and *Capnocytophaga spp.*) Ref.: 2006 *Red Book, 27th Ed., Amer Acad Pediatrics*	**Immunizations:** Ensure admin. of pneumococcal vaccine, H. influenzae B & quadrivalent meningococcal vaccines at recommended times. (*See Table 20*). In addition, asplenic children with sickle cell anemia, thalassemia, & perhaps others, daily antimicrobial prophylaxis until at least age 5—see *Comments*.	Antimicrobial prophylaxis until age 5: Amox 20 mg/kg/day or Pen V-K 125 mg bid. Over age 5: Consider Pen V-K 250 mg bid for at least 1 yr in children post-splenectomy. Some recommend prophylaxis until at least age 18. Maintain immunizations plus self-administer AM-CL with any febrile illness while seeking physician assistance. For self-administered therapy, respiratory FQ can be considered in beta lactam-allergic pt in appropriate populations. Pen. allergy: TMP-SMX or clarithro are options, but resistance in *S. pneumo* may be significant in some areas, particularly among pen-resistant isolates
Sexual Exposure		
Sexual assault survivor [likely agents and risks: see *NEJM* 332:234, 1995; *MMWR* 55(RR-11):1, 2006]	(**Ceftriaxone** 125 mg IM) + (**metronidazole** 2 gm po single dose) + [(**azithromycin** 1 gm po single dose) or (**doxycycline** 100 mg po bid times 7 days)] [*MMWR* 55(RR-11):1, 2006]	Obtain expert advice re: forensic exam & specimens, pregnancy, physical trauma, psychological support. If decision is to proceed with spec. collection, at initial exam: Test for gonococci & chlamydia, wet mount for T. vaginalis (& culture vaginal swab). Serologic evaluation for syphilis, Hep B, HIV, others as appropriate. Initiate post-exposure protocols for HIV & hepatitis B as appropriate (*see Table 15D*). Follow-up exam for STD at 1-2 wks. Retest syphilis & HIV serology at 6, 12, 24 wks if negative earlier.
Sexual contacts, likely agents: N. gonorrhoeae, C. trachomatis	[(**Ceftriaxone** 125 mg IM once) or (**cefixime** 400 mg po once)] for GC, plus [(**doxycycline** 100 mg bid, po times 7 days) or (**azithromycin** 1 gm po once)], for Chlamydia	Be sure to check for syphilis since all regimens may not eradicate incubating syphilis. Consider also T. vaginalis. Identify & rx contacts as appropriate to suspected STD [*see MMWR 55(RR-11):1, 2006 for other etiologies & rx options*]. Evaluate for HIV/HBV risks (*See Table 15D*).
Syphilis exposure		Presumptive rx for exposure within 3 mos., as tests may be negative. *See Table 1A, page 22.* Make effort to dx syphilis
Sickle-cell disease . Likely agent: S. pneumoniae (*see post-splenectomy, above*) Ref.: 2006 *Red Book, 27th Ed., Amer Acad Pediatrics*	Children <5 yrs: **Penicillin V** 125 mg po bid ≥5 yrs: **Penicillin V** 250 mg po bid. (Alternative in children: Amoxicillin 20 mg per kg per day)	Start prophylaxis by 2 mos. (*Pediatrics* 106:367, 2000). Age-appropriate vaccines, including pneumococcal,Hib, influenza, meningococcal. Treating infections, consider possibility of penicillin non-susceptible pneumococci.

* See page 3 for abbreviations

TABLE 15B – ANTIBIOTIC PROPHYLAXIS TO PREVENT SURGICAL INFECTIONS IN ADULTS*

(CID 38:1706, 2004; Am J Surg 189:395, 2005)

Surgical Procedures: To be optimally effective, **antibiotics must be started in the interval: 2 hrs before time of surgical incision** *(NEJM 326:281, 1992) or even closer to incision time (JAC 58:645, 2006).* For most procedures the number of doses needed for optimal coverage is not defined. Most applications employ a single dose *(Treat.Guide.Med.Lett. 4.83, 2006)* although FDA-approved product labeling is often for 2 or more doses. If the surgical procedure lasts >3 hrs, additional intraoperative doses of rapidly eliminated drugs should be given at approx. 3-hr intervals. A recent consensus statement from the National Surgical Infection Prevention Project *(CID 38:1706, 2004)* advises antibiotic prophylaxis be started within 1 hr before incision (except vancomycin & quinolones), be supplemented intraoperatively if the procedure lasts more than 2 half-lives of the prophylactic agent, and in most cases not be extended beyond 24 hrs. (Note: The dose/route/durations listed below for adults with normal renal function & not intolerant of these agents are for the most part those approved in FDA product labeling. For single dose regimens, the dosage & route are the same.) *See Table 15C for regimens to reduce risk of endocarditis.*

General Comments: (a) An evolving issue is when to use vancomycin for surgical prophylaxis, and whether to use it alone or in combination with another agent that extends the antimicrobial spectrum. In centers experiencing high rates of infections due to methicillin-resistant staphylococci, or for individual patients at high risk for surgical infection due to MRSA addition of vancomycin to the standard prophylaxis listed below may be justifiable. This may be especially true for those undergoing orthopedic surgery or cardiovascular (both cardiac and vascular) procedures. (b) In some centers, ↑ resistance in gram-negative organisms may render certain regimens (e.g., quinolones) unacceptable. (c) Pharmacokinetic considerations suggest that typical prophylaxis dosing may yield suboptimal serum/tissue levels in pts with high BMI *(see Surgery 136:738, 2004 for cefazolin; Eur J Clin Pharm 54:632, 1998 for vancomycin),* although clinical implications uncertain. (d) A potential risk of prophylaxis: during an outbreak of infection with hypervirulent C. difficile, 40 of 98 cases occurring in surgical pts had received no antibiotics other than peri-operative prophylaxis; no cases occurred among 389 surgical pts who had received no antibiotic *(CID 46:1838, 2008).* (e) For patients intolerant of penicillins or cephalosporins, vancomycin could be used to provide gram-positive coverage; clindamycin would be an alternative, but some staphylococci (esp. MRSA) are resistant. The recommended cephalosporins also provide activity against some gram-negative bacteria; when such activity is desirable, particularly for abdominal procedures, alternative gram-negative agents with gram-negative activity include fluoroquinolones or aminoglycosides, or aztreonam (in those without cross-sensitivity with the other β-lactams). Clindamycin or metronidazole might be included in prophylaxis regimens where activity against gram-negative anaerobes is desirable (e.g., hysterectomy). *(See Treat Guide Med Lett. 4.84, 2006).*

TYPE OF SURGERY	PROPHYLAXIS	COMMENTS
Cardiovascular Surgery Antibiotic prophylaxis in cardiovascular surgery has been proven beneficial only in the following procedures: • Reconstruction of abdominal aorta • Procedures on the leg that involve a groin incision • Any vascular procedure that inserts prosthesis/foreign body • Lower extremity amputation for ischemia • Cardiac surgery • Permanent Pacemakers *(see Comment)*	**Cefazolin** 1–2 gm IV as a single dose or q8h for 1–2 days, or **cefuroxime** 1.5 gm IV as a single dose or q12h for total of 6 gm or **vancomycin** 1 gm IV as single dose or q12h for 1–2 days. Consider **intranasal mupirocin** evening before, day of surgery & bid for 5 days post-op in pts with pos. nasal culture for S. aureus.	Single infusion just before surgery probably as effective as multiple doses. Not needed for cardiac catheterization. For prosthetic heart valves, customary to stop prophylaxis either after after removal of retrosternal drainage catheters or just a 2nd dose after coming off bypass. Vancomycin may be preferable in hospitals with ↑ freq of MRSA or in high-risk pts *(CID 38: 1555, 2004),* or those colonized with MRSA *(CID 38:1706, 2004);* however, does not cover gm-neg. bacilli; therefore would add cefazolin. Meta-analysis failed to demonstrate overall superiority of vancomycin over β-lactam prophylaxis for cardiac surgery *(CID 38: 1357, 2004).* A meta-analysis of 7 placebo-controlled randomized studies of prophylaxis for implantation of permanent pacemakers, sig. ↓ in incidence of infection *(Circulation 97: 1796, 1998).* Intranasal mupirocin ↓ sternal wound infections from S. aureus in 1850 pts; used historical controls *(An Thor Surg 71:1572, 2001);* in another trial, it ↓ nosocomial S. aureus infections only in nasal carriers *(NEJM 346:1871, 2002).* One study of 0.12% chlorhexidine gluconate gel to nares and oral rinse showed ↓ deep surg site and lower resp infections *(JAMA 296:2460, 2006).*
Gastric, Biliary and Colonic Surgery **Gastroduodenal/Biliary** Gastroduodenal, includes percutaneous endoscopic gastrostomy (high-risk only; see *Comments*). Biliary, includes laparoscopic cholecystectomy (high-risk only; see *Comments*).	**Cefazolin** or **cefoxitin** or **cefotetan** or **ceftizoxime** or **cefuroxime** 1.5 gm IV as a single dose or (some give additional doses q12h for 2–3 days). In biliary surgery, **cefazolin** 1 gm or **ceftizoxime** 1 gm (± repeat dosing at 12 & 24 hrs) were equivalent *(AAC 40:70, 1996).*	Gastroduodenal: High-risk is marked obesity, obstruction, ↓ gastric acid or ↓ motility. Meta-analysis supports use in percutaneous endoscopic gastrostomy *(Am J Gastro 95:3133, 2000).* Biliary high-risk: age > 70, acute cholecystitis, non-functioning gallbladder, obstructive jaundice or common duct stones. With cholangitis, treat as infection, not prophylaxis (e.g. PIP-TZ 3.375 gm q6h or 4.5 gm q8h IV, TC-CL 3.1 gm q4–6h IV, or AM-SB 3 gm q6h IV). (For guidelines of American Soc of Gastrointestinal Endoscopy, see *Gastroint Endosc 67:791, 2008*).
Endoscopic retrograde cholangiopancreatography Controversial: No data from single dose piperacillin in randomized placebo-controlled trial, *AnIM 125:442, 1996* (see *Comment*)	No rx without obstruction. If obstruction: **Ciprofloxacin** 500–750 mg po 2 hrs prior to procedure or **Ceftizoxime** 1.5 gm IV 1 hr prior to procedure or **PIP-TZ** 4.5 gm IV 1 hr prior to procedure	Most studies show that **achieving adequate drainage** will prevent postprocedural cholangitis or sepsis and no further benefit from prophylactic antibiotics. Meta-analysis suggested antibiotics may ↓ bacteremia, but not sepsis/cholangitis *(Endoscopy 31:718, 1999).* Oral CIP as effective as cephalosporins in 2 studies & less expensive but resistance increasing *(CID 23:380, 1996).* See *Gastroint Endosc 67:791, 2008* for Amer Soc Gastroint Endosc recommendations.

* See page 3 for abbreviations

TABLE 15B (2)

TYPE OF SURGERY	PROPHYLAXIS	COMMENTS
Gastric, Biliary and Colonic Surgery *(continued)*		
Colorectal	Oral antibiotics for elective surgery (see *Comments*) **Parenteral regimens** (emergency or elective): [**Cefazolin** 1-2 gm IV + **metronidazole** 0.5 gm IV] or **cefoxitin** or **cefotetan** 1-2 gm IV (if available) or **AM-SB** 3 gm IV or **ERTA** 1 gm IV (*NEJM 355:2640, 2006* study found ertapenem more effective than cefotetan, but associated with non-significant ↑ risk of C. difficile).	**Oral regimens: Neomycin + erythromycin** Pre-op day: (1) 10am 4L polyethylene glycol electrolyte solution (Colyte, GoLYTELY) po over 2hr. (2) Clear liquid diet only. (3) 1pm, 2pm & 11pm, neomycin 1 gm + erythro base 1 gm po. (4) NPO after midnight. Alternative regimens have been less well studied; GoLYTELY 1–6pm, then neomycin 2 gm po + metronidazole 2 gm po at 7pm & 11pm. Oral regimen as effective as parenteral; parenteral in add'n to oral not required but often used (*AmJSurg 189:395, 2005*). [*Alternative:* Neomycin + metronidazole: GoLYTELY 1-6 pm, then neomycin 2 gm PO + metronidazole 2 gm PO at 7 pm and 11 pm.]. Many used both parenteral + oral regimens for elective procedures (*AmJSurg 189:395, 2005*), but recent ↓ enthusiasm for mechanical bowel preparation. Meta-analysis did not support mech bowel prep in preventing anastomotic leaks with elective colorectal surg (*Cochr Database Syst Rev (3), 2007*)
Ruptured viscus: See Peritoneum/Peritonitis. Secondary, Table 1A, page 44.		
Head and Neck Surgery (*Ann Otol Rhinol Laryngol 101 Suppl:16, 1992*) **Cefazolin** 2 gm IV (single dose) or [**clindamycin** 600–900 mg IV (single dose) + **gentamicin** 1.5 mg per kg IV (single dose)]		Antimicrobial prophylaxis in head & neck surg appears efficacious only for procedures involving oral/ pharyngeal mucosa (e.g., laryngeal or pharyngeal tumor) but even with prophylaxis, wound infection rate high (41% in 1 center) (*Head Neck 23:447, 2001*). Uncontaminated head & neck surg does not require prophylaxis.
Neurosurgical Procedures [Prophylaxis not effective in ↓ infection rate with intracranial pressure monitors in retrospective analysis of 215 pts (*J Neurol Neurosurg Psych 69:381, 2000*)]		
Clean, non-implant: e.g., craniotomy	**Cefazolin** 1-2 gm IV once. Alternative: **vanco** 1 gm IV once	Reference: *Ln 344:1547, 1994.*
Clean, contaminated (cross sinuses, or naso/oropharynx)	**Clindamycin** 900 mg IV (single dose)	British recommend amoxicillin-clavulanate 1.2 gm IV[nus] or (cefuroxime 1.5 gm IV + metronidazole 0.5 gm IV).
CSF shunt surgery:	**Cefazolin** 1-2 gm IV once. Alternative: **vanco** 1 gm IV once.	Meta-analysis suggests benefit (*Cochrane Database (4) 2006*)
Obstetric/Gynecologic Surgery		
Vaginal or abdominal hysterectomy	**Cefazolin** 1–2 gm or **cefoxitin** 1–2 gm or **cefotetan** 1–2 gm or **cefuroxime** 1.5 gm all IV 30 min. before surgery.	1 study found cefotetan superior to cefazolin (*CID 20:677, 1995*). For prolonged procedures, doses can be repeated q4–8h for duration of procedure. Ampicillin–sulbactam is considered an acceptable alternative (*CID43:322, 2006*).
Cesarean section for premature rupture of membranes or active labor	**Cefazolin** once, administer IV as soon as umbilical cord clamped. (See *Comments*).	Prophylaxis decreases risk of endometritis/wound infection in elective as well as non-elective C-section; single dose equivalent to multiple dose regimens (*Cochrane Database System Rev 2002, issue 3, & 1999, issue 1*). Study suggests pre-incision cefazolin may be superior to post-clamp dosing in preventing endomyometritis (*Am J Obstet Gynecol 196:455.e1, 2007*). Larger studies needed to assess effect on neonates.
Abortion	1st trimester: aqueous **pen G** 2 mU IV or **doxycycline** 300 mg po. 2nd trimester: **Cefazolin** 1 gm IV	Meta-analysis showed benefit of antibiotic prophylaxis in all risk groups. One regimen was doxy 100 mg orally 1 hr before procedure, then 200 mg after procedure (*Ob Gyn 87:884, 1996*).

* See page 3 for abbreviations

TABLE 15B (3)

TYPE OF SURGERY	PROPHYLAXIS	COMMENTS
Orthopedic Surgery [Most pts with prosthetic joints do not require prophylaxis for routine dental procedures, but individual considerations prevail for high-risk procedures & prostheses (*J Am Dental Assn 134:895, 2003; Med Lett 47:59, 2005*)].		
Hip arthroplasty, spinal fusion	Same as cardiac	Customarily stopped after "Hemovac" removed. NSIPP workgroup recommends stopping prophylaxis within 24 hrs of surgery (*CID 38:1706, 2004*).
Total joint replacement (other than hip)	**Cefazolin** 1–2 gm IV pre-op (± 2nd dose) or **vancomycin** 1 gm IV on call to OR	NSIPP workgroup recommends stopping prophylaxis within 24 hrs of surgery (*CID 38:1706, 2004*). Recent study in total knee arthroplasty found dosing cefuroxime 1.5 gm just prior to tourniquet release (+ 2nd dose 6 hr after surgery) was not inferior to dosing before inflation (+ 2nd dose) (*CID 46:1009, 2008*).
Open reduction of closed fracture with internal fixation	**Ceftriaxone** 2 gm IV or IM once	3.6% vs 8.3% (for placebo) infection found in Dutch trauma trial (*Ln 347:1133, 1996*).
Peritoneal Dialysis Catheter Placement	**Vancomycin** single 1 gm IV dose 12 hrs prior to procedure	Effectively reduced peritonitis during 14 days post-placement in 221 pts: vanco 1%, cefazolin 7%, placebo 12% (p=0.02) (*Am J Kidney Dis 36:1014, 2000*).
Urologic Surgery/Procedures		
Antibiotics are not recommended in pts with sterile urine undergoing simple cystoscopy or cystography. A meta-analysis found prophylaxis (various, incl. fluoroquinolones) to reduce bacteriuria and sepsis after TURP even in pts with sterile urine (*J Urol 167:571, 2002*). (*Amer Urol Assoc's Best Practice Policy Statement discusses prophylaxis for various procedures in J Urol 179: 1379, 2008*; other meta-analyses are planned).		
Pts with pre-operative bacteriuria should be treated.	Recommended antibiotic to pts with pre-operative bacteriuria: **Cefazolin** 1 gm IV q8h times 1–3 doses perioperatively, followed by oral antibiotics (**nitrofurantoin** or **TMP-SMX**) until catheter is removed or for 10 days. Modify based on susceptibility test results. Prophylaxis usually given for GU implants (*Treat Guide Med Lett 4:83, 2006*).	
Transrectal prostate biopsy	**Ciprofloxacin** 500 mg po 12 hrs prior to biopsy and repeated 12 hrs after 1st dose	Bacteremia 7% with CIP vs 37% gentamicin (*Urology 38:84, 1991; review in JAC 39:115, 1997*). Levo 500 mg 30–60 min. before procedure was effective in low-risk pts; additional doses were given for ↑ risk (*J Urol 168:1021, 2002*). ↑ Fluoroquinolone resistance in enteric gram-negatives is a concern.
Other		
Breast surgery, herniorrhaphy	**P Ceph 1,2**, *dosage as Gynecologic Surgery, above*	Meta-analysis did not show clear evidence of benefit from prophylaxis in elective inguinal hernia repair (*Cochrane Database System Rev 2004, issue 4*).

* See page 3 for abbreviations

TABLE 15C – ANTIMICROBIAL PROPHYLAXIS FOR THE PREVENTION OF BACTERIAL ENDOCARDITIS IN PATIENTS WITH UNDERLYING CARDIAC CONDITIONS*

In 2007, the American Heart Association guidelines for the prevention of bacterial endocarditis were updated. The resulting document (*Circulation 2007; 115:1 and http://circ.ahajournals.org*), which was also endorsed by the Infectious Diseases Society of America, represents a significant departure from earlier recommendations.

- Antibiotic prophylaxis for dental procedures is now directed at individuals who are likely to suffer the most devastating consequences should they develop endocarditis.
- Prophylaxis to prevent endocarditis is no longer specified for gastrointestinal or genitourinary procedures. The following is adapted from and reflects the new AHA recommendations. See original publication for explanation and precise details.

SELECTION OF PATIENTS FOR ENDOCARDITIS PROPHYLAXIS

FOR PATIENTS WITH ANY OF THESE HIGH-RISK CARDIAC CONDITIONS ASSOCIATED WITH ENDOCARDITIS:	WHO UNDERGO DENTAL PROCEDURES INVOLVING:	WHO UNDERGO INVASIVE RESPIRATORY PROCEDURES INVOLVING:	WHO UNDERGO INVASIVE PROCEDURES OF THE GI OR GU TRACTS:	WHO UNDERGO PROCEDURES INVOLVING INFECTED SKIN AND SOFT TISSUES:
Prosthetic heart valves Previous infective endocarditis Congenital heart disease with any of the following: • Completely repaired cardiac defect using prosthetic material (Only for 1st 6 months) • Partially corrected but with residual defect near prosthetic material • Uncorrected cyanotic congenital heart disease • Surgically constructed shunts and conduits Valvulopathy following heart transplant	Any manipulation of gingival tissue, dental periapical regions, or perforating the oral mucosa. **PROPHYLAXIS RECOMMENDED‡** *(see Dental Procedures Regimens table below)* (Prophylaxis is *not* recommended for routine anesthetic injections (unless through infected area), dental x-rays, shedding of primary teeth, adjustment of orthodontic appliances or placement of orthodontic brackets or removable appliances.)	Incision of respiratory tract mucosa **CONSIDER PROPHYLAXIS** *(see Dental Procedures Regimens table)* Or For treatment of established infection **PROPHYLAXIS RECOMMENDED** *(see Dental Procedures Regimens table for oral flora, but include anti-staphylococcal coverage when S. aureus is of concern)*	PROPHYLAXIS is no longer recommended solely to prevent endocarditis, **but the following approach is reasonable:** For patients with enterococcal UTIs: • treat before elective GU procedures • include enterococcal coverage in peri-operative regimen for non-elective procedures† For patients with existing GU or GI infections or those who receive peri-operative antibiotics to prevent surgical site infections or sepsis • it is reasonable to include agents with anti-enterococcal activity in peri-operative coverage†	Include coverage against staphylococci and β-hemolytic streptococci in treatment regimens

† Agents with anti-enterococcal activity include penicillin, ampicillin, amoxicillin, piperacillin, vancomycin and others. Check susceptibility if available. (*See Table 5 for highly resistant organisms.*)
‡ 2008 AHA/ACC focused update of guidelines on valvular heart disease use term "is reasonable" to reflect level of evidence (*Circulation 118;887, 2008*).

PROPHYLACTIC REGIMENS FOR DENTAL PROCEDURES

SITUATION	AGENT	REGIMEN[1]
Usual oral prophylaxis	Amoxicillin	Adults 2 gm, children 50 mg per kg; orally, 1 hour before procedure
Unable to take oral medications	Ampicillin[2]	Adults 2 gm, children 50 mg per kg; IV or IM, within 30 min before procedure.
Allergic to penicillins	Cephalexin[3] OR	Adults 2 gm, children 50 mg per kg; orally, 1 hour before procedure
	Clindamycin OR	Adults 600 mg, children 20 mg per kg; orally, 1 hour before procedure
	Azithromycin or clarithromycin	Adults 500 mg, children 15 mg per kg; orally, 1 hour before procedure
Allergic to penicillins and unable to take oral medications	Cefazolin[3] OR	Adults 1 gm, children 50 mg per kg; IV or IM, within 30 min before procedure
	Clindamycin	Adults 600 mg, children 20 mg per kg; IV or IM, within 30 min before procedure

[1] Children's dose should not exceed adult dose. AHA document lists all doses as 30-60 min before procedure.
[2] AHA lists cefazolin or ceftriaxone (at appropriate doses) as alternatives here.
[3] Cephalosporins should not be used in individuals with immediate-type hypersensitivity reaction (urticaria, angioedema, or anaphylaxis) to penicillins or other β-lactams. AHA proposes ceftriaxone as potential alternative to cefazolin; and other 1st or 2nd generation cephalosporin in equivalent doses as potential alternatives to cephalexin.

* See page 3 for abbreviations

TABLE 15D – MANAGEMENT OF EXPOSURE TO HIV-1 AND HEPATITIS B AND C*

OCCUPATIONAL EXPOSURE TO BLOOD, PENILE/VAGINAL SECRETIONS OR OTHER POTENTIALLY INFECTIOUS BODY FLUIDS OR TISSUES WITH RISK OF TRANSMISSION OF HEPATITIS B/C AND/OR HIV-1 (E.G., NEEDLESTICK INJURY)

[Adapted from *MMWR 50(RR-11):1, 2001, NEJM 348:826, 2003* and *MMWR 54(RR-9)1: 2005; MMWR 55(RR-11), 2006* (available at *www.aidsinfo.nih.gov*).]
Free consultation for occupational exposures, call (PEPline) 1-888-448-4911.

General steps in management:
1. Wash clean wounds/flush mucous membranes immediately (use of caustic agents or squeezing the wound is discouraged; data lacking regarding antiseptics).
2. Assess risk by doing the following: (a) Characterize exposure; (b) Determine/evaluate source of exposure by medical history, risk behavior, & testing for hepatitis B/C, HIV; (c) Evaluate and test exposed individual for hepatitis B/C & HIV.

Hepatitis B Occupational Exposure *[Adapted from CDC recommendations: MMWR 50(RR-11), 2001]*

Exposed Person[§]	Exposure Source		
	HBs Ag+	HBs Ag–	Status Unknown or Unavailable for Testing[†]
Unvaccinated	Give HBIG 0.06 mL per kg IM & initiate HB vaccine	Initiate HB vaccine	Initiate HB vaccine
Vaccinated (antibody status unknown)	Do anti-HBs on exposed person: If titer ≥10 milli-International units per mL, no rx If titer <10 milli-International units per mL, give HBIG + 1 dose HB vaccine[†]	No rx necessary	Do anti-HBs on exposed person: If titer ≥10 milli-International units per mL, no rx If titer <10 milli-International units per mL, give 1 dose of HB vaccine

§ Persons previously infected with HBV are immune to reinfection and do not require postexposure prophylaxis.

For known vaccine series responder (titer ≥10 milli-International units per mL), monitoring of levels or booster doses not currently recommended. Known non-responder (<10 milli-International units per mL) to 1° series HB vaccine & exposed to either HBsAg+ source or suspected high-risk source—rx with HBIG & re-initiate vaccine series **or** give 2 doses HBIG 1 month apart. For non-responders after a 2ⁿᵈ vaccine series, 2 doses HBIG 1 month apart is preferred approach to new exposure *[MMWR 40(RR-13):21, 2001]*.

† If known high risk source, treat as if source were HBsAG positive

Hepatitis B Non-Occupational Exposure *[Adapted from CDC recommendations; MMWR 55(RR-11), 2006 and MMWR 55(RR-16), 2006]*

Post-exposure prophylaxis is recommended for persons with discrete nonoccupational exposure to blood or body fluids. Exposures include percutaneous (e.g., bite, needlestick or mucous membrane exposure to HBsAG-positive blood or sterile body fluids), sexual or needle-sharing contact of an HBsAG-positive person, or a victim of sexual assault or sexual abuse by a perpetrator who is HBsAg-positive. If immunoprophylaxis is indicated, it should be initiated ideally within the first 24h of exposure. Postexposure prophylaxis is unlikely to be effective if administered more than 7 days after a parenteral exposure or 14 days after a sexual exposure. The hepatitis B vaccine series should be completed regardless. The same guidelines for management of occupational exposures can also be used for nonoccupational exposures. For a previously vaccinated person (i.e., written documentation of being vaccinated) and no documentation of postvaccination titers with a discrete exposure to a HBsAG-positive source, it also is acceptable to administer a booster dose of hepatitis B vaccine without checking titers. No treatment is required for a vaccinated person exposed to a source of unknown HBsAG status.

Hepatitis C Exposure

Determine antibody to hepatitis C for both exposed person &, if possible, exposure source. If source + or unknownand exposed person negative, follow-up HCV testing for HCV RNA (detectable in blood in 1-3 weeks) and HCV antibody (90% who seroconvert will do so by 3 months) is advised. **No recommended prophylaxis;** immune serum globulin not effective. Monitor for early infection, as therapy may ↓ risk of progression to chronic hepatitis. Persons who remain viremic 8-12 weeks after exposure should be treated with a course of pegylated interferon (*Gastro 130:632, 2006 and Hpt 43:923, 2006*). See *Table 12*. Case-control study suggested risk factors for occupational HCV transmission include percutaneous exposure to needle that had been in artery or vein, deep injury, male sex of HCW, & was more likely when source VL >6 log10 copies/mL (*CID 41: 1423, 2005*).

* *See page 3 for abbreviations*

TABLE 15D(2)

HIV: Occupational exposure management *[Adapted from MMWR 54 (RR-9), 2005]* (available at www.cdc.gov/mmwr)

- The decision to initiate post-exposure prophylaxis (PEP) for HIV is a clinical judgment that should be made in concert with the exposed healthcare worker (HCW). It is based on:
  1. Likelihood of the source patient having HIV infection: ↑ with history of high-risk activity—injection drug use, sexual activity with known HIV+ person, unprotected sex with multiple partners (either hetero- or homosexual), receipt of blood products 1978–1985. ↑ with clinical signs suggestive of advanced HIV (unexplained wasting, night sweats, thrush, seborrheic dermatitis, etc.).
  2. Type of exposure (approx. 1 in 300–400 needlesticks from infected source will transmit HIV).
  3. Limited data regarding efficacy of PEP *(Cochrane Database Syst Rev. Jan 24;(1):CD002835, 2007)*.
  4. Significant adverse effects of PEP drugs & potential for drug interactions.
  5. Substances considered potentially infectious include: blood, tissues, semen, vaginal secretions, CSF, synovial, pleural, peritoneal, pericardial and amniotic fluids; and other visibly bloody fluids. Fluids normally considered low risk for transmission, unless visibly bloody, include: urine, vomitus, stool, sweat, saliva, nasal secretions, tears and sputum *(MMWR 54(RR-9), 2005)*
- If source person is **known positive for HIV** or **likely to be infected** and **status of exposure warrants PEP**, antiretroviral drugs should be started **immediately** (ASAP or within hours). If source person is HIV antibody negative, drugs can be stopped **unless source is suspected of having acute HIV infection**. The HCW should be re-tested at **3–4 weeks, 3 & 6 months whether PEP is used or not** (the vast majority of seroconversions will occur by 3 months; delayed conversions after 6 months are exceedingly rare). Tests for HIV RNA should not be used for dx of HIV infection in HCW because of false-positives (esp. at low titers) & these tests are only approved for established HIV infection [a possible exception is if pt develops signs of acute HIV (mononucleosis-like) syndrome within the 1ˢᵗ 4–6 wks of exposure when antibody tests might still be negative.]
- PEP for HIV is usually given for **4 wks** and monitoring of adverse effects recommended: baseline **complete blood count, renal and hepatic panel** to be **repeated at 2 weeks** (up to 50–75% of HCW on PEP demonstrate mild side-effects (nausea, diarrhea, myalgias, headache, etc.) but in up to ½ severe enough to discontinue PEP *(Antivir Ther 3:195, 2000)*. Consultation with infectious diseases/ HIV specialist valuable when questions regarding PEP arise. **Seek expert help in special situations, such as pregnancy, renal impairment, treatment-experienced source.**

3 Steps to HIV Post-Exposure Prophylaxis (PEP) After Occupational Exposure: *[For latest CDC recommendations, see MMWR 54(RR-9), 2005 available at www.aidsinfo.nih.gov]*

Step 1: Determine the exposure code (EC)

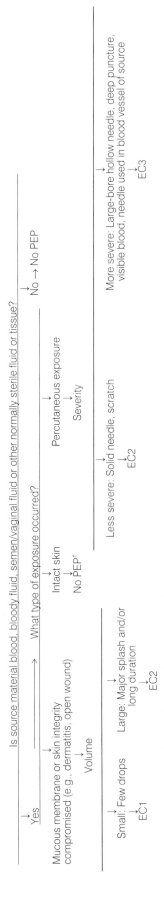

Is source material blood, bloody fluid, semen/vaginal fluid or other normally sterile fluid or tissue?

→ Yes

→ No → No PEP

What type of exposure occurred?

Mucous membrane or skin integrity compromised (e.g., dermatitis, open wound)

Intact skin
→ No PEP†

Percutaneous exposure
→ Severity

Volume

Small: Few drops
→ EC1

Large: Major splash and/or long duration
→ EC2

Less severe: Solid needle, scratch
→ EC2

More severe: Large-bore hollow needle, deep puncture, visible blood, needle used in blood vessel of source
→ EC3

† Exceptions can be considered when there has been prolonged, high-volume contact.

* See page 3 for abbreviations

TABLE 15D(3)

Step 2: Determine the HIV Status Code (HIV SC)

What is the HIV status of the exposure source?

HIV negative	HIV positive		Status unknown	Source unknown
→ No PEP	→ Low titer exposure: asymptomatic & high CD4 count, low VL (<1500 copies per mL)	→ High titer exposure: advanced AIDS, primary HIV, high viral load or low CD4 count	→ HIV SC unknown	→ HIV SC unknown
	HIV SC 1	HIV SC 2		

Step 3: Determine Post-Exposure Prophylaxis (PEP) Recommendation

EC	HIV SC	PEP
1	1	Consider basic regimen[1 a]
1	2	Recommend basic regimen[1 a,b]
2	1	Recommend basic regimen[1 b]
2	2	Recommend expanded regimen[1]
3	1 or 2	Recommend expanded regimen[1]
1, 2, 3	Unknown	If exposure setting suggests risks of HIV exposure, consider basic regimen[1 c]

[a] Based on estimates of ↓ risk of infection after mucous membrane exposure in occupational setting compared with needlestick.

Modification of CDC recommendations:

[b] Or, consider expanded regimen[1].

[c] In high risk circumstances, consider expanded regimen[1] on case-by-case basis.

Around the clock, urgent expert consultation available from: National Clinicians' Post-Exposure Prophylaxis Hotline (PEPline) at 1-888-448-4911 (1-888-HIV-4911)

Regimens: (Treat for 4 weeks; monitor for drug side-effects every 2 weeks)

Basic regimen: ZDV + 3TC, or FTC + TDF, or as an alternative d4T + 3TC.

Expanded regimen: Basic regimen + one of the following: lopinavir/ritonavir *(preferred)*, or *(as alternatives)* atazanavir/ritonavir or fosamprenavir/ritonavir. Efavirenz can be considered (except in pregnancy or potential for pregnancy—**Pregnancy Category D**), but CNS symptoms might be problematic. [**Do not use nevirapine**; serious adverse reactions including hepatic necrosis reported in healthcare workers (*MMWR 49:1153, 2001*).]

Other regimens can be designed. If possible, use antiretroviral drugs for which resistance is unlikely based on susceptibility data or treatment history of source pt (if known). Seek expert consultation if ARV-experienced source or in pregnancy or potential for pregnancy.

NOTE: Some authorities feel that an expanded regimen should be employed whenever PEP is indicated (*NEJM 349:1091, 2003; Eur J Epidemiol 19:577 2004*). Expanded regimens are likely to be advantageous with ↑ numbers of ART-experienced source pts or when there is doubt about exact extent of exposures in decision algorithm. Mathematical model suggests that under some conditions, completion of full course basic regimen is better than prematurely discontinued expanded regimen (*CID 39:395, 2004*). However, while expanded PEP regimens have ↑ adverse effects, there is not necessarily ↑ discontinuation (*CID 40:205, 2005*).

POST-EXPOSURE PROPHYLAXIS FOR NON-OCCUPATIONAL EXPOSURES TO HIV-1

From MMWR 54(RR-2):1, 2005—DHHS recommendations

Because the risk of transmission of HIV via sexual contact or sharing needles by injection drug users may reach or exceed that of occupational needlestick exposure, it is reasonable to consider PEP in persons who have had a non-occupational exposure to blood or other potentially infected fluids (e.g., genital/rectal secretions, breast milk) from an HIV+ source. Risk of HIV acquisition per exposure varies with the act (for needle sharing and receptive anal intercourse, ≥0.5%; approximately 10-fold lower with insertive vaginal or anal intercourse, 0.05–0.07%). Overt or occult traumatic lesions may ↑ risk in survivors of sexual assault.

For pts at risk of HIV acquisition through non-occupational exposure to HIV+ source material having occurred ≤72 hours before evaluation, DHHS recommendation is to treat for 28 days with an antiretroviral **expanded regimen**, using preferred regimens [efavirenz *(not in pregnancy or pregnancy risk—**Pregnancy Category D***) + (3TC or FTC) + (ZDV or TDF)] **or** [lopinavir/ritonavir + (3TC or FTC) + ZDV] or one of several alternative regimens [*see Table 14D & MMWR 54(RR-2):1, 2005*]. Failures of prophylaxis have been reported, and may be associated with longer interval from exposure to start of PEP (*CID 41:1507, 2005*); this supports prompt initiation of PEP if it is to be used.

Areas of uncertainty: (1) expanded regimens are not proven to be superior to 2-drug regimens, (2) while PEP not recommended for exposures >72 hours before evaluation, it may possibly be effective in some cases, (3) when HIV status of source patient is unknown, decision to treat and regimen selection must be individualized based on assessment of specific circumstances.

Evaluate for exposures to Hep B, Hep C (*see Occupational PEP above*), and bacterial sexually-transmitted diseases (*see Table 15A*) and treat as indicated. DHHS recommendations for sexual exposures to HepB and bacterial pathogens are available in *MMWR 55(RR-11), 2006*. Persons who are unvaccinated or who have not responded to full HepB vaccine series should receive hepB immune globulin preferably within 24-hours of percutaneous or mucosal exposure to blood or body fluids of an HBsAg-positive person, along with hepB vaccine, with follow-up to complete vaccine series. Unvaccinated or not-fully-vaccinated persons exposed to a source with unknown HepBsAg-status should receive vaccine and complete vaccine series. See *MMWR 55(RR-11), 2006* for details and recommendations in other circumstances.

* See page 3 for abbreviations

TABLE 15E – PREVENTION OF OPPORTUNISTIC INFECTION IN HUMAN STEM CELL TRANSPLANTATION (HSCT) OR SOLID ORGAN TRANSPLANTATION (SOT) FOR ADULTS WITH NORMAL RENAL FUNCTION*

General comments: Medical centers performing transplants will have detailed protocols for the prevention of opportunistic infections which are appropriate to the resources, patients and infections represented at those sites. Regimens continue to evolve and protocols adopted by an institution may differ from those of other centers. Care of transplant patients should be guided by physicians with expertise in this area. References: *MMWR 49(RR-10):1, 2000; CID 33:S26, 2001; COID 17:353, 2004.* For updated timeline of infections, see *NEJM 357:2601, 2007.*

OPPORTUNISTIC INFECTION (at risk)	TYPE OF TRANSPLANT	PROPHYLACTIC REGIMENS	COMMENTS/ REFERENCES
CMV (Recipient + OR Donor +/Recipient –)	HSCT	**Preemptive therapy:** Monitor ≥ 1x/wk (days 10–100) for CMV-antigenemia or viremia by PCR test (Note: culture alone not sufficiently sensitive), start rx when + [Ganciclovir 5 mg/kg IV q12h 7–14 days, then 5 mg/kg IV q24h 5 days/wk to day 100 or ≥ 3 wks (whichever longer) *[MMWR 49(RR-10):1, 2000]*. Some use oral ganciclovir 1 gm q8h after 7–14 day IV induction phase. Some use shorter courses; however, monitoring tests should be neg before stopping rx *(CID 35:999, 2002)*. Recent papers showed that 2 wks valganciclovir 900 mg po bid comp to ganciclovir 5 mg/kg IV bid as preemptive therapy in allo-HSCT *(BMTr 37:693, 2006)* & that valganciclovir 900 mg bid for 2 wks then 900 mg q24h for ≥ 7days after neg. assay was effective *(BMTr 37: 851, 2006)]* OR **Prophylaxis:** (for high-risk pts, see *CID 35:999, 2002,* or where CMV detection tests not available) From engraftment to day 100, rx with ganciclovir IV 5 mg per kg q12h for 7 days, then 5 mg per kg q24h 5–6 days per week. **General Comments:** Review in *CMR 16:647, 2003.* Role of valganciclovir in CMV prevention is under investigation.	
	SOT	**Kidney, kidney/pancreas, heart:** Valganciclovir 900 mg po q24h, start by day 10 & continue through day 100 of transplant. **Liver:** Ganciclovir 1 gm po q8h, start by day 10 & continue through day 100.[†] **Lung:** Ganciclovir 5 mg per kg q12h IV for 5–7 days, then valganciclovir 900 mg po q24h for 6 months (or at least 3 mos.)[†] Some centers have added CMV immune globulin 150 mg per kg within 72 hrs of transplant, & at 2, 4, 6, & 8 wks post-transplant, then 100 mg per kg at wk 12 & 16. **Comments:** For recs by US & Cndn transplantation societies, see *Am J Transpl 4 (Suppl.10):51, 2004 & 5:218, 2005.* For lung, see *Transpl 80:157, 2005.* Universal prophylaxis approach (above) favored by most; there are proponents of preemptive therapy in liver transplant *(CID 40:704 & 709, 2005: Transpl 79:85 & 1428, 2005).* Some add CMV Ig for other high-risk SOTs also. [†]*Note:* Valganciclovir not approved by FDA for liver or lung transplantation, but most centers use it *(Am J Transpl 8:158, 2008).* ↑ Bioavailability of valganciclovir may (?) ↓ risk of resistance *(CID 45: 448, 2007).* Recent review: *CID 47:702, 2008.*	
Hepatitis B	Liver	For antiviral therapy for HBV, see *Table 14A, page 138.* For discussion of hepB immune globulin in liver transplantation, *see J Viral Hepatitis (suppl 1:27, 2007).* For discussion of other investigational approaches, see *Amer. J Transplant 8:9, 2008.*	
	HSCT	An interesting phenomenon of "reverse seroconversion" has been described in pts with HBV reactivation in bone marrow transplantation: loss of HbsAb and appearance of HbsAg with viremia *(CID 41: 1277, 2005).*	
Herpes simplex (seropositive)	HSCT	Acyclovir 250 mg per meter-squared IV q12h or 200 mg po 3x/day from conditioning to engraftment or resolution of mucositis	
	SOT	Acyclovir 200 mg po 3x/day to 400 mg bid—start early post transplant *(ClinMicroRev 10:86, 1997)*	
		Comment: Higher doses have been used in both groups. Do not need acyclovir if receiving CMV prophylaxis. One study found pts receiving higher dose acyclovir or valacyclovir for ≥1 yr to prevent VZV reactivation in HSCT had ↓ HSV and ↓ acyclovir-resistant HSV than cohort treated for 30 days *(JID 196:266, 2007).*	
Aspergillus sp.	Lung/ Heart-lung	No controlled trials to determine optimal management, but regimens of an aerosolized lipid-based ampho B preparation & an oral anti-aspergillus agent have been used *[Am J Transpl 4(Suppl.10):110, 2004].* Randomized trial suggested nebulized ABLC better tolerated than nebul. ampho B deoxycholate *(Transpl 77:232, 2004).* Another study found nebulized liposomal amphotericin and nebul. amphotericin deoxycholate to be well tolerated and comparably effective in lung transplantation *(Transpl.Infect Dis. 9: 121, 2007).* Multi-nation survey showed wide variation in practices: best approach remains to be determined *(Transpl.Infect Dis 8: 213, 2006).*	
	HSCT	Itraconazole iv/po solution led to non-significant ↓ invasive aspergillus compared with fluconazole *(AnIM 138:705, 2003)* or significant ↓ infection with ↑ toxicity/intolerance *(Blood 103:1527, 2004).* Study of voriconazole vs fluconazole to prevent invasive fungal infections in progress *(CID 39:S176, 2004).* Vori assoc. with ↑ risk of zygomycosis *(JID 191:1350, 2005).* Posaconazole approved for prophylaxis of invasive Aspergillus and candida in high-risk, severely immunocompromised pts (eg, HSCT w/GVHD) at a dose of 200 mg three times daily. In comparative trial, posaconazole overall similar to fluconazole in preventing invasive fungal infections, but more effective in preventing Aspergillus *(NEJM 356: 335, 2007).*	

*See page 3 for abbreviations

TABLE 15E(2)

OPPORTUNISTIC INFECTION (at risk)	TYPE OF TRANSPLANT	PROPHYLACTIC REGIMENS	COMMENTS/ REFERENCES
Candida sp. (CID 38:161, 2004)	Liver	Fluconazole 200–400 mg IV/po 1 time per day starting before transplant & continuing up to 3 mos. in high-risk pts. Optimal duration unknown. Concerns for ↑ non-albicans candida with fluconazole prophylaxis (Transpl 75:2023, 2003). Liver Transpl 12: 850, 2006.	
	HSCT	Fluconazole 400 mg po 1 time per day from day 0 to engraftment or ANC >1000. Micafungin has also been approved for prophylaxis of Candida infections in HSCT (at recommended dose of 50 mg q24h. CID 39:1407. 2004). Posaconazole oral susp. 200 mg three times daily approved for prophylaxis in high-risk pts.	
Coccidioides immitis	Any	Fluconazole 400 mg po q24h (Transpl Inf Dis 5:3, 2003) or 200-400 mg po q24h (Am J Transpl 6:340, 2006) have been used in liver and renal transplant patients, respectively, with prior coccidioidomycosis. See COID 21:415, 2008 for approach by one center in endemic area.	
Pneumocystis carinii (P. jiroveci) & Toxoplasma gondii	All	TMP-SMX: 1 SS tab po q24h or 1 DS tab po 1x/day to 3–7days/wk. Dur: 6 mo–1yr renal; ≥6mo for allogenic HSCT; ≥1yr to life for heart, lung, liver [Am J Transpl 4(Suppl.10):135, 2004]. Breakthrough pneumocystis infections reported with atovaquone doses <1500 mg/day (CID 38:e76, 2004). For toxo D+/R– heart transplants, 3 mos pyrimethamine/sulfa prior to lifetime TMP-SMX prophylaxis has been suggested [see Am J Transpl 4(Suppl.10):142, 2004 for intensive pyri-sulfa regimen & alternatives].	
Trypanosoma cruzi	Heart	May be transmitted from organs or transfusions. Inspect peripheral blood smear of suspected cases for parasites (MMWR 55:798, 2006). Risk of reactivation during immunosuppression is variable (JAMA 298:2171, 2007 & JAMA 299:1134, 2008). If known Chagas' disease in donor or recipient, contact CDC for treatment options (phone 404-639-3670).	

* See page 3 for abbreviations

TABLE 16 – PEDIATRIC DOSAGES OF SELECTED ANTIBACTERIAL AGENTS*

[Adapted from: (1) Nelson's Pocket Book of Pediatric Antimicrobial Therapy, 2008–2009, 17th Ed., J. Bradley & J. Nelson, eds., Alliance for World Wide Editing, Buenos Aires, Argentina, and (2) 2006 Red Book, 27th Ed., American Academy of Pediatrics, pages 700–718]

DRUG	DOSES IN MG PER KG PER DAY OR MG PER KG AT FREQUENCY INDICATED[1]				
	BODY WEIGHT <2000 gm		BODY WEIGHT >2000 gm		>28 DAYS OLD
	0–7 days	8–28 days	0–7 days	8–28 days	
Aminoglycosides, IV or IM (check levels; some dose by gestational age + wks of life; *see Nelson's Pocket Book, p. 25*)					
Amikacin	7.5 q18–24h	7.5 q12h	10 q12h	10 q12h	10 q8h
Gent/tobra	2.5 q18–24h	2.5 q12h	2.5 q12h	2.5 q12h	2.5 q8h
Aztreonam, IV	30 q12h	30 q8h	30 q8h	30 q6h	30 q6h
Cephalosporins					
Cefaclor					20–40 div tid
Cefadroxil					30 div bid (max 2 gm per day)
Cefazolin	25 q12h	25 q12h	25 q12h	25 q8h	25 q8h
Cefdinir					7 q12h or 14 q24h
Cefepime	30 q12h	30 q12h	30 q12h	30 q12h	150 div q8h
Cefixime					8 as q24h or div bid
Cefotaxime	50 q12h	50 q8h	50 q12h	50 q8h	50 q8h (75 q6h for meningitis)
Cefoxitin			20 q12h		80–160 div q6h
Cefpodoxime					10 div bid (max 400 mg per day)
Cefprozil					15–30 div bid (max 1 gm per day)
Ceftazidime	50 q12h	50 q8h	50 q12h	50 q8h	50 q8h
Ceftibuten					4.5 bid
Ceftizoxime					33–66 q8h
Ceftriaxone	25 q24h	50 q24h	25 q24h	50 q24h	50 q24h (meningitis 100)
Cefuroxime IV	50 q12h	50 q8h	50 q8h	50 q8h	50 q8h (80 q8h for meningitis)
po					10–15 bid (max 1 gm per day)
Cephalexin					25–50 div q6h (max 4 gm per day)
Loracarbef					15–30 div bid (max 0.8 gm per day)
Chloramphenicol IV	25 q24h	25 q24h	25 q24h	15 q12h	12.5–25 q6h (max 2–4 gm per day)
Clindamycin IV po	5 q12h	5 q8h	5 q8h	5 q6h	7.5 q6h
Ciprofloxacin po[2]					20–30 div bid (max 1.5 gm per day)
Ertapenem IV	No data	No data	No data	No data	15 q12h (max. 1g/day)
Imipenem[3] IV			25 q12h	25 q8h	15–25 q6h (max 2–4 gm per day)
Linezolid	10 q12h	10 q8h	10 q8h	10 q8h	10 q8h to age 12
Macrolides					
Erythro IV & po	10 q12h	10 q8h	10 q12h	13 q8h	10 q6h
Azithro po/IV	5 q24h	10 q24h	5 q24h	10 q24h	10 q24h
Clarithro po					7.5 q12h (max. 1 gm per day)
Meropenem IV	20 q12h	20 q8h	20 q12h	20 q8h	60–120 div q8h (120 for meningitis)
Metro IV & po	7.5 q24h	7.5 q12h	7.5 q12h	15 q12h	7.5 q6h
Penicillins					
Ampicillin	50 q12h	50 q8h	50 q8h	50 q6h	50 q6h
AMP-sulbactam					100–300 div q6h
Amoxicillin po				30 div bid	25–50 div tid
Amox-Clav po			30 div bid	30 div bid	45 or 90 (AM/CL-HD) div bid if over 12wks
Dicloxacillin					12–25 div q6h
Mezlocillin	75 q12h	75 q8h	75 q12h	75 q8h	75 q6h
Nafcillin, oxacillin IV	25 q12h	25 q8h	25 q8h	37 q6h	37 q6h (to max. 8–12 gm per day)
Piperacillin, PIP-tazo IV	50 q12h	100 q12h	100 q12h	100 q8h	100 q6h
Ticarcillin, T.clav IV	75 q12h	75 q8h	75 q8h	75 q6h	75 q6h
Tinidazole					> Age 3: 50 mg/kg for 1 dose
Penicillin G, U/kg IV	50,000 q12h	75,000 q8h	50,000 q8h	50,000 q6h	50,000 units/kg per day
Penicillin V					25–50 mg per kg per day div q6–8h
Rifampin IV, po	10 q24h	10 q24h	10 q24h	10 q24h	10 q24h
Sulfisoxazole po					120–150 mg/kg per day div q4–6h
TMP-SMX po, IV; UTI: 8–12 TMP component div bid; Pneumocystis: 20 TMP component div q6h					
Tetracycline po (age 8 or older)					25–50 div q6h (>7yr old)
Doxycycline po, IV (age 8 or older)					2–4 div bid to max of 200 (>7yr old)
Vancomycin IV	12.5 q12h	15 q12h	18 q12h	22 q12h	40 div q6–8h; 60 for meningitis

[1] May need higher doses in patients with meningitis: *see CID 39:1267, 2004*
[2] With exception of cystic fibrosis, anthrax, and complicated UTI, not approved for use under age 18.
[3] Not recommended in children with CNS infections due to risk of seizures.

* *See page 3 for abbreviations*

TABLE 17A – DOSAGE OF ANTIMICROBIAL DRUGS IN ADULT PATIENTS WITH RENAL IMPAIRMENT

Adapted from a combination of DRUG PRESCRIBING IN RENAL FAILURE, 5th Ed., Aronoff et al (Eds.), American College of Physicians, 2007 and selected package inserts. For review of Continuous Renal Replacement Therapy: CID 41:1159, 2005.

UNLESS STATED, ADJUSTED DOSES ARE % OF DOSE FOR NORMAL RENAL FUNCTION.
Drug adjustments are based on the patient's estimated endogenous creatinine clearance, which can be calculated as:

$$\frac{(140 - \text{age})(\text{ideal body weight in kg})}{(72)(\text{serum creatinine, mg per dL})} \quad \text{for men (x 0.85 for women)}$$

Ideal body weight for men: 50.0 kg + 2.3 kg per inch over 5 feet
Ideal body weight for women: 45.5 kg + 2.3 kg per inch over 5 feet

For alternative methods to calculate estimated CrCl, see *NEJM 354:2473, 2006.*

NOTE: For summary of drugs requiring NO dosage adjustment with renal insufficiency, see Table 17B, page 186.

ANTIMICROBIAL	HALF-LIFE (NORMAL/ ESRD) hr	DOSE FOR NORMAL RENAL FUNCTION§	METHOD * (see footnote)	ADJUSTMENT FOR RENAL FAILURE — Estimated creatinine clearance (CrCl), mL/min — >50–90	10–50	<10	HEMODIALYSIS, CAPD+ (see footnote)	COMMENTS & DOSAGE FOR CRRT‡
ANTIBACTERIAL ANTIBIOTICS **Aminoglycoside Antibiotics:**		**Traditional multiple daily doses—adjustment for renal disease**						
Amikacin	1.4–2.3/17–150	7.5 mg per kg q12h or 15 mg per kg once daily (see below)	I	7.5 mg/kg q12h	7.5 mg/kg q24h **Same dose for CRRT‡**	7.5 mg/kg q48h	HEMO: ½ of normal renal function dose AD+ CAPD: 15–20 mg lost per L dialysate per day (see *Comment*)	High flux hemodialysis membranes lead to unpredictable aminoglycoside clearance. measure post-dialysis drug levels for efficacy and toxicity. With CAPD, pharmacokinetics highly variable—**check serum levels.** Usual method for CAPD: 2 liters of dialysis fluid placed qid or 8 liters per day (give 8Lx20 mg lost per L = 160 mg of amikacin supplement IV per day)
Gentamicin, Tobramycin	2–3/20–60	1.7 mg per kg q8h. Once daily dosing below	I	100% of q8h	100% of q12–24h **Same dose for CRRT‡**	100% of q48h	HEMO: ½ of normal renal function dose AD+ CAPD: 3–4 mg lost per L dialysate per day	
Netilmicin[NUS]	2–3/35–72	2.0 mg per kg q8h. Once daily dosing below	I	100% of q8h	100% of q12–24h **Same dose for CRRT‡**	100% of q48h	HEMO: ½ of normal renal function dose AD+ CAPD: 3–4 mg lost per L dialysate per day	Adjust dosing weight for obesity: [ideal body weight + 0.4(actual body weight – ideal body weight)] (*CID 25:112, 1997*).
Streptomycin	2–3/30–80	15 mg per kg (max. of 1.0 gm) q24h. Once daily dosing below	D, I	q24h	q24–72h **Same dose for CRRT‡**	q72–96h	HEMO: ½ of normal renal function dose AD+ CAPD: 20–40 mg lost per L dialysate per day	

ONCE-DAILY AMINOGLYCOSIDE THERAPY: ADJUSTMENT IN RENAL INSUFFICIENCY (see Table 10D for OD dosing/normal renal function)

Creatinine Clearance (mL per min.) Drug	>80	60–80	40–60	30–40	20–30	10–20	<10–0
	Dose q24h (mg per kg)				Dose q48h (mg per kg)		Dose q72h and AD+
Gentamicin/Tobramycin	5.1	4	3.5	2.5	4	3	
Amikacin/kanamycin/streptomycin	15	12	7.5	4	7.5	4	
Isepamicin[NUS]	8	8	8	8 q48h	8 q72h	8 q96h	
Netilmicin[NUS]	6.5	5	4	2	3	2.5	2

‡ **CRRT = Continuous renal replacement therapy.** Usually results in CrCl of approx 30 mL/min.   + **AD = after dialysis.** "Dose AD" refers only to timing of dose.
CAPD = Continuous ambulatory peritoneal dialysis.

TABLE 17A (2)

ANTIBACTERIAL ANTIBIOTICS (Continued)

ANTIMICROBIAL	HALF-LIFE (NORMAL/ESRD) hr	DOSE FOR NORMAL RENAL FUNCTION§	METHOD* (see footnote)	ADJUSTMENT FOR RENAL FAILURE, Estimated creatinine clearance (CrCl), mL/min >50–90	10–50	<10	HEMODIALYSIS, CAPD+ (see footnote)	COMMENTS & DOSAGE FOR CRRT‡
Carbapenem Antibiotics								
Doripenem	1/18	500 mg IV q8h	D&I	500 mg IV q8h	≥30 – ≤50: 250 mg IV q8h / >10 – <30: 250 mg IV q12h	No data	No data	
Ertapenem	4/>4	1.0 gm q24h	D	1.0 gm q24h	0.5 gm q24h (CrCl <30)	0.5 gm q24h	HEMO: Dose as for CrCl <10: if dosed <6 hrs prior to HD, give 150 mg supplement AD+	
Imipenem (see Comment)	1/4	0.5 gm q6h	D&I	250–500 mg q6–8h	250 mg q6–12h **Dose for CRRT‡: 0.5–1 gm bid** (AAC 49:2421, 2005)	125–250 mg q12h	HEMO: Dose AD+ / CAPD: Dose for CrCl <10	↑ potential for seizures if recommended doses exceeded in pts with CrCl <20 mL per min. See pkg insert, esp. for pts <70 kg
Meropenem	1/6–8	1.0 gm q8h	D&I	1.0 gm q8h	1.0 gm q12h / **Same dose for CRRT‡**	0.5 gm q24h	HEMO: Dose AD+ / CAPD: Dose for CrCl <10	
Cephalosporin Antibiotics: DATA ON SELECTED PARENTERAL CEPHALOSPORINS								
Cefazolin	1.9/40–70	1.0–2.0 gm q8h	I	1.0–2.0 gm q8h	q12h / **Same dose for CRRT‡**	q24–48h	HEMO: Extra 0.5–1 gm AD+ / CAPD: 0.5 gm q12h	
Cefepime	2.2/18	2.0 gm q8h (max. dose)	D&I	2 gm q8h	2 gm q12–24h / **Same dose for CRRT‡**	1 gm q24h	HEMO: Extra 1 gm AD+ / CAPD: 1–2 gm q48h	
Cefotaxime, Ceftizoxime	1.7/15–35	2.0 gm q8h	I	q8–12h	q12–24h / **Same dose for CRRT‡**	q24h	HEMO: Extra 1 gm AD+ / CAPD: 0.5–1 gm q24h	Active metabolite of cefotaxime in ESRD. ↓ dose further for hepatic & renal failure.
Cefotetan	3.5/13–25	1–2 gm q12h	D	100%	1–2 gm q24h / **Same dose for CRRT‡**	1–2 gm q48h	HEMO: Extra 1 gm AD+ / CAPD: 1 gm q24h	CRRT‡ dose: 750 mg q12h
Cefoxitin	0.8/13–23	2.0 gm q8h	I	q8h	q8–12h / **Same dose for CRRT‡**	q24–48h	HEMO: Extra 1 gm AD+ / CAPD: 1 gm q24h	May falsely increase serum creatinine by interference with assay.
Ceftazidime	1.2/13–25	2 gm q8h	I	q8–12h	Q12–24h / **Same dose for CRRT‡**	q24–48h	HEMO: Extra 1 gm AD+ / CAPD: 0.5 gm q24h	Volume of distribution increases with infection.
Ceftobiprole	2.9–3.3/No data	500 mg IV q8–12h	I	500 mg IV q8–12h	≥30 & ≤50: 500 mg q12h over 2 hrs / ≥10 & <30: 250 mg q12h over 2 hrs / **Same dose for CRRT‡**	No data	HEMO: No data	
Cefuroxime sodium	1.2/17	0.75–1.5 gm q8h	I	q8h	q8–12h / **Same dose for CRRT‡**	q24h	HEMO: Dose AD+ / CAPD: Dose for CrCl <10	
Fluoroquinolone Antibiotics								
Ciprofloxacin	3–6/6–9	500–750 mg po (or 400 mg IV) q12h	D	100%	50–75% CRRT 400 mg IV q24h	50%	HEMO: 250 mg po or 200 mg IV q12h / CAPD: 250 mg po or 200 mg IV q8h	
Gatifloxacin^NUS	7–14/11–40	400 mg po/IV q24h	D	400 mg q24h	400 mg, then 200 mg q24h / Same dose for CRRT‡	400 mg, then 200 mg q24h	HEMO: 200 mg q24h AD+ / CAPD: 200 mg q24h	

‡ **CRRT = continuous renal replacement therapy**; results in CrCl of approx 30 mL/min.   + **AD = after dialysis. "Dose AD" refers to timing of dose.**
CAPD = Continuous ambulatory peritoneal dialysis.
Supplement is to replace drug lost via dialysis; extra drug beyond continuation of regimen used for CrCl <10 mL per min.

TABLE 17A (3)

ANTIMICROBIAL	HALF-LIFE (NORMAL/ESRD) hr	DOSE FOR NORMAL RENAL FUNCTION§	METHOD* (see footnote)	ADJUSTMENT FOR RENAL FAILURE — Estimated creatinine clearance (CrCl), mL/min			HEMODIALYSIS, CAPD+ (see footnote)	COMMENTS & DOSAGE FOR CRRT‡
				>50-90	10-50	<10		
ANTIBACTERIAL ANTIBIOTICS/Fluoroquinolone Antibiotics *(continued)*								
Gemifloxacin	7/>7	320 mg po q24h	D	320 mg q24h	160 mg q24h	160 mg q24h	HEMO: 160 mg q24h AD+ CAPD: 160 mg q24h	
Levofloxacin	6-8/76	750 mg q24h IV, PO	D&I	750 mg q24h	**20-49:** 750 q48h	**<20:** 750 mg once, then 500 mg q48h	HEMO/CAPD: Dose for CrCl <20	CRRT‡ 750 mg once, then 500 mg q48h
Macrolide Antibiotics								
Clarithromycin	5-7/22	0.5-1.0 gm q12h	D	100%	75%	50-75%	HEMO: Dose AD+ CAPD: None	CRRT‡ as for CrCl 10-50
Erythromycin	1.4/5-6	250-500 mg q6h	D	100%	100%	50-75%	HEMO/CAPD/CRRT‡: None	Ototoxicity with high doses in ESRD
Miscellaneous Antibacterial Antibiotics								
Colistin	<6/≥48	80-160 mg q8h	D	160 mg q12h	160 mg q24h **Same dose for CRRT‡**	160 mg q36h	HEMO: 80 mg AD+	*LnID 6:589, 2006*
Daptomycin	9.4/30	4-6 mg per kg per day	I	4-6 mg per kg per day	CrCl <30, 4-6 mg per kg q48h	4-6 mg per kg q48h	HEMO & CAPD: 4-6 mg per kg q48h (after dialysis if possible)	
Linezolid	5-6/6-8	600 mg po/IV q12h	None	600 mg q12h	600 mg q12h **Same dose for CRRT‡**	600 mg q12h AD+	HEMO: As for CrCl <10 CAPD & CRRT: No dose adjustment	Accumulation of 2 metabolites—risk unknown (*JAC 56:172, 2005*)
Metronidazole	6-14/7-21	7.5 mg per kg q6h	D	100%	100% **Same dose for CRRT‡**	100%	HEMO: Dose AD+ CAPD: Dose for CrCl <10	
Nitrofurantoin	0.5/1	50-100 mg	D	100%	Avoid	Avoid	Not applicable	
Sulfamethoxazole	10/20-50	1.0 gm q8h	I	q12h	q18h Same dose for CAVH	q24h	HEMO: Extra 1 gm AD+ CAPD: 1 gm q24h	
Teicoplanin^NUS	45/62-230	6 mg per kg per day	I	q24h	q48h **Same dose for CRRT‡**	q72h	HEMO: Dose for CrCl <10 CAPD: Dose for CrCl <10	
Telithromycin	10/15	800 mg q24h	D	800 mg q24h	600 mg q24h (<30 mL per min.)	600 mg q24h	HEMO: 600 mg AD+ CAPD: No data	If CrCl <30, reduce dose to 600 mg once daily. If both liver and renal failure, dose is 400 mg once daily
Telavancin	7-8/17.9	10 mg/kg q24h	D&I	10 mg/kg q24h	**30-50:** 7.5 mg/kg q24h **10-30:** q18h **Same dose for CRRT‡**	**<30:** 10 mg/kg q48h	No data	No data
Trimethoprim (TMP)	11/20-49	100-200 mg q12h	I	q12h	**>30:** q12h **10-30:** q18h	q24h	HEMO: Dose AD+ CAPD: q24h	CRRT‡ dose: q18h
Trimethoprim-sulfamethoxazole-DS (Doses based on TMP component)								
Treatment (based on TMP component)	As for TMP	5-20 mg/kg/day divided q6-12h	D	5-20 mg/kg/d divided q6-12h	**30-50:** 5-7.5 mg/kg q8h (same dose for CRRT) **10-29:** 5-10 mg/kg q12h	Not recommended; but if used: 5-10 mg/kg per dose q24h	Not recommended; but if used: 5-10 mg/kg q24h	

‡ **CRRT** = continuous renal replacement therapy; results in CrCl of approx 30 mL/min.   + **AD** = after dialysis. **"Dose AD"** refers to timing of dose.
CAPD = Continuous ambulatory peritoneal dialysis.
Supplement is to replace drug lost via dialysis; extra drug beyond continuation of regimen used for CrCl <10 mL per min.

TABLE 17A (4)

ANTIMICROBIAL	HALF-LIFE (NORMAL/ ESRD) hr	DOSE FOR NORMAL FUNCTION§	METHOD * (see footnote)	ADJUSTMENT FOR RENAL FAILURE Estimated creatinine clearance (CrCl), mL/min			HEMODIALYSIS, CAPD+ (see footnote)	COMMENTS & DOSAGE FOR CRRT‡
				>50-90	10-50	<10		
ANTIBACTERIAL ANTIBIOTICS/Miscellaneous Antibacterial Antibiotics *(Continued)*								
Prophylaxis	As for TMP	1 tab po q24h or 3 times per week	No change	100%	100%	100%		
Vancomycin[1]	6/200-250	1 gm q12h	D&I	1 gm q12h	1 gm q24-96h	1 gm q4-7 days	HEMO/CAPD: Dose for CrCl <10	CAVH CVVH: 500 mg q24-48h. New hemodialysis membranes ↑ clear. of vanco; **check levels**
Penicillins								
Amoxicillin Ampicillin	1.0/5-20 1.0/7-20	250-500 mg q8h 250 mg-2 gm q6h	I	q8h q6h	q8-12h q6-12h	q24h q12-24h	HEMO: Dose AD+ CAPD: 250 mg q12h	IV amoxicillin not available in the U.S. CRRT‡ dose for CrCl 10-50
Amoxicillin/ Clavulanate[2]	1.3 AM/1.0	500/125 mg q8h (see Comments)	D&I	500/125 mg q8h	250-500 mg AM component q12h	250-500 mg AM component q24h	HEMO: As for CrCl <10; extra dose after dialysis	**If CrCl ≤30 per mL, do not use 875/125 or 1000/62.5 AM/CL**
Ampicillin (AM)/ Sulbactam(SB)	5-20/4.0 1.0 (AM)/1.0 (SB) 9.0 (AM)/10.0 (SB)	2 gm AM + 1.0 gm SB q6h	I	q6h	q8-12h	q24h	HEMO: Dose AD+ CAPD: 2 gm AM/1 gm SB q24h	CRRT‡ dose: 1.5 AM/0.75 SB q12h
Aztreonam	2.0/6-8	2 gm q8h	D	100%	50-75% **Same dose for CRRT‡**	25%	HEMO: Extra 0.5 gm AD+ CAPD: Dose for CrCl <10	Technically is a β-lactam antibiotic.
Penicillin G	0.5/6-20	0.5-4 million U q4h	D	100%	75% **Same dose for CRRT‡**	20-50%	HEMO: Dose AD+ CAPD: Dose for CrCl <10	1.7 mEq potassium per million units. ↑s potential of seizure. 10 million units per day max. dose in ESRD.
Piperacillin	1.0/3.3-5.1	3-4 gm q4-6h	I	q4-6h	q6-8h **Same dose for CRRT‡**	q8h	HEMO: 2 gm q8h plus 1 gm extra AD+ CAPD: Dose for CrCl <10	1.9 mEq sodium per gm
Pip (P)/Tazo(T)	0.71-1.2 (both)/2-6	3.375 – 4.5 gm q6-8h	D&I	100%	2.25 gm q6h <20: q8h **Same dose for CRRT‡**	2.25 gm q8h	HEMO: Dose for CrCl <10 + 0.75 gm AD+ CAPD: 4.5 gm q12h; CRRT: 4.5 gm q48h	
Ticarcillin	1.2/13	3 gm q4h	D&I	1-2 gm q4h	1-2 gm q8h **Same dose for CRRT‡**	1-2 gm q12h	HEMO: Extra 3.0 gm AD+ CAPD: Dose for CrCl <10	5.2 mEq sodium per gm
Ticarcillin/ Clavulanate[2]	1.2/11-16	3.1 gm q4h	D&I	3.1 gm q4h	3.1 gm q8-12h **Same dose for CRRT‡**	2.0 gm q12h	HEMO: Extra 3.1 gm AD+ CAPD: 3.1 gm q12h	See footnote 2
Tetracycline Antibiotics								
Tetracycline	6-10/57-108	250-500 mg qid	I	q8-12h	q12-24h **Same dose for CRRT‡**	q24h	HEMO/CAPD/CAVH: None	Avoid in ESRD

[1] If renal failure, use EMIT assay to measure levels; levels overestimated by RIA or fluorescent immunoassay.

[2] Clavulanate cleared by liver, not kidney. Hence as dose of combination decreased, a deficiency of clavulanate may occur (JAMA 285:386, 2001).

‡ **CRRT = continuous renal replacement therapy**; results in CrCl of approx 30 mL/min.   + **AD = after dialysis.** **"Dose AD" refers to timing of dose.**
CAPD = Continuous ambulatory peritoneal dialysis.
Supplement is to replace drug lost via dialysis; extra drug beyond continuation of regimen used for CrCl <10 mL per min.

TABLE 17A (5)

ANTIMICROBIAL	HALF-LIFE (NORMAL/ ESRD) hr	DOSE FOR NORMAL RENAL FUNCTION§	METHOD * (see footnote)	ADJUSTMENT FOR RENAL FAILURE — Estimated creatinine clearance (CrCl), mL/min >50–90	10–50	<10	HEMODIALYSIS, CAPD[+] (see footnote)	COMMENTS & DOSAGE FOR CRRT[‡]
ANTIFUNGAL ANTIBIOTICS								
Amphotericin B & Lipid-based ampho B	24h–15 days/unchanged	Non-lipid: 0.4–1.0 mg/kg/day ABLC: 5 mg/kg/day LAB: 3–5 mg/kg/day	I	q24h	q24h **Same dose for CRRT[‡]**	q24h	HEMO/CAPD/CRRT: No dose adjustment	For ampho B, toxicity lessened by saline loading; risk amplified by concomitant cyclosporine A, aminoglycosides, or pentamidine
Fluconazole	37/100	100–400 mg q24h	D	100%	50%	50%	HEMO: 100% of recommended dose AD[+] CAPD: Dose for CrCl <10	CRRT: 200–400 mg q24h
Flucytosine	3–6/75–200	37.5 mg per kg q6h	I	q12h	q12–24h **Same dose for CRRT[‡]**	q24h	HEMO: Dose AD[+] CAPD: 0.5–1.0 gm q24h	Goal is peak serum level >25 mcg per mL and <100 mcg per mL
Itraconazole, po soln	21/25	100–200 mg q12h	D	100%	100% **Same dose for CRRT[‡]**	50%	HEMO/CAPD: oral solution: 100 mg q12–24h	
Itraconazole, IV	21/25	200 mg IV q12h	–	200 mg IV bid	Do not use IV itra if CrCl <30 due to accumulation of carrier: cyclodextrin			
Terbinafine	36–200/?	250 mg po per day	–	q24h	Use has not been studied. Recommend avoidance of drug.		HEMO/CAPD: Dose for CrCl <10 due to accumulation of carrier: cyclodextrin	
Voriconazole, IV	Non-linear kinetics	6 mg per kg IV q12h times 2, then 4 mg per kg q12h	–	No change	If CrCl <50 mL per min, accum. of IV vehicle (cyclodextrin). Switch to po or DC **For CRRT:[‡]** 4 mg/kg po q12h			
ANTIPARASITIC ANTIBIOTICS								
Pentamidine	3–12/73–18	4 mg per kg per day	I	q24h	q24h **Same dose for CRRT[‡]**	q24–36h	HEMO: As for CrCl <10 plus 0.75 g AD. CAPD: Dose for CrCl <10	
Quinine	5–16/5–16	650 mg q8h	I	650 mg q8h	650 mg q8–12h **Same dose for CRRT[‡]**	650 mg q24h	HEMO: Dose AD[+] CAPD: Dose for CrCl <10	Marked tissue accumulation
ANTITUBERCULOUS ANTIBIOTICS *(Excellent review: Nephron 64:169, 1993)*								
Ethambutol	4/7–15	15–25 mg per kg q24h	I	q24h	q24–36h **Same dose for CRRT[‡]**	q48h	HEMO: Dose AD[+] CAPD: Dose for CrCl <10	25 mg per kg 4–6 hr prior to 3 times per wk dialysis. Streptomycin instead of ethambutol in renal failure.
Ethionamide	2.1/?	250–500 mg q12h	D	100%	100%	50%	HEMO/CAPD/CRRT[‡]: No dosage adjustment	
Isoniazid	0.7–4/8–17	5 mg per kg per day (max. 300 mg)	D	100%	100% **Same dose for CRRT[‡]**	100%	HEMO: Dose AD[+] CAPD/: Dose for CrCl <10	
Pyrazinamide	9/26	25 mg per kg q24h (max. dose 2.5 gm q24h)	D	100%	100% **Same dose for CRRT[‡]**	12–25 mg per kg q24h	HEMO: 40 mg/kg 24 hrs before each 3x/week dialysis CAPD: No reduction;	
Rifampin	1.5–5/1.8–11	600 mg per day	D	600 mg q24h	300–600 mg q24h **Same dose for CRRT[‡]**	300–600 mg q24h	HEMO: No adjustment CAPD/: Dose for CrCl <10	Biologically active metabolite

[‡] **CRRT = continuous renal replacement therapy**; results in CrCl of approx 30 mL/min.   [+] **AD = after dialysis.** "**Dose AD**" refers to timing of dose.
CAPD = Continuous ambulatory peritoneal dialysis.
Supplement is to replace drug lost via dialysis; extra drug beyond continuation of regimen used for CrCl <10 mL per min.

TABLE 17A (6)

ANTIMICROBIAL	HALF-LIFE (NORMAL/ ESRD) hr	DOSE FOR NORMAL RENAL FUNCTION§	METHOD * (see footnote)	ADJUSTMENT FOR RENAL FAILURE Estimated creatinine clearance (CrCl), mL/min			HEMODIALYSIS, CAPD+ (see footnote)	COMMENTS & DOSAGE FOR CRRT‡
				>50-90	10-50	<10		
ANTIVIRAL AGENTS For ANTIRETROVIRALS See CID 40:1559, 2005								
Acyclovir, IV	2-4/20	5-12.4 mg per kg q8h	D&I	100% q8h	100% q12-24h	50% q24h	HEMO: Dose AD+ CAPD: Dose for CrCl <10	Rapid IV infusion can cause ↑ Cr. CRRT‡ dose: 5-10 mg/kg q24h
Adefovir	7.5/15	10 mg po q24h	I	10 mg q24h	10 mg q48-72h[1]	10 mg q72h[1]	HEMO: 10 mg q week AD+	CAPD: No data; CRRT: Dose ?
Amantadine	12/500	100 mg po bid	I	q12h	q24-48h	q 7days	HEMO/CAPD: Dose for CrCl <10/	CRRT‡: Dose for CrCl 10-50
Atripla	See each drug	200 mg emtricitabine + 300 mg tenofovir + 600 mg efavirenz	I	Do not use if CrCl <50				
Cidofovir: **Complicated dosing—see package insert**								
Induction	2.5/unknown	5 mg per kg once per wk for 2 wks	–	5 mg per kg once per wk	Contraindicated in pts with CrCl ≤ 55 ml/min.			Major toxicity is renal. No efficacy, safety, or pharmacokinetic data in pts with moderate/severe renal disease.
Maintenance	2.5/unknown	5 mg per kg q2wks	–	5 mg per kg q2wks	Contraindicated in pts with CrCl ≤ 55 ml/min.			
Didanosine tablets[2]	0.6-1.6/4.5	125-200 mg q12h buffered tabs	D	200 mg q12h	200 mg q24h	<60 kg: 150 mg q24h >60 kg: 100 mg q24h	HEMO: Dose AD+ CAPD/CRRT‡: Dose for CrCl <10	Based on incomplete data. Data are estimates.
		400 mg q24h enteric-coated tabs	D	400 mg q24h	125-200 mg q24h	Do not use EC tabs	HEMO/CAPD: Dose for CrCl <10	**If <60 kg & CrCl <10 mL per min, do not use EC tabs**
Emtricitabine (CAPS)	10/>10	200 mg q24h	I	200 mg q24h	**30-49:** 200 mg q48h **10-29:** 200 mg q72h	200 mg q96h	HEMO: Dose for CrCl <10	See package insert for oral solution.
Emtricitabine + Tenofovir	See each drug	200-300 mg q24h	I	No change	**30-50:** 1 tab q48h	**CrCl <30:** Do not use		
Entecavir	128-149/?	0.5 mg q24h	D	0.5 mg q24h	0.15-0.25 mg q24h	0.05 mg q24h	HEMO/CAPD: 0.05 mg q24h	Give after dialysis on dialysis days
Famciclovir	2.3-3.0/10-22	500 mg q8h	D&I	500 mg q8h	500 mg q12-24h	250 mg q24h	HEMO: Dose AD+ CAPD: No data	CRRT‡: Not applicable

1 Ref: *Transplantation 80:1086, 2005*

2 Ref: for NRTIs and NNRTIs: *Kidney International 60:821, 2001*

‡ **CRRT = continuous renal replacement therapy**; results in CrCl of approx 30 mL/min. + **AD** = after dialysis. **"Dose AD" refers to timing of dose.**
CAPD = Continuous ambulatory peritoneal dialysis.
Supplement is to replace drug lost via dialysis; extra drug beyond continuation of regimen used for CrCl <10 mL per min.

TABLE 17A (7)

ANTIMICROBIAL	HALF-LIFE (NORMAL/ ESRD) hr	DOSE FOR NORMAL RENAL FUNCTION§	METHOD * (see footnote)	ADJUSTMENT FOR RENAL FAILURE Estimated creatinine clearance (CrCl), mL/min			HEMODIALYSIS, CAPD+ (see footnote)	COMMENTS & DOSAGE FOR CRRT‡
				>50-90	10-50	<10		
ANTIVIRAL AGENTS For ANTIRETROVIRALS See CID 40:1559, 2005. (continued)								
Ganciclovir	3.6/30	IV: Induction 5 mg per kg q12h IV	D&I	5 mg per kg q12h	1.25-2.5 mg per kg q24h	1.25 mg per kg 3 times per wk	HEMO: Dose AD+ CAPD: Dose for CrCl <10	
		IV: Maintenance 5 mg per kg q24h IV	D&I	2.5-5.0 mg per kg q24h	0.6-1.25 mg per kg q24h	0.625 mg per kg 3 times per wk	HEMO: 0.6 mg per kg AD+ CAPD: Dose for CrCl <10	
		po: 1.0 gm tid po	D&I	0.5-1 gm tid	0.5-1.0 gm q24h	0.5 gm 3 times per week	HEMO: 0.5 gm AD+	
Maraviroc	14-18/No data	300 mg bid		300 mg bid				Risk of side effects increased if concomitant CVP3A inhibitor
Lamivudine[1]	5-7/15-35	300 mg po q24h	D&I	300 mg po q24h	50-150 mg q24h	25-50 mg q24h	HEMO: Dose AD+; CAPD: Dose for CrCl<10. CRRT: 100 mg 1st days, then 50 mg/day.	
Oseltamivir, therapy	6-10/>20	75 mg po bid – treatment	I	75 mg q12h	30-50: 75 mg bid <30: 75 mg qod	No data	HEMO: 30 mg non-dialysis days; CAPD: 30 mg 1-2x/week	
Ribavirin		Use with caution in patients with creatinine clearance <50 mL per min.						
Rimantadine	13-65/Prolonged	100 mg bid po	I	100 mg bid	100 mg q24h-bid	100 mg q24h	HEMO/CAPD: No data	Use with caution, little data
Stavudine, po[1]	1-1.4/5.5-8	30-40 mg q12h	D&I	100%	50% q12-24h	≥60 kg: 20 mg per day <60 kg:15 mg per day	HEMO: Dose as for CrCl <10 AD+ CAPD: No data CRRT‡: Full dose	
Telbivudine	40-49/No data	600 mg po daily	I	600 mg q24h	30-49: 600 mg q48H <30: 600 mg q72h	600 mg q96h	HEMO: As for CrCl <10 AD	
Tenofovir, po	17/?	300 mg q24h		300 mg q24h	30-49: 300 mg q48h 10-29: 300 mg q72-96h	No data	HEMO: 300 mg q7d or after 12 hrs of HEMO.[2]	
Valacyclovir	2.5-3.3/14	1.0 gm q8h	D&I	1.0 gm q8h	1.0 gm q12-24h Same dose for CRRT‡	0.5 gm q24h	HEMO: Dose AD+ CAPD: Dose for CrCl <10	CAVH dose: As for CrCl 10-50
Valganciclovir	4/67	900 mg po bid	D&I	900 mg po bid	450 mg q24h to 450 mg every other day	DO NOT USE	See package insert	
Zalcitabine[1]	2.0/>8	0.75 mg q8h	D&I	0.75 mg q8h	0.75 mg q12h Same dose for CRRT‡	0.75 mg q24h	HEMO: Dose AD+ CAPD: No data	
Zidovudine[1]	1.1-1.4/1.4-3	300 mg q12h	D&I	300 mg q12h	300 mg q12h Same dose for CRRT‡	100 mg q8h	HEMO: Dose for CrCl <10 AD CAPD: Dose for CrCl <10	CRRT dose: As for CrCl 10-50

1 Ref. for NRTIs and NNRTIs: *Kidney International 60:821, 2001*

2 Acute renal failure and Fanconi syndrome reported.

‡ **CRRT = continuous renal replacement therapy**, results in CrCl of approx 30 mL/min.   + **AD = after dialysis. "Dose AD" refers to timing of dose.**
CAPD = Continuous ambulatory peritoneal dialysis.
Supplement is to replace drug lost via dialysis; extra drug beyond continuation of regimen used for CrCl <10 mL per min.

TABLE 17B – NO DOSAGE ADJUSTMENT WITH RENAL INSUFFICIENCY BY CATEGORY*

Antibacterials		Antifungals	Anti-TBc	Antivirals	
Azithromycin	Metronidazole	Andiulafngin	Rifabutin	Abacavir	Lopinavir
Ceftriaxone	Minocycline	Caspofungin	Rifapentine	Atazanavir	Nelfinavir
Chloramphenicol	Moxifloxacin	Itraconazole oral solution		Darunavir	Nevirapine
Ciprofloxacin XL	Nafcillin	Ketoconazole		Delavirdine	Raltegravir
Clindamycin	Pyrimethamine	Micafungin		Efavirenz	Ribavirin
Doxycycline	Rifaximin	Voriconazole, **po only**		Enfuvirtide[1]	Saquinavir
Linezolid	Tigecycline			Fosamprenavir	Tipranavir
				Indinavir	

[1] Enfuvirtide: Not studied in patients with CrCl <35 mL/min. DO NOT USE

TABLE 18 – ANTIMICROBIALS AND HEPATIC DISEASE DOSAGE ADJUSTMENT*

The following alphabetical list indicates antibacterials excreted/metabolized by the liver **wherein a dosage adjustment may be indicated** in the presence of hepatic disease. Space precludes details; consult the PDR or package inserts for details. List is **not** all-inclusive:

Antibacterials		Antifungals	Antivirals[§]	
Ceftriaxone	Nafcillin	Caspofungin	Abacavir	Indinavir
Chloramphenicol	Rifabutin	Itraconazole	Atazanavir	Lopinavir/ritonavir
Clindamycin	Rifampin	Voriconazole	Darunavir	Nelfinavir
Fusidic acid	Synercid**		Delavirdine	Nevirapine
Isoniazid	Telithromycin++		Efavirenz	Rimantadine
Metronidazole	Tigecycline		Enfuvirtide	Ritonavir
	Tinidazole		Fosamprenavir	

[§] Ref. on antiretrovirals: *CID 40:174, 2005*   ** Quinupristin/dalfopristin   ++ Telithro: reduce dose in renal & hepatic failure

TABLE 19 – TREATMENT OF CAPD PERITONITIS IN ADULTS*
(Periton Dial Intl 20:396, 2000)[2]

EMPIRIC Intraperitoneal Therapy:[3] Culture Results Pending

Drug		Residual Urine Output	
		<100 mL per day	**>100 mL per day**
Cefazolin +	Can mix in same bag	1 gm per bag, q24h	20 mg per kg BW per bag, q24h
Ceftazidime		1 gm per bag, q24h	20 mg per kg BW per bag, q24h

Drug Doses for SPECIFIC Intraperitoneal Therapy—Culture Results Known. NOTE: Few po drugs indicated

Drug	Intermittent Dosing (once per day)		Continuous Dosing (per liter exchange)	
	Anuric	**Non-Anuric**	**Anuric**	**Non-Anuric**
Gentamicin	0.6 mg per kg	↑ dose 25%	MD 8 mg	↑ MD by 25%
Cefazolin	15 mg per kg	20 mg per kg	LD 500 mg, MD 125 mg	LD 500 mg, ↑ MD 25%
Ceftazidime	1000–1500 mg	ND	LD 250 mg, MD 125 mg	ND
Ampicillin	250–500 mg po bid	ND	250–500 mg po bid	ND
Ciprofloxacin	500 mg po bid	ND	LD 50 mg, MD 25 mg	ND
Vancomycin	15–30 mg per kg q5–7 days	↑ dose 25%	MD 30–50 mg per L	↑ MD 25%
Metronidazole	250 mg po bid	ND	250 mg po bid	ND
Amphotericin B	NA	NA	MD 1.5 mg	NA
Fluconazole	200 mg q24h	ND	200 mg q24h	ND
Itraconazole	100 mg q12h	100 mg q12h	100 mg q12h	100 mg q12h
Amp-sulbactam	2 gm q12h	ND	LD 1 gm, MD 100 mg	ND
TMP-SMX	320/1600 mg po q1–2 days	ND	LD 320/1600 mg po, MD 80/400 mg po q24h	ND

CAPD = continuous ambulatory peritoneal dialysis

[1] Ref. for NRTIs and NNRTIs: *Kidney International 60:821, 2001*
[2] **All doses IP unless indicated otherwise.**
　LD = loading dose, **MD** = maintenance dose, **ND** = no data; **NA** = not applicable—dose as normal renal function.
　Anuric = <100 mL per day, **non-anuric** = >100 mL per day
[3] **Does not provide treatment for MRSA.** If Gram-positive cocci on Gram stain, include vancomycin.
* *See page 3 for other abbreviations*

TABLE 20A – RECOMMENDED CHILDHOOD & ADOLESCENT IMMUNIZATION SCHEDULE IN THE UNITED STATES, 2008.

Detailed information and all immunization tables may be accessed at:
http://www.cdc.gov/vaccines/pubs/vis/default.htm

TABLE 20B - ADULT IMMUNIZATION IN THE UNITED STATES
(MMWR 56 No.41:Q1–Q4, 2007) (Travelers: see Med Lett 38:17, 2006)

Recommended Adult Immunization Schedule, by vaccine and age group —United States, October 2007–September 2008

Vaccine	Age group (years)		
	19–49	50–64	≥65
Tetanus, diphtheria, pertussis (Td/Tdap)[1]*	1 dose booster every 10 years		
	Substitute 1 dose of Tdap for Td		
Human papillomavirus (HPV)[2]*	3 doses (females) (0, 2, 6 mos)		
Measles, mumps, rubella (MMR)[3]*	1 or 2 doses	1 dose	
Varicella[4]*	2 doses (0, 4–8 weeks)		
Influenza[5]*	1 dose annually	1 dose annually	
Pneumococcal (polysaccharide)[6,7]	1–2 doses		1 dose
Hepatitis A[8]*	2 doses (0, 6–12 mos, or 0, 6–18 mos)		
Hepatitis B[9]*	3 doses (0, 1–2, 4–6 mos)		
Meningococcal[10]	1 or more doses		
Zoster[11]			1 dose

* Covered by the Vaccine Injury Compensation Program.

▆ For all persons in this category who meet the age requirements and who lack evidence of immunity (e.g., lack documentation of vaccination or have no evidence of prior infection)

▢ Recommended if some other risk factor is present (e.g., on the basis of medical, occupational, lifestyle, or other indications).

NOTE: These recommendations must be read along with the footnotes.
Approved by the Advisory Committee on Immunization Practices (ACIP), the American Academy of Family Physicians, the American College of Obstetricians and Gynecologists, and the American College of Physicians. Complete statements from ACIP are available at http://www.cdc.gov/vaccines/pubs/acip-list.htm.

1. Tetanus, diphtheria, and acellular pertussis (Td/Tdap) vaccination

Tdap should replace a single dose of Td for adults aged <65 years who have not previously received a dose of Tdap. Only one of two Tdap products (Adacel® [Sanofi Pasteur]) is licensed for use in adults.

Adults with uncertain histories of a complete primary vaccination series with tetanus and diphtheria toxoid–containing vaccines should begin or complete a primary vaccination series. A primary series for adults is 3 doses of tetanus and diphtheria toxoid–containing vaccines; administer the first 2 doses at least 4 weeks apart and the third dose 6–12 months after the second. However, Tdap can substitute for any one of the doses of Td in the 3-dose primary series. The booster dose of tetanus and diphtheria toxoid–containing vaccine should be administered to adults who have completed a primary series and if the last vaccination was received ≥10 years previously. Tdap or Td vaccine may be used, as indicated.

If the person is pregnant and received the last Td vaccination ≥10 years previously, administer Td during the second or third trimester; if the person received the last Td vaccination in <10 years, administer Tdap during the immediate postpartum period. A one-time administration of 1 dose of Tdap with an interval as short as 2 years from a previous Td vaccination is recommended for postpartum women, close contacts of infants aged <12 months, and all health-care workers with direct patient contact. In certain situations, Td can be deferred during pregnancy and Tdap substituted in the immediate postpartum period, or Tdap can be administered instead of Td to a pregnant woman after an informed discussion with the woman.

Consult the ACIP statement for recommendations for administering Td as prophylaxis in wound management.

2. Human papillomavirus (HPV) vaccination

HPV vaccination is recommended for all females aged ≤26 years who have not completed the vaccine series. History of genital warts, abnormal Papanicolaou test, or positive HPV DNA test is not evidence of prior infection with all vaccine HPV types; HPV vaccination is still recommended for these persons.

Ideally, vaccine should be administered before potential exposure to HPV through sexual activity; however, females who are sexually active should still be vaccinated. Sexually active females who have not been infected with any of the HPV vaccine types receive the full benefit of the vaccination. Vaccination is less beneficial for females who have already been infected with one or more of the HPV vaccine types. A complete series consists of 3 doses. The second dose should be administered 2 months after the first dose; the third dose should be administered 6 months after the first dose.

Although HPV vaccination is not specifically recommended for females with the medical indications described in Figure 2, "Vaccines that might be indicated for adults based on medical and other indications," it is not a live-virus vaccine and can

TABLE 20B (2)

be administered. However, immune response and vaccine efficacy might be less than in persons who do not have the medical indications described or who are immunocompetent.

3. Measles, mumps, rubella (MMR) vaccination

Measles component: adults born before 1957 can be considered immune to measles. Adults born during or after 1957 should receive ≥1 dose of MMR unless they have a medical contraindication, documentation of ≥1 dose, history of measles based on health-care provider diagnosis, or laboratory evidence of immunity.

A second dose of MMR is recommended for adults who 1) have been recently exposed to measles or are in an outbreak setting; 2) have been previously vaccinated with killed measles vaccine; 3) have been vaccinated with an unknown type of measles vaccine during 1963–1967; 4) are students in postsecondary educational institutions; 5) work in a health-care facility; or 6) plan to travel internationally.

Mumps component: adults born before 1957 can generally be considered immune to mumps. Adults born during or after 1957 should receive 1 dose of MMR unless they have a medical contraindication, history of mumps based on health-care provider diagnosis, or laboratory evidence of immunity.

A second dose of MMR is recommended for adults who 1) are in an age group that is affected during a mumps outbreak; 2) are students in postsecondary educational institutions; 3) work in a health-care facility; or 4) plan to travel internationally. For unvaccinated healthcare workers born before 1957 who do not have other evidence of mumps immunity, consider administering 1 dose on a routine basis and strongly consider administering a second dose during an outbreak.

Rubella component: administer 1 dose of MMR vaccine to women whose rubella vaccination history is unreliable or who lack laboratory evidence of immunity. For women of childbearing age, regardless of birth year, routinely determine rubella immunity and counsel women regarding congenital rubella syndrome. Women who do not have evidence of immunity should receive MMR vaccine on completion or termination of pregnancy and before discharge from the health-care facility.

4. Varicella vaccination

All adults without evidence of immunity to varicella should receive 2 doses of single-antigen varicella vaccine unless they have a medical contraindication. Special consideration should be given to those who 1) have close contact with persons at high risk for severe disease (e.g., health-care personnel and family contacts of immunocompromised persons) or 2) are at high risk for exposure or transmission (e.g., teachers; child care employees; residents and staff members of institutional settings, including correctional institutions; college students; military personnel; adolescents and adults living in households with children; nonpregnant women of childbearing age; and international travelers).

Evidence of immunity to varicella in adults includes any of the following: 1) documentation of 2 doses of varicella vaccine at least 4 weeks apart; 2) U.S.-born before 1980 (although for health-care personnel and pregnant women, birth before 1980 should not be considered evidence of immunity); 3) history of varicella based on diagnosis or verification of varicella by a health-care provider (for a patient reporting a history of or presenting with an atypical case, a mild case, or both, health-care providers should seek either an epidemiologic link with a typical varicella case or to a laboratory-confirmed case or evidence of laboratory confirmation, if it was performed at the time of acute disease); 4) history of herpes zoster based on health-care provider diagnosis; or 5) laboratory evidence of immunity or laboratory confirmation of disease.

Assess pregnant women for evidence of varicella immunity. Women who do not have evidence of immunity should receive the first dose of varicella vaccine upon completion or termination of pregnancy and before discharge from the health-care facility. The second dose should be administered 4–8 weeks after the first dose.

5. Influenza vaccination

Medical indications: chronic disorders of the cardiovascular or pulmonary systems, including asthma; chronic metabolic diseases, including diabetes mellitus, renal or hepatic dysfunction, hemoglobinopathies, or immunosuppression (including immunosuppression caused by medications or human immunodeficiency virus [HIV]); any condition that compromises respiratory function or the handling of respiratory secretions or that can increase the risk of aspiration (e.g., cognitive dysfunction, spinal cord injury, or seizure disorder or other neuromuscular disorder); and pregnancy during the influenza season. No data exist on the risk for severe or complicated influenza disease among persons with asplenia; however, influenza is a risk factor for secondary bacterial infections that can cause severe disease among persons with asplenia.

Occupational indications: health-care personnel and employees of long-term–care and assisted-living facilities. *Other indications:* residents of nursing homes and other long-term–care and assisted-living facilities; persons likely to transmit influenza to persons at high risk (e.g., in-home household contacts and caregivers of children aged 0–59 months, or persons of all ages with high-risk conditions); and anyone who would like to be vaccinated. Healthy, nonpregnant adults aged ≤49 years without high-risk medical conditions who are not contacts of severely immunocompromised persons in special care units can receive either intranasally administered live, attenuated influenza vaccine (FluMist®) or inactivated vaccine. Other persons should receive the inactivated vaccine.

6. Pneumococcal polysaccharide vaccination

Medical indications: chronic pulmonary disease (excluding asthma); chronic cardiovascular diseases; diabetes mellitus; chronic liver diseases, including liver disease as a result of alcohol abuse (e.g., cirrhosis); chronic alcoholism, chronic renal failure, or nephrotic syndrome; functional or anatomic asplenia (e.g., sickle cell disease or splenectomy [if elective splenectomy is planned, vaccinate at least 2 weeks before surgery]); immunosuppressive conditions; and cochlear implants and cerebrospinal fluid leaks. Vaccinate as close to HIV diagnosis as possible.

Other indications: Alaska Natives and certain American Indian populations and residents of nursing homes or other long-term–care facilities.

7. Revaccination with pneumococcal polysaccharide vaccine

One-time revaccination after 5 years for persons with chronic renal failure or nephrotic syndrome; functional or anatomic asplenia (e.g., sickle cell disease or splenectomy); or immunosuppressive conditions. For persons aged ≥65 years, one-time revaccination if they were vaccinated ≥5 years previously and were aged <65 years at the time of primary vaccination.

8. Hepatitis A vaccination

Medical indications: persons with chronic liver disease and persons who receive clotting factor concentrates.

Behavioral indications: men who have sex with men and persons who use illegal drugs.

Occupational indications: persons working with hepatitis A virus (HAV)-infected primates or with HAV in a research laboratory setting.

TABLE 20B (3)

Other indications: persons traveling to or working in countries that have high or intermediate endemicity of hepatitis A (a list of countries is available at http://wwwn.cdc.gov/travel/contentdiseases.aspx) and any person seeking protection from HAV infection.

Single-antigen vaccine formulations should be administered in a 2-dose schedule at either 0 and 6–12 months (Havrix®), or 0 and 6–18 months (Vaqta®). If the combined hepatitis A and hepatitis B vaccine (Twinrix®) is used, administer 3 doses at 0, 1, and 6 months.

9. Hepatitis B vaccination

Medical indications: persons with end-stage renal disease, including patients receiving hemodialysis; persons seeking evaluation or treatment for a sexually transmitted disease (STD); persons with HIV infection; and persons with chronic liver disease.

Occupational indications: health-care personnel and public-safety workers who are exposed to blood or other potentially infectious body fluids.

Behavioral indications: sexually active persons who are not in a long-term, mutually monogamous relationship (e.g., persons with more than one sex partner during the previous 6 months); current or recent injection-drug users; and men who have sex with men.

Other indications: household contacts and sex partners of persons with chronic hepatitis B virus (HBV) infection; clients and staff members of institutions for persons with developmental disabilities; international travelers to countries with high or intermediate prevalence of chronic HBV infection (a list of countries is available at http://wwwn.cdc.gov/travel/contentdiseases.aspx); and any adult seeking protection from HBV infection.

Settings where hepatitis B vaccination is recommended for all adults: STD treatment facilities; HIV testing and treatment facilities; facilities providing drug-abuse treatment and prevention services; health-care settings targeting services to injection-drug users or men who have sex with men; correctional facilities; end-stage renal disease programs and facilities for chronic hemodialysis patients; and institutions and nonresidential day care facilities for persons with developmental disabilities.

Special formulation indications: for adult patients receiving hemodialysis and other immunocompromised adults, 1 dose of 40 μg/mL (Recombivax HB®) or 2 doses of 20 μg/mL (Engerix-B®), administered simultaneously.

10. Meningococcal vaccination

Medical indications: adults with anatomic or functional asplenia or terminal complement component deficiencies.

Other indications: first-year college students living in dormitories; microbiologists who are routinely exposed to isolates of *Neisseria meningitidis*; military recruits; and persons who travel to or live in countries in which meningococcal disease is hyperendemic or epidemic (e.g., the "meningitis belt" of sub-Saharan Africa during the dry season [December–June]), particularly if their contact with local populations will be prolonged. Vaccination is required by the government of Saudi Arabia for all travelers to Mecca during the annual Hajj.

Meningococcal conjugate vaccine is preferred for adults with any of the preceding indications who are aged ≤55 years, although meningococcal polysaccharide vaccine (MPSV4) is an acceptable alternative. Revaccination after 3–5 years might be indicated for adults previously vaccinated with MPSV4 who remain at increased risk for infection (e.g., persons residing in areas in which disease is epidemic).

11. Herpes zoster vaccination

A single dose of zoster vaccine is recommended for adults aged ≥60 years regardless of whether they report a prior episode of herpes zoster. Persons with chronic medical conditions may be vaccinated unless a contraindication or precaution exists for their condition.

12. Selected conditions for which *Haemophilus influenzae* type b (Hib) vaccine may be used

Hib conjugate vaccines are licensed for children aged 6 weeks–71 months. No efficacy data are available on which to base a recommendation concerning use of Hib vaccine for older children and adults with the chronic conditions associated with an increased risk for Hib disease. However, studies suggest good immunogenicity in patients who have sickle cell disease, leukemia, or HIV infection or who have had splenectomies; administering vaccine to these patients is not contraindicated.

13. Immunocompromising conditions

Inactivated vaccines generally are acceptable (e.g., pneumococcal, meningococcal, and influenza [trivalent inactivated influenza vaccine]) and live vaccines generally are avoided in persons with immune deficiencies or immune suppressive conditions. Information on specific conditions is available at http://www.cdc.gov/vaccines/pubs/acip-list.htm.

TABLE 20B (4)

Vaccines that might be indicated for adults based on medical and other indications — United States, October 2007– September 2008

Vaccine	Pregnancy	Immuno-compromising conditions (excluding human immunodeficiency virus [HIV]), medications[13], radiation	HIV infection[3,12,13] CD4+ T lymphocyte count <200 cells/µL	HIV infection[3,12,13] CD4+ T lymphocyte count ≥200 cells/µL	Diabetes, heart disease, chronic pulmonary disease, chronic alcoholism	Asplenia[12] (including elective splenectomy and terminal complement component deficiencies)	Chronic liver disease	Kidney failure, end-stage renal disease, receipt of hemodialysis	Health-care personnel
Tetanus, diphtheria, pertussis (Td/Tdap)[1]*	1 dose Td booster every 10 yrs (Substitute 1 dose of Tdap for Td)								
Human papillomavirus (HPV)[2]*	3 doses for females through age 26 yrs (0, 2, 6 mos)								
Measles, mumps, rubella (MMR)[3]*		Contraindicated	Contraindicated	1 or 2 doses					
Varicella[4]*	Contraindicated	Contraindicated	Contraindicated	2 doses (0, 4–8 wks)					
Influenza[5]*					1 dose TIV annually				1 dose TIV or LAIV annually
Pneumococcal (polysaccharide)[6,7]					1–2 doses				
Hepatitis A[8]*					2 doses (0, 6–12 mos, or 0, 6–18 mos)				
Hepatitis B[9]*					3 doses (0, 1–2, 4–6 mos)				
Meningococcal[10]*					1 or more doses				
Zoster[11]	Contraindicated	Contraindicated	Contraindicated		1 dose				

Indication: Pregnancy · Immuno-compromising conditions · HIV infection · Diabetes, heart disease, chronic pulmonary disease, chronic alcoholism · Asplenia · Chronic liver disease · Kidney failure, end-stage renal disease, receipt of hemodialysis · Health-care personnel

* Covered by the Vaccine Injury Compensation Program.

☐ For all persons in this category who meet the age requirements and who lack evidence of immunity (e.g., lack documentation of vaccination or have no evidence of prior infection)

▨ Recommended if some other risk factor is present (e.g., on the basis of medical, occupational, lifestyle, or other indications)

TABLE 20C – ANTI-TETANUS PROPHYLAXIS, WOUND CLASSIFICATION, IMMUNIZATION

WOUND CLASSIFICATION			IMMUNIZATION SCHEDULE				
Clinical Features	Tetanus Prone	Non-Tetanus Prone	History of Tetanus Immunization	Dirty, Tetanus-Prone Wound		Clean, Non-Tetanus Prone Wound	
				Td[1,2]	TIG	Td	TIG
Age of wound	> 6 hours	≤ 6 hours	Unknown or < 3 doses	Yes	Yes	Yes	No
Configuration	Stellate, avulsion	Linear					
Depth	> 1 cm	≤ 1 cm	3 or more doses	No[3]	No	No[4]	No
Mechanism of injury	Missile, crush, burn, frostbite	Sharp surface (glass, knife)	[1] Td = Tetanus & diphtheria toxoids adsorbed (adult) TIG = Tetanus immune globulin (human) [2] Yes if wound >24 hr old. For children <7yr, DPT (DT if pertussis vaccine contraindicated); For persons ≥7yr, Td preferred to tetanus toxoid alone. [3] Yes if >5 years since last booster [4] Yes if >10 years since last booster				
Devitalized tissue	Present	Absent					
Contaminants (dirt, saliva, etc.)	Present	Absent					
(From ACS Bull. 69:22,23, 1984, No. 10)			*[From MMWR 39:37, 1990; MMWR 46(SS-2):15, 1997]*				

TABLE 20D – RABIES POST-EXPOSURE PROPHYLAXIS

All wounds should be cleaned immediately & thoroughly with soap & water. This has been shown to protect 90% of experimental animals![1]

Post-Exposure Prophylaxis Guide, United States, 2000

(CID 30:4, 2000; NEJM 351:2626, 2004; MMWR 57: RR-3, 2008)

Animal Type	Evaluation & Disposition of Animal	Recommendations for Prophylaxis
Dogs, cats, ferrets	Healthy & available for 10-day observation Rabid or suspected rabid Unknown (escaped)	Don't start unless animal develops sx, then immediately begin HRIG + HDCV or RVA Immediate vaccination Consult public health officials
Skunks, raccoons, bats,* foxes, coyotes, most carnivores	Regard as rabid	Immediate vaccination
Livestock, rodents, rabbits; includes hares, squirrels, hamsters, guinea pigs, gerbils, chipmunks, rats, mice, woodchucks		Almost never require anti-rabies rx. Consult public health officials.

* Most recent cases of human rabies in U.S. due to contact (not bites) with silver-haired bats or rarely big brown bats *(MMWR 46:770, 1997; AnIM 128:922, 1998)*. For more detail, *see CID 30:4, 2000; JAVMA 219:1687, 2001; CID 37:96, 2003 (travel medicine advisory); Ln 363:959, 2004; EID 11:1921, 2005; MMWR 55 (RR-5), 2006*.

Post-Exposure Rabies Immunization Schedule

IF NOT PREVIOUSLY VACCINATED

Treatment	Regimen[2]
Local wound cleaning	**All post-exposure treatment should begin with immediate, thorough cleaning of all wounds with soap & water.**
Human rabies immune globulin (HRIG)	20 units per kg body weight given once on day 0. If anatomically feasible, the full dose should be infiltrated around the wound(s), the rest should be administered IM in the gluteal area. HRIG should **not** be administered in the **same syringe, or** into the **same anatomical site** as vaccine, or more than 7 days after the initiation of vaccine. Because HRIG may partially suppress active production of antibody, no more than the recommended dose should be given.[3]
Vaccine	Human diploid cell vaccine (HDCV), rabies vaccine adsorbed (RVA), or purified chick embryo cell vaccine (PCECV) 1.0 mL **IM (deltoid area[4])**, one each days 0, 3, 7, 14, & 28.

IF PREVIOUSLY VACCINATED[5]

Treatment	Regimen[2]
Local wound cleaning	All post-exposure treatment should begin with immediate, thorough cleaning of all wounds with soap & water.
HRIG	HRIG should **not** be administered
Vaccine	HDCV, RVA or PCEC, 1.0 mL **IM (deltoid area[4])**, one each on days 0 & 3

CORRECT VACCINE ADMINISTRATION SITES

Age Group	Administration Site
Children & adults	**DELTOID[4]** only (**NEVER** in gluteus)
Infants & young children	Outer aspect of thigh (anterolateral thigh) may be used (**NEVER** in gluteus)

[1] From *MMWR 48:RR-1, 1999; CID 30:4, 2000;* B.T. Matyas, Mass. Dept. of Public Health

[2] These regimens are applicable for all age groups, including children.

[3] In most reported post-exposure treatment failures, only identified deficiency was failure to infiltrate wound(s) with HRIG *(CID 22:228, 1996)*. However, several failures reported from SE Asia in patients in whom WHO protocol followed *(CID 28:143, 1999)*.

[4] The **deltoid** area is the **only** acceptable site of vaccination for adults & older children. For infants & young children, outer aspect of the thigh (anterolateral thigh) may be used. Vaccine should **NEVER** be administered in gluteal area.

[5] Any person with a history of pre-exposure vaccination with HDCV, RVA, PCECV; prior post-exposure prophylaxis with HDCV, RVA, PCEC; or previous vaccination with any other type of rabies vaccine & a documented history of antibody response to the prior vaccination

TABLE 21 SELECTED DIRECTORY OF RESOURCES

ORGANIZATION	PHONE/FAX	WEBSITE(S)

ANTIPARASITIC DRUGS & PARASITOLOGY INFORMATION *(CID 37:694, 2003)*
CDC Drug Line	Weekdays: 404-639-3670	www.cdc.gov/ncidod/srp/drugs/drug-service.html
	Evenings, weekends, holidays: 404-639-2888	
DPDx: Lab ID of parasites		www.dpd.cdc.gov/dpdx/default.htm
Gorgas Course Tropical Medicine		http://info.dom.uab.edu/gorgas
Malaria	daytime: 770-488-7788	www.cdc.gov/malaria
	other: 770-488-7100	
Panorama Compound. Pharm.	800-247-9767/818-787-7256	www.uniquerx.com
World Health Organization (WHO)		www.who.org
Parasites & Health		www.dpd.cdc.gov/dpdx/HTML/Para_Health.htm

BIOTERRORISM
Centers for Disease Control & Prevention	770-488-7100	www.bt.cdc.gov
Infectious Diseases Society of America	703-299-0200	www.idsociety.org
Johns Hopkins Center Civilian Biodefense		www.jhsph.edu
Center for Biosecurity of the Univ. of Pittsburgh Med. Center		www.upmc-biosecurity.org
US Army Medical Research Institute of Inf. Dis.		www.usamriid.army.mil

HEPATITIS B
| ACT-HBV | | www.act-hbv.com |

HEPATITIS C *(CID 35:754, 2002)*
CDC		www.cdc.gov/ncidod/diseases/hepatitis/C
Individual		http://hepatitis-central.com
Medscape		www.medscape.com

HIV
General
| HIV InSite | | http://hivinsite.ucsf.edu |
| Johns Hopkins AIDS Service | | www.hopkins-aids.edu |
Drug Interactions
Johns Hopkins AIDS Service		www.hopkins-aids.edu
Liverpool HIV Pharm. Group		www.hiv-druginteractions.org
Other		http://AIDS.medscape.com
Prophylaxis/Treatment of Opportunistic Infections; HIV Treatment		www.aidsinfo.nih.gov

IMMUNIZATIONS *(CID 36:355, 2003)*
CDC, Natl. Immunization Program	404-639-8200	www.cdc.gov/vaccines/
FDA, Vaccine Adverse Events	800-822-7967	www.fda.gov/cber/vaers/vaers.htm
National Network Immunization Info.	877-341-6644	www.immunizationinfo.org
Influenza vaccine, CDC	404-639-8200	www.cdc.gov/vaccines/
Institute for Vaccine Safety		www.vaccinesafety.edu

OCCUPATIONAL EXPOSURE, BLOOD-BORNE PATHOGENS (HIV, HEPATITIS B & C)
| National Clinicians' Post-Exposure Hotline | 888-448-4911 | www.ucsf.edu/hivcntr |

Q-Tc INTERVAL PROLONGATION BY DRUGS
| | | www.qtdrugs.org |

SEXUALLY TRANSMITTED DISEASES
| | | www.cdc.gov/std/treatment/TOC2002TG.htm |
| | Slides: http://www.phac-aspc.gc.ca/slm-maa/slides/index.html | |

TRAVELERS' INFO: Immunizations, Malaria Prophylaxis, More
Amer. Soc. Trop. Med. & Hyg.		www.astmh.org
CDC, general	877-394-8747/888-232-3299	http://wwwn.cdc.gov/travel/default.asp
CDC, Malaria:		www.cdc.gov/malaria
Prophylaxis		http://wwwn.cdc.gov/travel/default.asp
Treatment	770-488-7788	www.who.int/health_topics/malaria
MD Travel Health		www.mdtravelhealth.com
Pan American Health Organization		www.paho.org
World Health Organization (WHO)		www.who.int/home-page

VACCINE & IMMUNIZATION RESOURCES *(CID 36:355, 2003)*
American Academy of Pediatrics		www.cispimmunize.org
CDC, National Immunization Program		www.cdc.gov/vaccines/
National Network for Immunization Information		www.immunizationinfo.org

TABLE 22A – ANTI-INFECTIVE DRUG-DRUG INTERACTIONS
Importance: ± = theory/anecdotal; + = of probable importance; ++ = of definite importance

ANTI-INFECTIVE AGENT (A)	OTHER DRUG (B)	EFFECT	IMPORT
Amantadine (Symmetrel)	Alcohol	↑ CNS effects	+
	Anticholinergic and anti-Parkinson agents (ex. Artane, scopolamine)	↑ effect of B: dry mouth, ataxia, blurred vision, slurred speech, toxic psychosis	+
	Trimethoprim	↑ levels of A & B	+
	Digoxin	↑ levels of B	±
Aminoglycosides—parenteral (amikacin, gentamicin, kanamycin, netilmicin, sisomicin, streptomycin, tobramycin)	Amphotericin B	↑ nephrotoxicity	++
	Cis platinum (Platinol)	↑ nephro & ototoxicity	+
	Cyclosporine	↑ nephrotoxicity	+
	Neuromuscular blocking agents	↑ apnea or respiratory paralysis	+
	Loop diuretics (e.g., furosemide)	↑ ototoxicity	++
	NSAIDs	↑ nephrotoxicity	+
	Non-polarizing muscle relaxants	↑ apnea	+
	Radiographic contrast	↑ nephrotoxicity	+
	Vancomycin	↑ nephrotoxicity	+
Aminoglycosides— oral (kanamycin, neomycin)	**Oral anticoagulants (dicumarol, phenindione, warfarin)**	↑ prothrombin time	+
Amphotericin B and ampho B lipid formulations	Antineoplastic drugs	↑ nephrotoxicity risk	+
	Digitalis	↑ toxicity of B if K⁺ ↓	+
	Nephrotoxic drugs: aminoglycosides, cidofovir, cyclosporine, pentamidine	↑ nephrotoxicity of A	++
Ampicillin, amoxicillin	Allopurinol	↑ frequency of rash	++
Fosamprenavir	Antiretrovirals—see Table 22B & Table 22C		
	Contraceptives, oral	↓ levels of A & B; use other contraception	++
	Lovastatin/simvastatin	↑ **levels of B—avoid**	++
	Rifabutin	↑ levels of B (↓ dose by 50–75%)	++
	Rifampin	↓ **levels of A—avoid**	++
Atazanavir	See protease inhibitors and Table 22B & Table 22C		
Atovaquone	Rifampin (perhaps rifabutin)	↓ serum levels of A; ↑ levels of B	+
	Metoclopramide	↓ levels of A	+
	Tetracycline	↓ levels of A	++

Azole Antifungal Agents[1]   [**Flu** = fluconazole; **Itr** = itraconazole; **Ket** = ketoconazole; **Posa** = posaconazole **Vor** = voriconazole; + = occurs; **blank space** = either studied & no interaction OR no data found (may be in pharm. co. databases)]

Flu	Itr	Ket	Posa	Vor	OTHER DRUG (B)	EFFECT	IMPORT
+	+				Amitriptyline	↑ levels of B	+
+	+	+		+	Calcium channel blockers	↑ levels of B	++
		+		+	Carbamazepine (vori contraindicated)	↓ levels of A	++
+	+	+	+	+	Cyclosporine	↑ levels of B, ↑ risk of nephrotoxicity	+
	+	+			Didanosine	↓ absorption of A	+
+	+	+		+	Efavirenz	↓ levels of A, ↑ levels of B	++ (avoid)
	+	+	+		H₂ blockers, antacids, sucralfate	↓ absorption of A	+
+	+	+	+	+	Hydantoins (phenytoin, Dilantin)	↑ levels of B, ↓ levels of A	++
	+	+			Isoniazid	↓ levels of A	+
	+			+	Lovastatin/simvastatin	Rhabdomyolysis reported; ↑ levels of B	++
				+	Methadone	↑ levels of B	+
+	+	+	+	+	Midazolam/triazolam, po	↑ levels of B	++
+	+	+		+	Oral anticoagulants	↑ effect of B	++
+	+			+	Oral hypoglycemics	↑ levels of B	++
		+	+		Pimozide	↑ levels of B—**avoid**	++
	+	+		+	Protease inhibitors	↑ levels of B	++
	+	+	+	+	Proton pump inhibitors	↓ levels of A, ↑ levels of B	++
+	+	+	+	+	Rifampin/rifabutin (vori contraindicated)	↑ levels of B, ↓ serum levels of A	++
			+	+	Sirolimus (vori and posa contraindicated)	↑ levels of B	++
+		+	+	+	Tacrolimus	↑ levels of B with toxicity	++
+		+			Theophyllines	↑ levels of B	+
		+			Trazodone	↑ levels of B	++
+					Zidovudine	↑ levels of B	+

TABLE 22A (2)

Caspofungin	Cyclosporine	↑ levels of A	++
	Tacrolimus	↓ levels of B	++
	Carbamazepine, dexamethasone, efavirenz, nevirapine, phenytoin, rifamycin	↓ levels of A; ↑ dose of caspofungin to 70 mg/d	++
Cephalosporins with methyl-tetrathiozolethiol side-chain	Oral anticoagulants (dicumarol, warfarin), heparin, thrombolytic agents, platelet aggregation inhibitors	↑ effects of B, bleeding	+
Chloramphenicol	Hydantoins	↑ toxicity of B, nystagmus, ataxia	++
	Iron salts, Vitamin B12	↓ response to B	++
	Protease inhibitors—HIV	↑ levels of A & B	++
Clindamycin (Cleocin)	Kaolin	↓ absorption of A	+
	Muscle relaxants, e.g., atracurium, baclofen, diazepam	↑ frequency/duration of respiratory paralysis	+
Cycloserine	Ethanol	↑ frequency of seizures	+
	INH, ethionamide	↑ frequency of drowsiness/dizziness	+
Dapsone	Didanosine	↓ absorption of A	+
	Oral contraceptives	↓ effectiveness of B	+
	Pyrimethamine	↑ in marrow toxicity	+
	Rifampin/Rifabutin	↓ serum levels of A	+
	Trimethoprim	↑ levels of A & B (methemoglobinemia)	+
	Zidovudine	May ↑ marrow toxicity	+
Daptomycin	HMG-CoA inhibitors (statins)	DC statin while on dapto	++
Delavirdine (Rescriptor)	*See Non-nucleoside reverse transcriptase inhibitors (NNRTIs) and Table 22C*		
Didanosine (ddI) (Videx)	Allopurinol	↑ levels of A—**AVOID**	++
	Cisplatin, dapsone, INH, metronidazole, nitrofurantoin, stavudine, vincristine, zalcitabine	↑ risk of peripheral neuropathy	+
	Ethanol, lamivudine, pentamidine	↑ risk of pancreatitis	+
	Fluoroquinolones	↓ absorption 2° to chelation	+
	Drugs that need low pH for absorption: dapsone, indinavir, itra/ketoconazole, pyrimethamine, rifampin, trimethoprim	↓ absorption	+
	Methadone	↓ levels of A	++
	Ribavirin	↑ levels ddI metabolite—**avoid**	++
	Tenofovir	↑ levels of A **(reduce dose of A)**	++
Doripenem	Probenecid	↑ levels of A	++
	Valproic acid	↓ levels of B	++
Doxycycline	Aluminum, bismuth, iron, Mg^{++}	↓ absorption of A	+
	Barbiturates, hydantoins	↓ serum t/2 of A	+
	Carbamazepine (Tegretol)	↓ serum t/2 of A	+
	Digoxin	↑ serum levels of B	+
	Warfarin	↑ activity of B	++
Efavirenz (Sustiva)	*See non-nucleoside reverse transcriptase inhibitors (NNRTIs) and Table 22C*		
Ertapenem (Invanz)	Probenecid	↑ levels of A	++
Ethambutol (Myambutol)	Aluminum salts (includes didanosine buffer)	↓ absorption of A & B	+
Etravirine	*See non-nucleoside reverse transcriptase inhibitors (NNRTIs) and Table 22C*		

Fluoroquinolones (***Cipro*** = ciprofloxacin; ***Gati*** = gatifloxacin; ***Gemi*** = gemifloxacin; ***Levo*** = levofloxacin; ***Moxi*** = moxifloxacin; ***Oflox*** = ofloxacin)

NOTE: Blank space = either studied and no interaction OR no data found (*pharm. co. may have data*)

Cipro	Gati	Gemi	Levo	Moxi	Oflox			
	+		+	+		**Antiarrhythmics (procainamide, amiodarone)**	↑ Q-T interval (torsade)	++
+	+		+	+	+	Insulin, oral hypoglycemics	↑ & ↓ blood sugar	++
+						Caffeine	↑ levels of B	+
+					+	Cimetidine	↑ levels of A	+
+					+	Cyclosporine	↑ levels of B	±
+	+		+	+	+	Didanosine	↓ absorption of A	++
+	+	+	+	+	+	**Cations: Al+++, Ca++, Fe++, Mg++, Zn++ (antacids, vitamins, dairy products), citrate/citric acid**	↓ absorption of A (some variability between drugs)	++
+						Methadone	↑ levels of B	++
+		+			+	**NSAIDs**	↑ risk CNS stimulation/seizures	++
+						Phenytoin	↑ or ↓ levels of B	+
+	+	+			+	Probenecid	↓ renal clearance of A	+
+						Rasagiline	↑ levels of B	++

Fluoroquinolones (continued)

Cipro	Gati	Gemi	Levo	Moxi	Oflox			
						NOTE: Blank space = either studied and no interaction OR no data found (pharm. co. may have data)		
					+	Rifampin	↓ levels of A *(CID 45:1001, 2007)*	++
+	+	+	+		+	**Sucralfate**	↓ absorption of A	++
+						Theophylline	↑ levels of B	++
+						Thyroid hormone	↓ levels of B	++
+						Tizanidine	↑ levels of B	++
+		+	+		+	Warfarin	↑ prothrombin time	+

Ganciclovir (Cytovene) & **Valganciclovir** (Valcyte)	Imipenem	↑ risk of seizures reported	+
	Probenecid	↑ levels of A	+
	Zidovudine	↓ levels of A, ↑ levels of B	+
Gentamicin	*See Aminoglycosides—parenteral*		
Indinavir	*See protease inhibitors and Table 22B & Table 22C*		
Isoniazid	**Alcohol, rifampin**	**↑ risk of hepatic injury**	++
	Aluminum salts	↓ absorption (take fasting)	++
	Carbamazepine, phenytoin	↑ levels of B with nausea, vomiting, nystagmus, ataxia	++
	Itraconazole, ketoconazole	↓ levels of B	+
	Oral hypoglycemics	↓ effects of B	+
Lamivudine	Zalcitabine	**Mutual interference—do not combine**	++
Linezolid (Zyvox)	Adrenergic agents	Risk of hypertension	++
	Aged, fermented, pickled or smoked foods —↑ tyramine	Risk of hypertension	+
	Rasagiline (MAO inhibitor)	Risk of serotonin syndrome	+
	Rifampin	↓ levels of A	++
	Serotonergic drugs (SSRIs)	Risk of serotonin syndrome	++
Lopinavir	*See protease inhibitors*		

Macrolides [*Ery* = erythromycin; *Azi* = azithromycin; *Clr* = clarithromycin; + = occurs; **blank space** = either studied and no interaction OR no data (pharm. co. may have data)]

Ery	Azi	Clr			
+		+	Carbamazepine	↑ serum levels of B, nystagmus, nausea, vomiting, ataxia	**++ (avoid w/ erythro)**
+		+	Cimetidine, **ritonavir**	↑ levels of B	+
+			Clozapine	↑ serum levels of B, CNS toxicity	+
		+	**Colchicine**	**↑ levels of B (potent, fatal)**	**++ (avoid)**
+			Corticosteroids	↑ effects of B	+
+	+	+	Cyclosporine	↑ serum levels of B with toxicity	+
+	+	+	Digoxin, digitoxin	↑ serum levels of B (10% of cases)	+
		+	Efavirenz	↓ levels of A	++
+		+	Ergot alkaloids	↑ levels of B	++
+		+	Lovastatin/simvastatin	↑ levels of B; rhabdomyolysis	++
+			Midazolam, triazolam	↑ levels of B, ↑ sedative effects	+
+		+	Phenytoin	↑ levels of B	+
+	+	+	Pimozide	**↑ Q-T interval**	++
+		+	Rifampin, rifabutin	↓ levels of A	+
+		+	Tacrolimus	↑ levels of B	++
+		+	Theophylline	↑ serum levels of B with nausea, vomiting, seizures, apnea	++
+		+	Valproic acid	↑ levels of B	+
+		+	Warfarin	May ↑ prothrombin time	+
		+	Zidovudine	↓ levels of B	+

Maraviroc	Clarithromycin	↑ serum levels of A	++
	Delavirdine	↑ levels of A	++
	Itaconazoler/ketoconazole	↑ levels of A	++
	Nefazodone	↑ levels of A	++
	Protease Inhibitors (not tipranavir/ritonavir)	↑ levels of A	++
	Anticonvulsants: carbamazepine, phenobarbital, phenytoin	↓ levels of A	++
	Efavirenz	↓ levels of A	++
	Rifampin	↓ levels of A	++

TABLE 22A (4)

Mefloquine	ß-adrenergic blockers, calcium channel blockers, quinidine, quinine	↑ arrhythmias	+
	Divalproex, valproic acid	↓ level of B with seizures	++
	Halofantrine	Q-T prolongation	++ (avoid)
Methenamine mandelate or hippurate	Acetazolamide, sodium bicarbonate, thiazide diuretics	↓ antibacterial effect 2° to ↑ urine pH	++
MetronidazoleTinidazole	**Alcohol**	Disulfiram-like reaction	+
	Cyclosporin	↑ levels of B	++
	Disulfiram (Antabuse)	Acute toxic psychosis	+
	Lithium	↑ levels of B	++
	Oral anticoagulants	↑ anticoagulant effect	++
	Phenobarbital, hydantoins	↑ levels of B	++
Micafungin	Nifedipine	↑ levels of B	+
	Sirolimus	↑ levels of B	+
Nelfinavir	*See protease inhibitors and Table 22B & Table 22C*		
Nevirapine (Viramune)	*See non-nucleoside reverse transcriptase inhibitors (NNRTIs) and Table 22C*		
Nitrofurantoin	Antacids	↓ absorption of A	+

Non-nucleoside reverse transcriptase inhibitors (NNRTIs): For interactions with protease inhibitors, *see Table 22C*.
Del = delavirdine; **Efa** = efavirenz; **Etr** = etravirine; **Nev** = nevirapine

Del	Efa	Etr	Nev	**Co-administration contraindicated:**		
+		+		Anticonvulsants: carbamazepine, phenobarbital, phenytoin		++
+		+		Antimycobacterials: rifabutin, rifampin		++
+				Antipsychotics: pimozide		++
+	+	+		Benzodiazepines: alprazolam, midazolam, triazolam		++
+	+			Ergotamine		++
+	+	+		HMG-CoA inhibitors (statins): lovastatin, simvastatin, atorvastatin, pravastatin		++
+	+			St. John's wort		++
				Dose change needed:		
+				Amphetamines	↑ levels of B—**caution**	++
+	+	+		Antiarrhythmics: amiodarone, lidocaine, others	↓ or ↑ levels of B—**caution**	++
+	+	+	+	Anticonvulsants: carbamazepine, phenobarbital, phenytoin	↓ levels of A and/or B	++
+	+	+	+	Antifungals: itraconazole, ketoconazole, voriconazole, posaconazole	Potential ↓ levels of B, ↑ levels of A	++ (avoid)
+		+		Antirejection drugs: cyclosporine, rapamycin, sirolimus, tacrolimus	↑ levels of B	++
+			+	Calcium channel blockers	↑ levels of B	++
+	+	+		Clarithromycin	↑ levels of B metabolite, ↑ levels of A	++
+	+	+		Cyclosporine	↑ levels of B	++
+	+			Dexamethasone	↓ levels of A	++
+	+	+	+	Sildenafil, vardenafil, tadalafil	↑ levels of B	++
+	+			Fentanyl, methadone	↑ levels of B	++
+				Gastric acid suppression: antacids, H-2 blockers, proton pump inhibitors	↓ levels of A	++
	+	+	+	Methadone, fentanyl	↓ levels of B	++
	+		+	Oral contraceptives	↑ or ↓ levels of B	++
+	+	+	+	Protease inhibitors—*see Table 22C*		
+	+	+	+	**Rifabutin, rifampin**	↑ or ↓ levels of rifabutin; ↓ levels of A—**caution**	++
+	+	+	+	St. John's wort	↓ levels of B	
+		+	+	Warfarin	↑ levels of B	++

Pentamidine, IV	Amphotericin B	↑ risk of nephrotoxicity	+
	Pancreatitis-assoc drugs, eg, alcohol, valproic acid	↑ risk of pancreatitis	+
Piperacillin	Cefoxitin	Antagonism vs pseudomonas	++
Pip-tz	Methotrexate	↑ levels of B	++
Primaquine	Chloroquine, dapsone, INH, probenecid, quinine, sulfonamides, TMP/SMX, others	**↑ risk of hemolysis in G6PD-deficient patients**	++

TABLE 22A (5)

Protease Inhibitors—Anti-HIV Drugs. (**Atazan** = atazanavir; **Darun** = darunavir; **Fosampren** = fosamprenavir; **Indin** = indinavir; **Lopin** = lopinavir; **Nelfin** = nelfinavir; **Saquin** = saquinavir; **Tipran** = tipranavir). For interactions with antiretrovirals, *see Table 22B & Table 22C* **Only a partial list—check package insert**
Also see http://aidsinfo.nih.gov

Atazan	Darun	Fosampren	Indin	Lopin	Nelfin	Saquin	Tipran	Drug	Effect	
								Analgesics:		
							+	1. Alfentanil, fentanyl, hydrocodone, tramadol	↑ levels of B	+
	+		+			+	+	2. Codeine, hydromorphone, morphine, methadone	↓ levels of B (*JAIDS 41:563, 2006*)	+
+	+	+	+	+	+		+	**Anti-arrhythmics: amiodarone, lidocaine, mexiletine, flecainide**	↑ levels of B; **do not co-administer**	++
	+		+	+	+	+		**Anticonvulsants: carbamazepine, clonazepam, phenobarbital**	↓ levels of A, ↑ levels of B	++
+		+	+				+	Antidepressants, all tricyclic	↑ levels of B	++
+	+						+	Antidepressants, all other	↑ levels of B; do not use pimozide	++
	+							Antidepressants: SSRIs	↓ levels of B - avoid	++
							+	Antihistamines	**Do not use**	++
+	+	+	+	+	+		+	**Benzodiazepines, e.g., diazepam, midazolam, triazolam**	**↑ levels of B—do not use**	++
+	+	+	+	+	+	+	+	Calcium channel blockers (all)	↑ levels of B	++
+	+		+	+	+	+		Clarithro, erythro	↑ levels of B if renal impairment	+
+	+		+	+			+	Contraceptives, oral	↓ levels of A & B	++
	+	+	+					Corticosteroids: prednisone, dexamethasone	↓ levels of A, ↑ levels of B	+
+	+	+	+	+	+	+	+	Cyclosporine	↑ levels of B, monitor levels	+
							+	Digoxin	↑ levels of B	++
+	+	+	+	+	+	+	+	Ergot derivatives	**↑ levels of B—do not use**	++
		+	+			+	+	Erythromycin, clarithromycin	↑ levels of A & B	+
			+			+		Grapefruit juice (>200 mL/day)	↓ indinavir & ↑ saquinavir levels	++
+	+	+	+	+	+	+		H2 receptor antagonists	↓ levels of A	++
+	+	+	+	+	+	+	+	**HMG-CoA reductase inhibitors (statins): lovastatin, simvastatin**	**↑ levels of B—do not use**	++
+								Irinotecan	**↑ levels of B—do not use**	++
*	+	+	+	+	+	+	+	Ketoconazole, itraconazole, ? vori.	↑ levels of A, ↑ levels of B	+
	+	+	+	+	+	+	+	Posaconazole	↑ levels of A, no effect on B	++
				+			+	Metronidazole	Poss. disulfiram reaction, alcohol	+
				+				Phenytoin (*JAIDS 36:1034, 2004*)	↑ levels of A & B	++
+	+	+	+	+	+	+	+	**Pimozide**	**↑ levels of B—do not use**	++
+	+		+	+	+	+		Proton pump inhibitors	↓ levels of A	++
+	+	+	+	+	+	+	+	Rifampin, rifabutin	↓ levels of A, ↑ levels of B **(avoid)**	++ **(avoid)**
+	+	+	+	+	+	+	+	Sildenafil (Viagra), tadalafil, vardenafil	Varies, some ↑ & some ↓ levels of B	++
+	+	+	+	+	+	+	+	**St. John's wort**	**↓ levels of A—do not use**	++
+	+	+	+	+	+	+	+	Sirolimus, tracrolimus	↑ levels of B	++
+								Tenofovir	↓ levels of A—add ritonavir	++
	+		+	+				Theophylline	↓ levels of B	+
+		+		+			+	Warfarin	↑ levels of B	+
Pyrazinamide								INH, rifampin	May ↑ risk of hepatotoxicity	±
Pyrimethamine								Lorazepam	↑ risk of hepatotoxicity	+
								Sulfonamides, TMP/SMX	↑ risk of marrow suppression	+
								Zidovudine	↑ risk of marrow suppression	+
Quinine								Digoxin	↑ digoxin levels; ↑ toxicity	++
								Mefloquine	↑ arrhythmias	+
								Oral anticoagulants	↑ prothrombin time	++

TABLE 22A (6)

Quinupristin- dalfopristin (Synercid)	Anti-HIV drugs: NNRTIs & PIs	↑ levels of B	++
	Antineoplastic: vincristine, docetaxel, paclitaxel	↑ levels of B	++
	Calcium channel blockers	↑ levels of B	++
	Carbamazepine	↑ levels of B	++
	Cyclosporine, tacrolimus	↑ levels of B	++
	Lidocaine	↑ levels of B	++
	Methylprednisolone	↑ levels of B	++
	Midazolam, diazepam	↑ levels of B	++
	Statins	↑ levels of B	++
Raltegravir	Rifampin	↓ levels of A	++
Ribavirin	Didanosine	↑ levels of B → toxicity—**avoid**	++
	Stavudine	↓ levels of B	++
	Zidovudine	↓ levels of B	++
Rifamycins (rifampin, rifabutin) *See note below for less severe or less common interactions* Ref.: *ArIM 162:985, 2002* **The following is a partial list of drugs with rifampin-induced ↑ metabolism and hence lower than anticipated serum levels: ACE inhibitors, dapsone, diazepam, digoxin, diltiazem, doxycycline, fluconazole, fluvastatin, haloperidol, moxifloxacin, nifedipine, progestins, triazolam, tricyclics, voriconazole, zidovudine** *(Clin Pharmocokinet 42:819, 2003).*	Al OH, ketoconazole, PZA	↓ levels of A	+
	Atovaquone	↑ levels of A, ↓ levels of B	+
	Beta adrenergic blockers (metoprolol, propranolol)	↓ effect of B	+
	Caspofungin	↓ levels of B—increase dose	++
	Clarithromycin	↑ levels of A, ↓ levels of B	++
	Corticosteroids	↑ replacement requirement of B	++
	Cyclosporine	↓ effect of B	++
	Delavirdine	**levels of A, ↓ levels of B—avoid**	++
	Digoxin	↓ levels of B	++
	Disopyramide	↓ levels of B	++
	Fluconazole	↑ levels of A[1]	+
	Amprenavir, indinavir, nelfinavir, ritonavir	↑ levels of A (↓ dose of A), ↓ levels of B	++
	INH	Converts INH to toxic hydrazine	++
	Itraconazole[2], ketoconazole	↓ levels of B, ↑ levels of A[1]	++
	Linezolid	↓ levels of B	++
	Methadone	↓ serum levels (withdrawal)	+
	Nevirapine	**↓ levels of B—avoid**	++
	Oral anticoagulants	Suboptimal anticoagulation	++
	Oral contraceptives	↓ effectiveness; spotting, pregnancy	+
	Phenytoin	↓ levels of B	+
	Protease inhibitors	**↓ levels of A, ↑ levels of B—CAUTION**	++
	Qunidine	↓ effect of B	+
	Sulfonylureas	↓ hypoglycemic effect	+
	Tacrolimus	**↓ levels of B**	++
	Theophylline	↑ levels of B	+
	TMP/SMX	↓ levels of A	+
	Tocainide	↓ effect of B	+
Rimantadine	*See Amantadine*		
Ritonavir	*See protease inhibitors and Table 22B & Table 22C*		
Saquinavir	*See protease inhibitors and Table 22B & Table 22C*		
Stavudine	Dapsone, INH	May ↑ risk of peripheral neuropathy	±
	Ribavirin	↓ levels of A—**avoid**	++
	Zidovudine	Mutual interference—do not combine	++

TABLE 22A (7)

Sulfonamides	Cyclosporine	↓ cyclosporine levels	+
	Methotrexate	↑ antifolate activity	+
	Oral anticoagulants	↑ prothrombin time; bleeding	+
	Phenobarbital, rifampin	↓ levels of A	+
	Phenytoin	↑ levels of B; nystagmus, ataxia	+
	Sulfonylureas	↑ hypoglycemic effect	+
Telithromycin (Ketek)	Carbamazine	↓ levels of A	+ +
	Digoxin	↑ levels of B—do digoxin levels	+ +
	Ergot alkaloids	↑ **levels of B—avoid**	+ +
	Itraconazole; ketoconazole	↑ levels of A; no dose change	+
	Metoprolol	↑ levels of B	+ +
	Midazolam	↑ levels of B	+ +
	Oral anticoagulants	↑ prothrombin time	+
	Phenobarbital, phenytoin	↓ levels of A	+ +
	Pimozide	↑ **levels of B; QT prolongation— AVOID**	+ +
	Rifampin	↓ **levels of A—avoid**	+ +
	Simvastatin & other "statins"	↑ levels of B (↑ risk of myopathy)	+ +
	Sotalol	↓ levels of B	+ +
	Theophylline	↑ levels of B	+ +
Tenofovir	Atazanavir	↓ levels of B—add ritonavir	+ +
	Didanosine (ddI)	↑ **levels of B (reduce dose)**	+ +
Terbinafine	Cimetidine	↑ levels of A	+
	Phenobarbital, rifampin	↓ levels of A	+
Tetracyclines	*See Doxycycline, plus:*		
	Atovaquone	↓ levels of B	+
	Digoxin	↑ toxicity of B (may persist several months—up to 10% pts)	+ +
	Methoxyflurane	↑ toxicity; polyuria, renal failure	+
	Sucralfate	↓ absorption of A (separate by ≥2 hrs)	+
Thiabendazole	Theophyllines	↑ serum theophylline, nausea	+
Tigecycline	Oral contraceptives	↓ levels of B	+ +
Tinidazole (Tindamax)	*See Metronidazole—similar entity, expect similar interactions*		
Tobramycin	*See Aminoglycosides*		
Trimethoprim	Amantadine, dapsone, digoxin, methotrexate, procainamide, zidovudine	↑ serum levels of B	+ +
	Potassium-sparing diuretics	↑ serum K⁺	+ +
	Thiazide diuretics	↓ serum Na⁺	+
Trimethoprim-Sulfameth-oxazole	Azathioprine	Reports of leukopenia	+
	Cyclosporine	↓ levels of B, ↑ serum creatinine	+
	Loperamide	↑ levels of B	+
	Methotrexate	Enhanced marrow suppression	+ +
	Oral contraceptives, pimozide, and 6-mercaptopurine	↓ effect of B	+
	Phenytoin	↑ levels of B	+
	Rifampin	↑ levels of B	+
	Warfarin	↑ activity of B	+
Valganciclovir (Valcyte)	See Ganciclovir		
Vancomycin	Aminoglycosides	↑ frequency of nephrotoxicity	+ +
Zalcitabine (ddC) (HIVID)	Valproic acid, pentamidine (IV), alcohol, lamivudine	↑ pancreatitis risk	+
	Cisplatin, INH, metronidazole, vincristine, nitrofurantoin, d4T, dapsone	↑ risk of peripheral neuropathy	+
Zidovudine (ZDV) (Retrovir)	Atovaquone, fluconazole, methadone	↑ levels of A	+
	Clarithromycin	↓ levels of A	±
	Indomethacin	↑ levels of ZDV toxic metabolite	+
	Nelfinavir	↓ levels of A	+ +
	Probenecid, TMP/SMX	↑ levels of A	+
	Rifampin/rifabutin	↓ levels of A	+ +
	Stavudine	**Interference—DO NOT COMBINE!**	+ +
	Valproic Acid	↑ levels of A	+ +

TABLE 22B – DRUG-DRUG INTERACTIONS BETWEEN PROTEASE INHIBITORS

(Adapted from Guidelines for the Use of Antiretroviral Agents in HIV-Infected Adults & Adolescents; see *www.aidsinfo.nih.gov*)

NOTE WELL: THERE IS NO EVIDENCE THAT USING TWO BOOSTED PI AGENTS TOGETHER HAVE ANY ADDITIONAL ANTIVIRAL ACTIVITY THAN ONE BOOSTED PI. DO NOT COUNT 2 BOOSTED PIs AS 2 ACTIVE AGENTS IN A NEW REGIMEN!

NAME (Abbreviation, Trade Name)	Atazanavir (ATV, Reyataz)	Darunavir (DRV, Prezista)	Fosamprenavir (FOS-APV, Lexiva)	Indinavir (IDV, Crixivan)	Lopinavir/Ritonavir (LP/R, Kaletra)	Nelfinavir (NFV, Viracept)	Saquinavir (SQV, Invirase)	Tipranavir (TPV)
Atazanavir (ATV, Reyataz)		ATV 300 mg once daily with (DRV 600 mg + ritonavir 100 mg bid)		Do not co-administer; risk of additive ↑ in indirect bilirubin	RTV 100 mg ↑ ATV AUC[1] 238%		SQV (Invirase) 1600 mg + ATV 300 mg + RTV 100 mg, all q24h	
Darunavir (DRV, Prezista)	ATV 300 mg once daily with (DRV 600 mg + ritonavir 100 mg bid)		No data	Dose unclear	DO NOT co-administer; Doses not established	No data	DO NOT co-administer; Doses not established	No data
Fosamprenavir (FOS-APV, Lexiva)	No data	No data			↓ serum conc. both drugs: do not co-administer		Insufficient data	Fos APV levels ↓. Do not co-administer
Indinavir (IDV, Crixivan)	Do not co-administer; risk of additive ↑ in bilirubin	Dose unclear			IDV AUC[1] ↑; IDV dose 600 mg q12h	↑ IDV & NFV levels. Dose: IDV 1200 mg q12h, NFV 1250 mg q12h	SQV levels ↑ 4–7 fold. Dose: Insufficient data	No data
Lopinavir/Ritonavir (LP/R, Kaletra)	RTV 100 mg ↑ ATV. AUC[3] 238%	DO NOT co-administer; Doses not established	↓ serum conc. both drugs; do not co-administer	IDV AUC[1] ↑. IDV dose 600 mg q12h		Dose: LP/R 533/133 mg q12h; NFV 1000 mg q12h	SQV levels ↑. Dose: SQV 1000 mg b.i.d.; LP/R standard	LPV levels ↓ Do not co-administer
Nelfinavir (NFV, Viracept)		No data		↑ IDV & NFV levels. Dose: IDV 1200 mg q12h, NFV 1250 mg q12h	LP levels ↓; NFV levels ↑. Dose: LP/R 533/133 mg q12h; NFV 1000 mg q12h		Dose:SQV 1200 mg b.i.d., NFV 1250 mg b.i.d.	No data
Saquinavir (SQV, Invirase)	SQV (Invirase) 1600 mg + ATV 300 mg + RTV 100 mg, all q24h	DO NOT co-administer; Doses not established	SQV (Invirase) 1000 mg q12h + RTV 100–200 mg q12h + FOS-APV 700 mg q12h	SQV levels ↑ 4–7 fold. Dose: Insufficient data	SQV levels ↑. Dose: SQV 1000 mg b.i.d., LP/R-standard	Dose SQV 1200 mg b.i.d., NFV 1250 mg b.i.d.		SQV ↓ Do not co-administer
Tipranavir (TPV)		No data	Fos-APV levels ↓. Do not co-administer	No data	LPV levels ↓. Do not co-administer	No data	SQV ↓. Do not co-administer	

TABLE 22C – DRUG-DRUG INTERACTIONS BETWEEN NON-NUCLEOSIDE REVERSE TRANSCRIPTASE INHIBITORS (NNRTIS) AND PROTEASE INHIBITORS
(Adapted from Guidelines for the Use of Antiretroviral Agents in HIV-Infected Adults & Adolescents; see *www.aidsinfo.nih.gov*)

NAME (Abbreviation, Trade Name)	Atazanavir (ATV, Reyataz)	DARUNAVIR (DRV, Prezista)	Fosamprenavir (FOS-APV, Lexiva)	Indinavir (IDV, Crixivan)	Lopinavir/Ritonavir (LP/R, Kaletra)	Nelfinavir (NFV, Viracept)	Saquinavir (SQV, Invirase)	Tipranavir (TPV)
Delavirdine (DLV, Rescriptor)	No data	No data	**Co-administration not recommended**	IDV levels ↑ 40%. Dose: IDV 600 mg q8h. DLV standard	Expect LP levels to ↑. No dose data	NFV levels ↑ 2X; DLV levels ↓ 50%. Dose: No data	SQV levels ↑ 5X. Dose: SQV 800 mg q8h. DLV standard	No data
Efavirenz (EFZ, Sustiva)	ATV AUC[1] ↓ 74%. Dose: EFZ standard; ATA/RTV 300/100 mg q24h with food	Standard doses of both drugs	FOS-APV levels ↓. Dose: EFZ standard; FOS-APV 1400 mg + RTV 300 mg q24h or 700 mg FOS-APV + 100 mg RTV q12h	Levels: IDV ↓ 31%. Dose: IDV 1000 mg q8h. EFZ standard	Level of LP ↓ 40%. Dose: LP/R 533/133 mg q12h, EFZ standard	Standard doses	Level: SQV ↓ 62%. Dose: SQV 400 mg + RTV 400 mg q12h	No dose change necessary
Etravirine (ETR, Intelence)	↑ATV & ↑ETR levels. **Avoid combination.**	No data	↑ levels of FOS-APV. **Avoid combination.**	↓ level of IDV. **Avoid combination.**	↑ levels of ETR, ↓ levels of **LP/R. Use caution if combined.**	↑ levels of NFV. **Avoid combination.**	↓ ETR levels 33%; SQV/R no change. Standard dose of both drugs.	↓ levels of ETR, ↑ levels of TPV & RTV. **Avoid combination.**
Nevirapine (NVP, Viramune)	No data. Avoid combination	Standard doses of both drugs	No data	IDV levels ↓ 28%. Dose: IDV 1000 mg q8h or combine with RTV; NVP standard	LP levels ↓ 53%. Dose: LP/R 533/133 mg q12h; NVP standard	Standard doses	Dose: SQV + RTV 400/400 mg, both q12h	Standard doses

TABLE 23 – LIST OF GENERIC AND COMMON TRADE NAMES

GENERIC NAME: TRADE NAMES	GENERIC NAME: TRADE NAMES	GENERIC NAME: TRADE NAMES
Abacavir: Ziagen	Efavirenz/Emtricitabine/Tenofovir: Atripla	Oseltamivir: Tamiflu
Abacavir+Lamivudine: Epzicom	Emtricitabine: Emtriva	Oxacillin: Prostaphlin
Abacavir+Lamivudine+Zodovudine: Trizivir	Emtricitabine + tenofovir: Truvada	Palivizumab: Synagis
Acyclovir: Zovirax	Enfuvirtide (T-20): Fuzeon	Paromomycin: Humatin
Adefovir: Hepsera	Entecavir: Baraclude	Pentamidine: NebuPent, Pentam 300
Albendazole: Albenza	Ertapenem: Invanz	Piperacillin: Pipracil
Amantadine: Symmetrel	Etravirine: Intelence	Piperacillin/tazobactam: Zosyn
Amikacin: Amikin	Erythromycin(s): Ilotycin	Piperazine: Antepar
Amoxicillin: Amoxil, Polymox	*Ethyl succinate:* Pediamycin	Podophyllotoxin: Condylox
Amox./clav.: Augmentin, Augmentin ES-600; Augmentin XR	*Glucoheptonate:* Erythrocin	Posaconazole: Noxafil
Amphotericin B: Fungizone	*Estolate:* Ilosone	Praziquantel: Biltricide
Ampho B-liposomal: AmBisome	Erythro/sulfisoxazole: Pediazole	Primaquine: Primachine
Ampho B-lipid complex: Abelcet	Ethambutol: Myambutol	Proguanil: Paludrine
Ampicillin: Omnipen, Polycillin	Ethionamide: Trecator	Pyrantel pamoate: Antiminth
Ampicillin/sulbactam: Unasyn	Famciclovir: Famvir	Pyrimethamine: Daraprim
Atazanavir: Reyataz	Fluconazole: Diflucan	Pyrimethamine/sulfadoxine: Fansidar
Atovaquone: Mepron	Flucytosine: Ancobon	Quinupristin/dalfopristin: Synercid
Atovaquone + proguanil: Malarone	Fosamprenavir: Lexiva	Raltegravir: Isentress
Azithromycin: Zithromax	Fosfomycin: Monurol	Retapamulin: Altabax
Azithromycin ER: Zmax	Ganciclovir: Cytovene	Ribavirin: Virazole, Rebetol
Aztreonam: Azactam	Gatifloxacin: Tequin	Rifabutin: Mycobutin
Caspofungin: Cancidas	Gemifloxacin: Factive	Rifampin: Rifadin, Rimactane
Cefaclor: Ceclor, Ceclor CD	Gentamicin: Garamycin	Rifapentine: Priftin
Cefadroxil: Duricef	Griseofulvin: Fulvicin	Rifaximin: Xifaxan
Cefazolin: Ancef, Kefzol	Halofantrine: Halfan	Rimantadine: Flumadine
Cefdinir: Omnicef	Idoxuridine: Dendrid, Stoxil	Ritonavir: Norvir
Cefditoren pivoxil: Spectracef	INH + RIF: Rifamate	Saquinavir: Invirase
Cefepime: Maxipime	INH + RIF + PZA: Rifater	Spectinomycin: Trobicin
Cefixime[NUS]: Suprax	Interferon alfa: Intron A	Stavudine: Zerit
Cefoperazone-sulbactam: Sulperazon[NUS]	Interferon, pegylated: PEG-Intron, Pegasys	Stibogluconate: Pentostam
Cefotaxime: Claforan	Interferon + ribavirin: Rebetron	Silver sulfadiazine: Silvadene
Cefotetan: Cefotan	Imipenem + cilastatin: Primaxin, Tienam	Sulfamethoxazole: Gantanol
Cefoxitin: Mefoxin	Imiquimod: Aldara	Sulfasalazine: Azulfidine
Cefpodoxime proxetil: Vantin	Indinavir: Crixivan	Sulfisoxazole: Gantrisin
Cefprozil: Cefzil	Itraconazole: Sporanox	Telbivudine : Tyzeka
Ceftazidime: Fortaz, Tazicef, Tazidime	Iodoquinol: Yodoxin	Telithromycin: Ketek
Ceftibuten: Cedax	Ivermectin: Stromectol	Tenofovir: Viread
Ceftizoxime: Cefizox	Kanamycin: Kantrex	Terbinafine: Lamisil
Ceftobiprole: Zevtera	Ketoconazole: Nizoral	Thalidomide: ThalomidThiabendazole: Mintezol
Ceftriaxone: Rocephin	Lamivudine: Epivir, Epivir-HBV	Ticarcillin: Ticar
Cefuroxime: Zinacef, Kefurox, Ceftin	Lamivudine + abacavir: Epzicom	Tigecycline: Tygacil
Cephalexin: Keflex	Levofloxacin: Levaquin	Tinidazole: Tindamax
Cephradine: Anspor, Velosef	Linezolid: Zyvox	Tipranavir: Aptivus
Chloroquine: Aralen	Lomefloxacin: Maxaquin	Tobramycin: Nebcin
Cidofovir: Vistide	Lopinavir/ritonavir: Kaletra	Tretinoin: Retin A
Ciprofloxacin: Cipro, Cipro XR	Loracarbef: Lorabid	Trifluridine: Viroptic
Clarithromycin: Biaxin, Biaxin XL	Mafenide: Sulfamylon	Trimethoprim: Proloprim, Trimpex
Clindamycin: Cleocin	Maraviroc: Selzentry	Trimethoprim/sulfamethoxazole: Bactrim, Septra
Clofazimine: Lamprene	Mebendazole: Vermox	Valacyclovir: Valtrex
Clotrimazole: Lotrimin, Mycelex	Mefloquine: Lariam	Valganciclovir: Valcyte
Cloxacillin: Tegopen	Meropenem: Merrem	Vancomycin: Vancocin
Colistimethate: Coly-Mycin M	Mesalamine: Asacol, Pentasa	Voriconazole: Vfend
Cycloserine: Seromycin	Methenamine: Hiprex, Mandelamine	Zalcitabine: HIVID
Daptomycin: Cubicin	Metronidazole: Flagyl	Zanamivir: Relenza
Darunavir: Prezista	Micafungin: Mycamine	Zidovudine (ZDV): Retrovir
Delavirdine: Rescriptor	Minocycline: Minocin	Zidovudine + 3TC: Combivir
Dicloxacillin: Dynapen	Moxifloxacin: Avelox	Zidovudine + 3TC + abacavir: Trizivir
Didanosine: Videx	Mupirocin: Bactroban	
Diethylcarbamazine: Hetrazan	Nafcillin: Unipen	
Diloxanide furoate: Furamide	Nelfinavir: Viracept	
Doripenem: Doribax	Nevirapine: Viramune	
Doxycycline: Vibramycin	Nitazoxanide: Alinia	
Drotrecogin alfa: Xigris	Nitrofurantoin: Macrobid, Macrodantin	
Efavirenz: Sustiva	Nystatin: Mycostatin	
	Ofloxacin: Floxin	

TABLE 23 (2)
LIST OF COMMON TRADE AND GENERIC NAMES

TRADE NAME: GENERIC NAME	TRADE NAME: GENERIC NAME	TRADE NAME: GENERIC NAME
Abelcet: Ampho B-lipid complex	Halfan: Halofantrine	Retin A: Tretinoin
Albenza: Albendazole	Hepsera: Adefovir	Retrovir: Zidovudine (ZDV)
Aldara: Imiquimod	Herplex: Idoxuridine	Reyataz: Atazanavir
Alinia: Nitazoxanide	Hiprex: Methenamine hippurate	Rifadin: Rifampin
Altabax: Retapamulin	HIVID: Zalcitabine	Rifamate: INH + RIF
AmBisome: Ampho B-liposomal	Humatin: Paromomycin	Rifater: INH + RIF + PZA
Amikin: Amikacin	Ilosone: Erythromycin estolate	Rimactane: Rifampin
Amoxil: Amoxicillin	Ilotycin: Erythromycin	Rocephin: Ceftriaxone
Ancef: Cefazolin	Intelence: Etravirine	Selzentry: Maraviroc
Ancobon: Flucytosine	Intron A: Interferon alfa	Septra: Trimethoprim/sulfa
Anspor: Cephradine	Invanz: Ertapenem	Seromycin: Cycloserine
Antepar: Piperazine	Invirase: Saquinavir	Silvadene: Silver sulfadiazine
Antiminth: Pyrantel pamoate	Isentress: Raltegravir	Spectracef: Cefditoren pivoxil
Aptivus: Tipranavir	Kantrex: Kanamycin	Sporanox: Itraconazole
Aralen: Chloroquine	Kaletra: Lopinavir/ritonavir	Stoxil: Idoxuridine
Asacol: Mesalamine	Keflex: Cephalexin	Stromectol: Ivermectin
Atripla:	Kefurox: Cefuroxime	Sulfamylon: Mafenide
Efavirenz/emtricitabine/tenofovir	Ketek: Telithromycin	Sulperazon[NUS]: Cefoperazone-sulbactam
Augmentin, Augmentin ES-600	Lamisil: Terbinafine	Suprax: Cefixime[NUS]
Augmentin XR: Amox./clav.	Lamprene: Clofazimine	Sustiva: Efavirenz
Avelox: Moxifloxacin	Lariam: Mefloquine	Symmetrel: Amantadine
Azactam: Aztreonam	Levaquin: Levofloxacin	Synagis: Palivizumab
Azulfidine: Sulfasalazine	Lexiva: Fosamprenavir	Synercid: Quinupristin/dalfopristin
Bactroban: Mupirocin	Lorabid: Loracarbef	Tamiflu: Oseltamivir
Bactrim: Trimethoprim/sulfamethoxa-zole	Macrodantin, Macrobid: Nitrofurantoin	Tazicef: Ceftazidime
Baraclude: Entecavir	Malarone: Atovaquone + proguanil	Tegopen: Cloxacillin
Biaxin, Biaxin XL: Clarithromycin	Mandelamine: Methenamine mandel.	Tequin: Gatifloxacin
Biltricide: Praziquantel	Maxaquin: Lomefloxacin	Thalomid: Thalidomide
Cancidas: Caspofungin	Maxipime: Cefepime	Ticar: Ticarcillin
Ceclor, Ceclor CD: Cefaclor	Mefoxin: Cefoxitin	Tienam: Imipenem
Cedax: Ceftibuten	Mepron: Atovaquone	Timentin: Ticarcillin-clavulanic acid
Cefizox: Ceftizoxime	Merrem: Meropenem	Tinactin: Tolnaftate
Cefotan: Cefotetan	Minocin: Minocycline	Tindamax: Tinidazole
Ceftin: Cefuroxime axetil	Mintezol: Thiabendazole	Trecator SC: Ethionamide
Cefzil: Cefprozil	Monocid: Cefonicid	Trizivir: Abacavir + ZDV + 3TC
Cipro, Cipro XR: Ciprofloxacin & extended release	Monurol: Fosfomycin	Trobicin: Spectinomycin
Claforan: Cefotaxime	Myambutol: Ethambutol	Truvada: Emtricitabine + tenofovir
Coly-Mycin M: Colistimethate	Mycamine: Micafungin	Tygacil: Tigecycline
Combivir: ZDV + 3TC	Mycobutin: Rifabutin	Tyzeka: Telbivudine
Crixivan: Indinavir	Mycostatin: Nystatin	Unasyn: Ampicillin/sulbactam
Cubicin: Daptomycin	Nafcil: Nafcillin	Unipen: Nafcillin
Cytovene: Ganciclovir	Nebcin: Tobramycin	Valcyte: Valganciclovir
Daraprim: Pyrimethamine	NebuPent: Pentamidine	Valtrex: Valacyclovir
Diflucan: Fluconazole	Nizoral: Ketoconazole	Vancocin: Vancomycin
Doribax: Doripenem	Norvir: Ritonavir	Vantin: Cefpodoxime proxetil
Duricef: Cefadroxil	Noxafil: Posaconazole	Velosef: Cephradine
Dynapen: Dicloxacillin	Omnicef: Cefdinir	Vermox: Mebendazole
Emtriva: Emtricitabine	Omnipen: Ampicillin	Vfend: Voriconazole
Epivir, Epivir-HBV: Lamivudine	Pediamycin: Erythro. ethyl succinate	Vibramycin: Doxycycline
Epzicom: Lamivudine + abacavir	Pediazole: Erythro. ethyl succinate + sulfisoxazole	Videx: Didanosine
Factive: Gemifloxacin	Pegasys, PEG-Intron: Interferon, pegylated	Viracept: Nelfinavir
Famvir: Famciclovir		Viramune: Nevirapine
Fansidar: Pyrimethamine + sulfadoxine	Pentam 300: Pentamidine	Virazole: Ribavirin
Flagyl: Metronidazole	Pentasa: Mesalamine	Viread: Tenofovir
Floxin: Ofloxacin	Pipracil: Piperacillin	Vistide: Cidofovir
Flumadine: Rimantadine	Polycillin: Ampicillin	Xifaxan: Rifaximin
Fortaz: Ceftazidime	Polymox: Amoxicillin	Xigris: Drotrecogin alfa
Fulvicin: Griseofulvin	Prezista: Darunavir	Yodoxin: Iodoquinol
Fungizone: Amphotericin B	Priftin: Rifapentine	Zerit: Stavudine
Furadantin: Nitrofurantoin	Primaxin: Imipenem + cilastatin	Zevtera: Ceftobiprole
Fuzeon: Enfuvirtide (T-20)	Proloprim: Trimethoprim	Ziagen: Abacavir
Gantanol: Sulfamethoxazole	Prostaphlin: Oxacillin	Zinacef: Cefuroxime
Gantrisin: Sulfisoxazole	Rebetol: Ribavirin	Zithromax: Azithromycin
Garamycin: Gentamicin	Rebetron: Interferon + ribavirin	Zmax: Azithromycin ER
	Relenza: Zanamivir	Zovirax: Acyclovir
	Rescriptor: Delavirdine	Zosyn: Piperacillin/tazobactam
		Zyvox: Linezolid

PAGES (page numbers bold if major focus)   PAGES (page numbers bold if major focus)

Bold numbers indicate major considerations. Antibiotic selection often depends on modifying circumstances and alternative agents.